The Ultimate Fertility Guidebook

DR. CHRISTINA BURNS

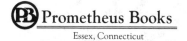

Prometheus Books

Essex, Connecticut

Ⓟ Prometheus Books

An imprint of Globe Pequot, the trade division of
The Rowman & Littlefield Publishing Group, Inc.
4501 Forbes Blvd., Ste. 200
Lanham, MD 20706
www.rowman.com

Distributed by NATIONAL BOOK NETWORK

British Library Cataloguing in Publication Information Available

Library of Congress Cataloging-in-Publication Data

Names: Burns, Christina, author.
Title: The ultimate fertility guidebook / Christina Burns.
Description: Lanham, MD : Prometheus, An imprint of Globe Pequot, the trade
  division of The Rowman & Littlefield Publishing Group, Inc., [2023] |
  Includes bibliographical references and index. | Summary: "The principal
  mission of this book is to provide a simple and easy guidebook with
  proven tactics to help women tune into their body's natural 'language'
  and increase their chances of conceiving."—Provided by publisher.
Identifiers: LCCN 2022033727 (print) | LCCN 2022033728 (ebook) | ISBN
  9781633888852 (paper) | ISBN 9781633888869 (epub)
Subjects: LCSH: Infertility. | Infertility—Alternative treatment. |
  Fertility, Human.
Classification: LCC RC889 .B83 2023 (print) | LCC RC889 (ebook) | DDC
  616.6/92—dc23/eng/20220912
LC record available at https://lccn.loc.gov/2022033727
LC ebook record available at https://lccn.loc.gov/2022033728

∞™ The paper used in this publication meets the minimum requirements of American
National Standard for Information Sciences—Permanence of Paper
for Printed Library Materials, ANSI/NISO Z39.48-1992.

Contents

APPENDIXES

Abbreviations

ADD	attention deficit disorder
ADHD	attention-deficit hyperactivity disorder
AFC	antral follicle count
AMH	anti-Müllerian hormone
ANA	antinuclear antibody
APA	antiphospholipid antibody
ART	assisted reproductive technology
BBT	basal body temperature
BMI	body mass index
BPA	bisphenol A
CDC	Centers for Disease Control and Prevention
CHM	Chinese herbal medicine
CNS	central nervous system
CoQ10	coenzyme Q10
CRH	corticotropin-releasing hormone
CRP	C-reactive protein
CSA	Community Supported Agriculture
D&C	dilation and curettage
DHA	docosahexaenoic acid
DHEA	dehydroepiandrosterone
DIM	diindolylmethane
DOR	diminished ovarian reserve
E2	estradiol
EMF	electromagnetic field
ENS	enteric nervous system
EPA	eicosapentaenoic acid
ERA	endometrial receptivity assay
FDA	Food and Drug Administration

FET	frozen embryo transfer
FSC	Forest Stewardship Council
FSH	follicle-stimulating hormone
GABA	gamma-aminobutyric acid
GI	gastrointestinal
GMO	genetically modified organism
GnRH	gonadotropin-releasing hormone
GOTS	Global Organic Textile Standard
HCG	human chorionic gonadotropin
HEPA	high-efficiency air particulate absorbing
HgA1c	hemoglobin A1c
HIIT	high-intensity interval training
HIV	human immunodeficiency virus
HPA	hypothalamic–pituitary–adrenal
HPO	hypothalamic–pituitary–ovarian
HSG	hysterosalpingogram
I3C	indole-3-carbinol
IBS	irritable bowel syndrome
ICSI	intracytoplasmic sperm injection
IU	international units
IUI	intrauterine insemination
IV	intravenous
IVF	in vitro fertilization
IVIG	intravenous immunoglobulin
LEEP	loop electrosurgical excision procedure
LPD	luteal phase defect
LH	luteinizing hormone
MACH	macrophage-activating Chinese mixed herbs
MSG	monosodium glutamate
NAC	N-acetyl cysteine
NHANES	National Health and Nutrition Examination Survey
NK	natural killer
NSAID	nonsteroidal anti-inflammatory drug
OGTT	oral glucose tolerance test
OHSS	ovarian hyperstimulation syndrome
OPK	ovulation predictor kit
P4	progesterone
PCB	polychlorinated biphenyl
PCOS	polycystic ovarian syndrome
PGT-A	preimplantation genetic testing for aneuploidies
PID	pelvic inflammatory disease

PNS	parasympathetic nervous system
POA	premature ovarian aging
POF	premature ovarian failure
PMDD	premenstrual dysphoric disorder
PMS	premenstrual syndrome
PVC	polyvinyl chloride
REI	reproductive endocrinologist
REM	rapid eye movement
RPL	recurrent pregnancy loss
SDF	sperm DNA fragmentation
SNS	sympathetic nervous system
TCM	traditional Chinese medicine
TM	Transcendental Meditation
TPO	thyroid peroxidase
TSH	thyroid-stimulating hormone
T3	triiodothyronine
T4	thyroxine
VOC	volatile organic compound

Introduction

INFERTILITY IS TRENDING

Women are making serious moves in this day and age. Approximately 74.6 million of us are active members of the civilian workforce in the United States. As of 2018, four out of every 10 U.S. businesses are women owned, which accounts for 12.3 million businesses netting approximately $1.8 *trillion* per year. That's a 58 percent increase from 2007, and it's likely to keep rising. We've never had more independence—financially or otherwise.

There's a price for progress, however: the modern woman has more on her plate than ever before. We hustle every day to balance the growing demands of family, friends, career, health, and home. There is a self-imposed need to get everything done *now*, including getting pregnant. The pressure we place on ourselves is not only stressful and unrealistic but also counterproductive to our fertility efforts.

Why Not Me?!

Infertility is a confusing and upsetting thing for any woman, but it hits type A personalities especially hard. Alpha-wired females always plan ahead and strive to have every aspect of life under control. After months of peeing on ovulation sticks to determine precisely when to jump your partner, that negative pregnancy test is horribly disheartening. For many, it's even panic inducing ("Why isn't it working?"). You do internet searches for so-called fertility-boosting vitamins and health foods and follow all the guidelines, yet that single line keeps taunting you. After trying for a while to no avail, the fear and the mistrust of your own body set in. The mind says, "WTF?! What's going on? This should be easy!" Having a baby is our God-given right as women after all, isn't it?

Everywhere you look, it's like everyone's preggo. Social media amplify the assault—all your pals are posting bump and baby photos. Why not you? Well, first of all, Facebook is a big fat fibber. The photos aren't telling the entire story, only snippets. The pregnant women you see waddling around? You can't know what kind of journey they had. Most of us keep our fertility struggles tightly under wraps.

YOU ARE NOT ALONE

When you can't get pregnant despite your efforts, all sense of control slips away—and that, in and of itself, is frightening, not to mention disorienting. This incredibly important aspect of your life now seems unattainable, and you're at a loss for how to reach out and reclaim it. You may feel embarrassed that you cannot figure out this thing that is supposed to come naturally. You withdraw from family and friends. You shy away from anything that might remind you of what you consider to be your failings. You can't relax until you're *pregnant*.

You are not alone. In 2015, the Centers for Disease Control and Prevention found that 12 percent of all U.S. women experienced infertility, meaning they were unable to get pregnant after 12 months of regular, unprotected sex. Twelve percent doesn't sound like a lot out of context, but that's actually about 38.5 million women. Of these, 20 percent are deemed "unexplained infertility." No answers, no direction. What's a girl to do?

Exploring the Why

Today's lifestyle is demanding on everyone but arguably more so for ambitious women. Because of self-imposed expectations and a tendency for perfectionism, we are easily stressed and frustrated. We are constantly rushing, constantly busy, and constantly under pressure. Stretching ourselves in so many directions leaves us more stressed out than ever before. Women everywhere are experiencing mental burnout and a slew of internal imbalances. The health of our reproductive system (or lack thereof) is intimately tied to our daily choices. In today's world, we make rapid-fire decisions all day long. A lot of the "shortcuts" modern women take to get through their hectic days have negative, unseen impacts on their reproductive health.

FOR STARTERS, LOOK AT OUR DAILY GRIND

When it comes to meals, we often reach for what's convenient over more nourishing options. With our fast-paced lifestyles, we eat on the fly. Processed foods are easily accessible, but they are also the most unhealthy options. "Quick and easy" essentially translates into high-carb, sugary eats. This messes with our blood sugar and insulin, which knocks several other hormones askew.

Despite our feeling constantly rushed, we're more sedentary than ever. If you're a woman pushing to meet a career goal, that probably means you're sitting down for the majority of your life. Without movement, hormonal balance and blood circulation are negatively impacted. Worse still, our bodies then struggle to detoxify myriad garbage that we ingest via polluted air, poor-quality food, cosmetics, and the like. Even drinking tap water has chemicals and heavy metals! Junk accumulates and causes inflammatory responses that wreak havoc with our egg quality, uterine receptivity, and overall hormonal wellness.

It also doesn't help that conventional farming practices have led to more genetically modified and chemical-filled foods. Globalization has given us the gift of variety, but that food often has low nutrient density because it's not local and fresh. Animals like chickens and cows are pumped full of hormones, fed grain-based diets, and given regular doses of antibiotics due to poor living conditions and inhumane farming practices. Then we ingest their ill health.

THE TICKING CLOCK

As if the ticking sound of our biological clock wasn't already deafening, those of us trying to conceive are always reminded of the danger of our aging ovaries. However, there's more to the story. Chronological and ovarian age are not always one and the same. For some women, their ovaries (i.e., egg count) sync with their number of years on the planet. However, other women's ovaries appear to age much faster or much slower than their birthdays suggest. There are tests to explore your unique fertility "profile," which we will cover in the pages of this book.

As a general rule (meaning "statistics say"), female fertility starts declining around age 32 and decreases more rapidly after age 37. Those are our prime earning years! Due to demanding careers, increased opportunities, and noble aspirations, women are having children later in life, when fertility is already in decline. Everything comes with a price—unfair but true.

THE DISCONNECT

The difficulties of getting knocked up often stem from a disconnect between the desire to conceive and basic conception know-how. Many women aren't sure when they ovulate or how their hormones function. So, they don't have the proper tools to become pregnant on their own. It's not their fault. Women aren't educated on their bodies. Personally, I can't recall ever being taught about my fertile window or anything related to my lady parts or reproduction. Everything vagina related was (and still is) kept so hush-hush. Frankly, it's nonsensical.

Early understanding of how our female bodies operate would allow us to tune into our cycle and quicken the path to baby. Tuning into our rhythm also helps us understand how hormonal changes affect moods and tendencies. This would have been especially helpful during our teenage years, when we were undergoing some of the biggest and most confusing changes! This same education would help us avoid pregnancy in the years it is more unwanted. I have met women in their forties who still pop the morning-after pill after an "oops" one-night stand when the "oops" was nowhere near their fertile window! A check for sexually transmitted disease? Yes. Morning-after pill? Not really necessary.

Nutrition, lifestyle, and natural remedies aside, knowing your body is a very important starting point on your fertility journey. If you can't "nail" the window, you are missing the opportunity to do this the old-fashioned way. In this book, I'm going to impart the body know-how you need to get it done.

Been there, done that? If you've already got the basics down *or* the basics don't fit the bill for your story, you can fast-track your read by hopping over to chapter 3 for a deep dive into a litany of causes underlying infertility. Of course, it couldn't hurt to skim chapters 1 and 2 for a refresher.

Sometimes It Takes a Village

Between 2011 and 2015, about 7.3 million U.S. women sought infertility treatments. They saw their doctors for help ranging from a variety of diagnostic tests to artificial insemination and in vitro fertilization (IVF). About one in six couples today seek assisted reproductive techniques such as intrauterine insemination (IUI) or IVF, and the numbers are on the rise.

Among those 7.3 million women and their doctors, there is a growing movement of combining Eastern and Western medicinal practices, such as adding acupuncture to their IVF treatment. Acupuncture users increased from 8.19 million to 14.01 million in the United States between 2002 and 2007, and experts expect that the number has only increased in recent years. The integration of these natural and complementary methods with conventional methods often produces better results than conventional methods on their own and can help reduce many of the unpleasant side effects. It's no surprise that many couples experiencing infertility are going this route. Fertility doctors increasingly refer their patients to specialists like me—in fact, a good deal of my patients find me via their fertility centers.

Complementary medicine supports you both emotionally and physically during your efforts to conceive, providing you with concrete steps to enhance your fertility as well as relaxation techniques to keep you calm throughout. Better still, a lot of them can be added to your daily routine without a hitch.

So you've picked up this book. You're ready to do what it takes to get your baby. The women who come to see me want to know what they can do to improve the odds. These amazing women are willing to take on an entirely new "fertility-friendly" lifestyle to make it happen. In the pages to follow, I break down all the tools in my arsenal to help you take charge of your fertility. I've compiled research and insight from more than 18 years of practice, thousands of patients, and various experts in the fields of fertility, natural medicine, sex, and nutrition to give you a comprehensive do-it-yourself guide to getting pregnant. *The Ultimate Fertility Guidebook* is your how-to guide to boosting your fertility through natural and integrative approaches.

This Book Is for You If . . .

- You are looking for natural, holistic approaches to enhancing your fertility.
- You want to understand the mechanics of your body and get informed about all things fertility.
- You are in the process of conventional treatments such as IVF or IUI and want to add complementary, natural medicine and lifestyle changes to boost your chances of success.
- You have been diagnosed with a preexisting medical condition that makes it harder for you to get pregnant, and you want to know what you can do to improve your odds.
- You are a busy, modern woman seeking actionable tips to quicken your path to conception.

If you put a mental check mark beside any of the reasons above, you're going to find answers in these pages. Although fertility is an expansive and complicated topic, this book boils it down to an easily navigable guide containing the information you're seeking with none of the fluff. Are some aspects of your fertility beyond your control? Yes. However, this book can teach you proven, effective steps to take control of what *is* within your power to change. Best of all, this book provides you with natural, holistic options that can also be integrated with conventional techniques to give you the widest range of solutions.

I have tried to anticipate all your questions based on those I've been asked during my years of clinical practice as a licensed doctor of Eastern medicine, an acupuncturist, and an integrative fertility expert. However, everyone's story is unique, so if you reach the end of this book and still have questions, please reach out to me at Drchristina@naturnalife.com.

Now let's jump in because you're a busy woman and you have things to do!

CHAPTER 1

Hormone Basics

We've all experienced those days when something inside feels "off." You don't feel sick per se, but you don't feel your best. Something's hinky. The jeans that fit you perfectly yesterday are somehow extra tight today. Even though you got eight hours of sleep, all you want to do is lay your head on your desk and nap. Or maybe you feel super anxious and can't get a handle on why.

At times, it feels like you need x-ray vision to see what's going on inside that body of yours. What could be responsible for the seemingly random highs and lows of your physical and emotional well-being? They're called hormones, and on top of playing vital roles in baby making, they determine how you look and feel much of the time.

Our hormones are in constant flux, and many (most) women are entirely unaware of what is happening behind the scenes. The natural hormonal rhythms signal our fertile window with changes in cervical fluid and libido. Our period is often preceded by dips in energy or changes in appetite. The cyclical changes in our hormones trigger both physical and emotional sensations. You might say that women are somewhat ruled by their hormones, so much so that we try, for much of our lives, to suppress them with birth control. "So *what?*" you say. Well, if you are currently struggling to get pregnant, getting in touch with the nuances of your cycle can illuminate the path to a baby.

Putting the Cart before the Horse

Basics are often overlooked in favor of complex, time-consuming medical exams and invasive procedures. However, in some cases, an understanding of your body is all you actually need to get knocked up. Even if something more complex *is* going on, dealing with the basics (your hormones, your cycle, and the main signs

1

of fertility) first creates a stronger foundation, empowering you to take on more complicated problems with fewer headaches down the line.

Now, if you've picked up this book because you've tried and tried the basic techniques to no avail, you may already know some of the things discussed in both this chapter and the next. However, I encourage you to at least take the time to speed-read both chapters, pausing if some new information catches your eye, because there will be tips and insights that can't be gleaned from internet searches or your average "mommy blog." There are also a number of topics and terms introduced here that will continue to pop back up in later chapters, and I want you to stay in the loop.

Since we are living in an age of information, it makes sense that we begin this book with a factual dissection of body mechanics. From there, you can learn to tune into sensations that will help you make the best choices for your hormonal health and fertility. When you know what to look for, you can take action to optimize your fertility and get your body on track. It's time to get savvy about your cycle!

Mapping Your Cycle

All your fertility hormones are supposed to work in harmony, like a coordinated dance. One hormone leads during each phase of your cycle, and then it steps aside for the next when the "song" changes. If something interrupts the rhythm of your phases, the hormones get out of step. Essentially, your brain and ovaries stop communicating properly. This is when difficulties arise.

To take control of your fertility, it's helpful to recognize the signs of these hormonal imbalances and know which steps will help you glide back into proper rhythm. In this chapter, we'll explore the hormones present in your body, the role each one plays, and how an imbalance of one or more hormones might manifest. You'll see these themes cropping up throughout the coming chapters, so learning the patterns will be the foundation on which you get in touch with your body's unique rhythms and your most fertile days.

IN THE FLOW

The menstrual phase is the forerunner we're all most familiar with because it has a flashing red sign attached. Entering the menstrual phase means your hormones are rapidly declining, causing your uterine lining to shed. Day 1 is considered the first day of flow, which can be confusing since it has to be full "flow" rather than "spotting." Think of day 1 as the first day of actual bleeding, not the brown or pink spotting that can occur in the days before flow comes to town. During days 1 to 3, doctors test your follicle-stimulating hormone (FSH) levels, which works together with estrogen to grow an egg. It is also a very important data point to assess the health of your ovaries. To understand the important role this hormone plays, it's helpful to know that your ovaries are lined with follicles, which (mostly) contain eggs inside them. FSH stimulates follicles to grow, allowing the egg to begin maturing under the influence of estrogen (secreted by the follicles).

> An FSH test is administered on day 2 of your cycle because, in the menstrual phase, estrogen is at its lowest and FSH is at its highest in order to stimulate the release of estrogen needed for the next phases. Once your estrogen levels go up, the FSH number isn't reliable anymore.

Your brain sends a signal that triggers FSH to "tickle" your follicles, but this occurs only if your levels are within the designated healthy ranges. If not, the eggs could grow too slow, arrest (i.e., stop growing), or even grow too fast. Each of these scenarios poses problems for egg quality and the eggs' ability to mature, fertilize, and develop properly.

If your FSH is too high (registering higher than 10 on days 2 or 3 of your cycle), it is an indication that your ovaries might be a tad on the fritz. Essentially, your brain keeps signaling your body to produce FSH, which should signal your ovaries to produce an egg, but your ovaries are not responding to the rise in FSH. So you continue producing more FSH with little or no result (i.e., an egg won't grow and mature). Most commonly, this happens naturally as you age, but it can also be related to things like excess toxin exposure, chronic stress, autoimmune issues, or chemotherapy.

Take my patient Marie, for example. Marie was an ambitious 41-year-old tech mogul. She and her husband had embarked on an IVF journey after trying naturally to no avail for six months. The fertility clinic ran her "day 2 numbers" and found her FSH was slightly elevated at 14. She was told to sit the IVF cycle out in hopes of a better number to start the next cycle. Her fertility doctor told her that an elevated FSH is associated with poor IVF outcomes and suggested Chinese medicine as a means to bring the number down, sending her my way.

Marie was quite the sugar-fiend workaholic and had trouble slowing down. I explained that FSH can spike when there is too much stress in the body and that she needed to cool it on the sweets and tone down her type A task list for the few weeks leading up to her next cycle. I combined two Chinese herbal formulas that are commonly used for menopausal symptoms, anxiety, and premature ovarian failure. I'm not implying that Marie was menopausal, but this particular herbal combination had qualities that reversed the premature aging of her ovaries. I also used acupuncture twice per week, focusing on specific acupoints that target the FSH. When she went in for her next day 2 testing, her FSH was down to 9, and she was given the go-ahead to start IVF.

GROW, EGG(S), GROW!

As your period starts to taper, you enter the follicular phase. It marks the beginning of the slow rise of estrogen that triggers the follicles in your ovaries to begin growing an egg or eggs in preparation for ovulation. During this phase, you're getting a steady "drip" of estrogen, helping you feel clear, inspired, and energetic.

Estrogen is the lady hormone everyone is familiar with. Sadly, it's used in a negative context quite commonly, due in part to the lingering effects of misogyny. Maybe your first time hearing it went something like, "There's way too much estrogen in this room." It gets blamed for crying fits and anything emotional. But what estrogen also does is boost your libido and collagen, keeping you perky in more ways than one. It keeps your lady parts lubricated, and in healthy ratios, it actually keeps you clearheaded. Without it, you may feel saggy, dry, foggy, and crabby. In terms of fertility, estrogen is essential to grow both an egg and a thick uterine lining. You can't make a baby without it.

> Estrogen makes us feel feminine and beautiful! In optimal levels, it promotes collagen production in the skin (fighting off wrinkles), makes our boobs perky, and prevents skin sag.

If your estrogen levels are less than adequate, you may feel a somewhat dry down yonder with little to no sex drive. Not great for the baby-making mission. Low levels of estrogen or estrogen that is slow to climb are associated with a late ovulation (20 or more days into your cycle). Late ovulation can at times be associated with lesser egg quality when it occurs in conjunction with an elevated FSH or polycystic ovarian syndrome (PCOS). That said, many of my patients ovulate late and still get pregnant, but it takes longer than if we were working with more abundant estrogen levels.

> Estrogen lubricates your lady parts, grows your egg(s), and thickens your lining. Baby making can't happen without it!

Prolonged low estrogen levels can cause discomforts like body aches, hot flashes, and intense mood swings. You basically experience menopausal-type symptoms, including an irregular or absent period. It's quite unpleasant and totally unnecessary. I've been there. When I was 27, I moved to China, and my previously regular 28-day period went AWOL. It could have been the stress, the pollution, a parasite, or a combination (the Orient bestowed all of these gifts during my stay). When I was also diagnosed with PCOS by a doctor in India who saw multiple cysts on my ovaries, it made sense. PCOS is a hormonal disorder closely tied to improper hormone production. Regardless of which factor was most responsible, my period remained absent until I went on a meditation retreat one and a half years later. When I returned to Canada, the first nurse who saw my blood work was confused. Brow furrowed, she told me, "Your hormones are in the postmenopausal ranges" (i.e., flatlined). I wasn't producing eggs, my breasts were a little limp, and I felt frenzied. Although it should have been alarming, I knew there must be a way to mend my lady parts. Out of concern for my future fertility, I took action. As a clinician focused on women's health, I was excited to take on the challenge of a total body-healing experiment. I put myself on a Chinese herbal cocktail and did acupuncture twice per week with a colleague. It took only one month for my period to return, but my hormones needed a bit more time to fully regulate.

> Insanely heavy periods? Your estrogen levels are likely causing the crime scene.

Much of the time, low estrogen, or estrogen deficiency, is caused by simple aging. But low estrogen can also be caused by factors like being underweight, overexercising, chronic stress, premature ovarian failure, PCOS, and toxins floating in the air or lurking in your daily beauty routine.

One of my past patients, Mary, wasn't ovulating because her body wasn't producing enough estrogen to grow an egg. Her levels were so low that she was noticing droopy breasts and a nonexistent sex drive. In addition, she was lacking fertile signs, such as clear cervical mucus in her underwear. After a long chat in my office, we pinpointed the cause as a recent stressful event in her life that had caused her to lose weight very rapidly. This shock to her system had slowed her estrogen production. My prescription? Rest, meditation, herbs, acupuncture, and nutritious meals. It's often a combination of many little things remedied by simple but often overlooked day-to-day habit changes.

> Estrogen is commonly low in women with PCOS, POA, perimenopause, amenorrhea, and menopause.

Too Much of a Good Thing

Too much estrogen can also be devastating to our bodies. Estrogen is meant to be your dominant hormone only for the two weeks leading up to ovulation. After that, the hormone progesterone is meant to take the lead, keeping estrogen in balance. If progesterone is deficient or if you have excess estrogens in your system, you can develop estrogen dominance and experience symptoms such as horribly painful periods, mood swings, weight gain, and migraines. There are many circumstances that can lead to estrogen dominance. Some women aren't producing enough progesterone naturally. Sometimes, it's brought on by an anovulatory cycle, meaning a cycle where you don't ovulate. Other contributors are excess weight, immune disorders, a low-fiber diet, and too much stress. Much of the time, excess estrogen is linked to issues like fibroids or endometriosis. These conditions are exacerbated by ingesting too much estrogen-heavy food (e.g., soy) or overexposure to environmental estrogens (e.g., xenoestrogens found in plastics and pesticides). The catch is that conditions like fibroids also *produce* excess estrogens that proliferate symptoms. The best approach here is to make sure the liver and guts are healthy enough to effectively eliminate the estrogens. More on that in chapters 4 and 7.

READY, SET, GO!

The ovulation phase begins once the egg has matured. Ovulation is triggered by a surge in luteinizing hormone (LH) around the middle of your cycle. The spike in LH makes the egg drop out of the follicle into the ovary to travel down the fallopian tubes and meet with the sperm. Preceding this surge, you were likely feeling extra frisky thanks to your peaking estrogen levels. Men can actually smell your fertile pheromones, so don't be surprised if you are getting more attention than usual during this time. During ovulation and in the days leading up, your vaginal discharge begins to turn clear, thin out, and become extra slippery. You're basically creating natural "lube" during this phase. Your skyrocketing sex hormones are trying to urge you to get between the sheets because your egg is moving into prime position.

Without the LH surge, the egg likely doesn't drop. LH essentially pulls the trigger that gets your egg moving. Even with the aid of ovulation predictor kits (OPKs), many women have issues tracking their fertile window (i.e., the time at which they ovulate) because their LH levels don't perform as they should. Sometimes the surge doesn't happen because the egg didn't reach maturation, and sometimes (as in PCOS or premature ovarian failure [POF]) the LH is continuously elevated, so you never get a clear read. Or perhaps the "half-life" of your surge was too short, and the LH left your system before you tested in the morning. To combat this, I suggest testing twice a day. You can use cheap OPK dip sticks off Amazon (Clinical Guard is one such brand) so you don't feel the financial burn. Although most women can use an ovulation predictor stick with good success, this method is not the best for some. In the next chapter, we explore all the ways you can identify your fertile window.

My patient Carlene came to me holding a box of ovulation sticks, a scowl on her face. She couldn't get a clear reading. The sticks were signaling that she was in the fertile zone, but they never confirmed ovulation. Carlene's LH was failing to spike. She often had long cycles up to 45 days and could never fully pinpoint her fertile window. Her system was a bit sluggish and slow to produce estrogen to mature the egg. Once her egg finally got there, her ovary wouldn't give it the boot. In her case, it ended up being a simple fix. I suspected insulin resistance (chapter 5)

> If your LH isn't spiking naturally, you have a few options to trigger ovulation manually. You can try out acupuncture for a more natural stimulation or ask your doctor for a "trigger shot" to release the egg. Optimal nutrition can also help you ovulate regularly.

and asked her to lay off heavy, fatty foods and excess carbs and exercise for 20 minutes four times per week. We added acupuncture to induce ovulation, and she was pregnant within two months.

Once an LH spike has gotten your egg in transit, it will slowly make its way down your fallopian tube over the next couple days. If one of your part-

> The technical term for a fertilized egg is an embryo.

ner's sperms manages to wriggle up the tube and fertilize the egg, the cells start dividing rapidly, working to create life.

INCUBATION

The luteal phase begins after the egg drops. If the egg is fertilized, it will become an embryo and travel through the fallopian tube to the uterus. Once there, it will burrow in. The sac left inside the empty follicle becomes a progesterone-secreting structure called the corpus luteum. While estrogen is the key player in producing an egg, progesterone is the VIP when it comes to maintaining a pregnancy. That's because after estrogen thickens your uterine lining, progesterone keeps it fluffed up and intact so that the embryo stays in place. Progesterone also warms your body, which is why you'll see your body temperature stay above 98°F throughout your luteal phase (more on this in the next chapter).

Eastern medicine purports that many cases of infertility are due to a "cold uterus." Theoretically, the modern translation could be low body temps due to low progesterone, low thyroid, or both. Many women struggling with infertility report cold feet, so it's not too surprising that Eastern medicine relates this to the state of the uterus. Eastern tradition says to keep your feet toasty with foot baths or warm socks when you are trying to get pregnant.

This increase in temperature is sort of like incubation, helping to create an ideal environment for an implanted egg.

My patient Suzie came to me with all the symptoms of progesterone deficiency. She had a mean case of premenstrual insomnia in addition to her fertility struggles. She felt absolutely nuts with anxiety and rage leading up to her period. To boot, she also felt fat and bloated and had freezing-cold feet between ovulation and menstruation. She told me she wore wool socks to bed, even in the summer. Suzie's body temperature never went above 97.2°F, even in her ovulation window and afterward. It sounded to me as if her progesterone was too low. It was also plausible that she wasn't ovulating at all. Without adequate progesterone, she couldn't relax or sleep, and her symptoms with premenstrual syndrome (PMS) were hellish. Most of all, a healthy pregnancy would be unlikely in this scenario.

Adequate progesterone is essential for quality sleep, a balanced mood, and minimal PMS symptoms. It makes you feel skinny and relaxed. If you feel bloated and anxious or if you have trouble sleeping before your period, you may be progesterone deficient.

Progesterone deficiency, like Suzie was experiencing, is the partner syndrome of estrogen dominance, and it's equally as detrimental to fertility. Progesterone plays a crucial role in getting and staying pregnant. Between approximately the seventh and tenth day of your luteal phase, a fertilized egg should burrow into the wall of the uterus. If you're undergoing IVF, the time frame is accelerated to implant three to five days after the fertilized embryo is placed in your uterus. If you don't have enough progesterone, the uterine lining will break apart and drop the burrowing embryo before it properly latches, causing an early miscarriage. One telltale symptom of low progesterone is spotting leading up to the period, caused by

Progesterone deficiency and fluctuations are associated with premenstrual dysphoric disorder (PMDD). This is essentially a severe form of PMS that can produce serious issues like depression and extreme anxiety in the two weeks leading up to your period.

the lining dissolving too early, though this could also be caused by growths such as fibroids or polyps. Period-like bleeding around the time of ovulation could signify luteal phase defect (LPD), a syndrome in which your progesterone isn't functioning properly (or at all). LPD also likely indicates an issue with ovulation.

The luteal phase is the final phase before menstruation begins again. Around 10 to 12 days into this phase, if sperm and egg have not united, your hormones will begin to decline. The uterine lining will shed, and the remnants pass through as a period. However, if you *are* pregnant at this point, the progesterone keeps pumping, and the lining stays intact—hence no bleeding—and then you enter the "prego" phase.

Unraveling the System

There is so much power in learning the nuances of our monthly cycle and mastering our body's rhythms. Now that you have a full picture of how your hormones interact with each other, you can pinpoint which of your hormones might be on the fritz. Getting a handle on hormone basics is an essential first step to taking charge of your fertility. Being cycle savvy also sets you up for success in the next foundational step: honing in on your fertile window. No one is getting knocked up without "doing the deed" at the right time. Every woman will have a unique rhythm, but luckily, the basic steps to uncovering it are mostly the same for everybody. So, next, let's talk about how to perfect your timing.

CHAPTER 2

Finding Your Fertile Window

I don't know about you, but I didn't learn jack about my hormones as a teen. The arrival of our womanhood is quite hush-hush and perhaps still even somewhat "taboo." Unfortunately, the result is that many women are never taught about their bodies. Many women I encounter have never heard of their fertile window and aren't aware that their hormones change several times throughout the month. Without an understanding of your body, taking the proper steps to get pregnant at the proper time becomes blind luck. Learning hormone fundamentals opened my eyes to how much more women could accomplish if we just understood our natural rhythms. I place great emphasis on educating women about their monthly cycle because in many cases, it's getting in tune that makes all the difference. Understanding and tracking fertility signs takes the guesswork out of getting busy.

Charting Your Fertility Signs

Body Basics 101: It's tricky to make a baby if you don't know when you ovulate. Technically, you could accidentally have sex at the right time, but you picked up this book because you want to make sure you are taking your best shot. Let's explore how listening to your body's signals enhances your ability to conceive.

There are three main signs of ovulation that you can observe and chart to give yourself a visual representation of your cycle (i.e., a map to guide you). First up, we have cervical mucus, that lovely goo that appears in your underwear. The other two are a little harder to see but can still be easily tracked. Many women don't know their cervix lengthens and shortens each month like clockwork, but testing your cervical position is actually a highly reliable indicator you're ovulating. Finally, your basal body temperature (BBT) (your body's resting internal temperature) can be taken and charted to pinpoint the drop of your egg. Tracking these major indicators and noting the place where all the signs overlap predicts your prime ovulation days, aka your "fertile window."

Charting may sound tedious at first, but it really takes only a few minutes every day, and it's a heck of a lot cheaper (and often more accurate) than buying one-time-use ovulation sticks. In the age of apps, it's even simpler. No need to draw out graphs; you can quickly record and store all the data together and then have a graph generated for you.

Recommended Apps

There are a zillion apps out there, some with sophisticated graphics and some that keep it super bare bones. Some you'll have to pay for, but others are free. A number of my patients use Glow, Ovia, FMC, and Kindara. They are all good, in my opinion, and they'll get the job done. When app shopping, check for the ability to record notes on daily moods, sensations, sexual activity, and cervical fluid on top of merely recording temperature to generate a graph.

Your prime time to get between the sheets is before and during ovulation, not after. Yes, there are other variables at play, like the strength of the sperm, but in general, when your egg drops, you have a short time frame in which to get pregnant. So you want your partner's sperm already in transit toward your fallopian tube. If you miss that narrow window of opportunity and your egg does not unite with sperm, it will start to dissolve. Thanks to your fertile mucus, the sperm are a little more resilient; they can live inside your lady cave for 48 hours. So, if you have sex a day or two before you ovulate, the sperm are basically sitting at the starting line, waiting for the race to the egg to begin. Of course, to have those sperm ready and waiting, you need to predict when that egg will drop. That's where efficient, thorough charting, and a reliable app come in.

What's Your pH Down There?

Sometimes sperm doesn't make it to the egg because your vaginal and cervical environments are too acidic for the sperm to thrive. You essentially have what I call an "angry vag." Most of the time, it's simple lifestyle factors causing the trouble. You'll learn more later in this book, but for starters, I recommend getting a simple pH kit from Amazon to test your acidity. If your pH is skewing more acidic than alkaline, then try eating more alkaline foods than acidic foods to achieve a more sperm-friendly pH— i.e., more plant foods (veggies)—and avoid coffee, booze, and stress, which are some leading causes of "angry (acidic) vag."

For example, one of my patients, Lindsay, had been trying to get pregnant for six months. She was 28, newly married, and hoping to avoid going to a fertility doctor. She came to me, frustrated, a few months after her wedding. She had quit taking birth control on her honeymoon, but three months had lapsed with no luck. She said she was following her app to find her fertile window and was having sex on day 14 of her cycle. When I asked her how long her cycles were, she said sometimes 27 days and sometimes 33 days. Well, that irregularity meant her fertile window would shift around each month, meaning she was likely missing it if she was narrowly focused on day 14. The most basic "menstrual apps" use your last period as the main indicator of your ovulation, but that leaves room for inaccuracies when your cycles aren't precisely 28 days. These kinds of apps aren't taking in enough variables, and thus their predictions are less than superb. In fact, even if you have a solid 28-day cycle each month, it doesn't mean the app is correct. It's guesstimating based on very limited data. It's best to track all your body's changes to get an accurate read.

I asked Lindsay if she had any symptoms around her ovulation. She hadn't noticed anything and couldn't really tell me much detail about her vaginal discharge. I then asked if she had tried an OPK (the stick that you pee on to see if you are ovulating). She said she had tried, but they stressed her out because she didn't know when to start them and wasn't getting a "positive" on the days she used them. I told her that a good, cheap, and easy at-home option to explore was to track her three main fertility signs and log them into an app. All she'd have to buy was a digital thermometer.

I had Lindsay take her temperature orally each morning at the same time, then log it into a new app daily. I then told her to keep a close eye out for when the temperature suddenly shot up. At the same time, she needed to pay attention

> ## Did You Know?
>
> It is possible to have your period without ovulating.

to her libido, discharge, and, if she was feeling adventurous, the position of her cervix. After tracking for a month, we took a look at the chart and saw that the new "cycle tracking" system was not at all matching up with that first menstrual app's predictions. She'd been having sex either too early or too late every month. The next month, she tracked again and started to notice more of the fertility signs coming together. She didn't have to do any charting after that because she and her husband got the timing right. She was pregnant!

So you've learned about the four phases of your cycle, and you're starting to get a better handle on the timing of your fertile window. Lindsay got knocked up by getting in tune with her body's natural cues. Rather than just relying on expensive and frustrating OPKs, let's look at how you can master your own natural cues to identify your ovulation and optimize your fertile time.

Ovulation Predictor Kits (OPKs)— Are They Worth It?

Seeing that positive result "smiley face" on an ovulation stick is a reassuring feeling, making their use worthwhile. However, many women complain that the tests indicated they were in the fertile window, but they never got a strong positive indicating ovulation. To avoid this frustration and save your money, it's best to chart your cycle in conjunction with using an OPK. That way, you'll have more information about the state of your hormone levels, and you'll have an additional way to determine ovulation in case the stick fails you. Also worth noting is that a lot of women have much more success using an OPK when they have already started charting their cycle. They realize that before charting, they were testing on the wrong days. Keep in mind that you don't *need* the expensive, fancy ones with the smiley faces. But if having the more advanced gadget makes you feel more comfortable, go for it. The best method is to use the OPK as confirmation that your chart is accurate and as one final check mark indicating ovulation.

CERVICAL MUCUS

It's an unpleasant word, "mucus," but it's important to talk about the egg white–like goo that appears around this time each month. You may have noticed that it changes in color, consistency, and quantity as you move through your cycle. This is because the changes in estrogen and progesterone are what dictate the state of your cervical mucus. If you are getting funky colors, odors, or textures, then the conversation is more about bacteria and yeast. More on that later.

When your period is drawing to an end, it's time to start checking your underwear and examining your cervical mucus. I recommend checking a few times a day since the timing for the arrival of the "goo" isn't the same for everyone. For instance, modern women are often drier in the evenings thanks to long, stressful days.

At times, you may find little to no mucus in your panties, so a little extra effort is involved in order to effectively chart. Sit on the toilet or squat, insert your (clean) index finger into your hoo-ha, and rub the sides to get a little something. If you're too dry for even this technique, then your estrogen may be low, or there may be other hormonal factors that lifestyle changes and natural medicine can address. The fertility drug Clomid can also have a drying effect. Chat with

Did You Know?

Stress can dry up your cervical mucus.

your practitioner if your cervical mucus is on the dry side. A fertility specialist or OB/GYN may suggest a lubricant such as "preseed," and/or an acupuncturist or naturopath can help address it with natural methods to regulate hormones, reduce stress, and the like.

Tips for Stellar Cervical Fluid

Not noticing much going on down there? Perhaps you're a little dry. Here are some simple tips to get the healthy moisture flowing:

1. Quit coffee.
2. Reduce intense exercise.
3. Relax more.
4. Hydrate.
5. Get quality sleep.
6. Try maca or a Chinese formula containing rehmannia and Dang Gui.

When your estrogen levels are rising, in the follicular phase, you get the clear or slightly milky fluid that makes your underwear damp. When estrogen is at its peak, nearing the ovulation phase, you have fertile mucus—that slippery, thicker, clear mucus that looks like egg whites. It's actually very stretchy, so if you're unsure whether you've switched from follicular-phase fluid to fertile ovulation mucus, take a little between your fingers, pinch them together, and then slowly separate them. If the mucus stretches about one or two inches between two fingers before it separates, you're in the fertile zone, either ovulating or just about to ovulate. When you move into the luteal phase and progesterone takes over, your mucus turns milky white and more opaque.

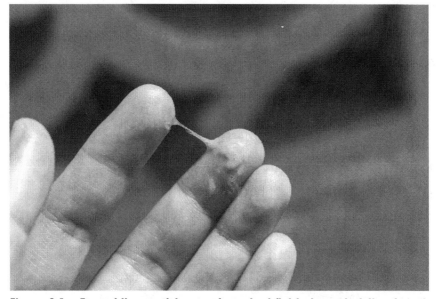

Figure 2.1. Egg white consistency of cervical fluid characteristic of peak fertility and ovulation. *Kckate16*

Ideally, you want to see three to five days of fertile mucus. It builds up before you ovulate so that the sperm enter into a hospitable environment. Fertile mucus acts as a source of nourishment, allowing the sperm to sit around in your uterus or fallopian tubes and patiently wait for the egg to arrive. Your egg survives for only 12 hours after being released, so that slippery consistency allows the sperm to swim faster and reach the egg in time. It's also a natural lubricant that makes sex more enjoyable.

Best of all, charting your cervical fluid can help you pinpoint your peak day, which is essentially the day you are the most likely to conceive. The quantity of mucus continues building right up until the egg is released from the ovary, and then it quickly changes consistency. So, when you notice a pattern in your fertile mucus chart, you can predict your peak day by identifying which day is going to be the last day you produce fertile mucus. Once the mucus changes consistency to its more opaque form after ovulation, you and your hubby can take a break because the window has passed.

You need to do a full month of charting before your app can properly predict your peak day. Also keep in mind that you actually want to start getting busy two to three days before you ovulate, the reason being that knowing your peak day doesn't mean you know exactly when the egg will drop. If your partner has a low sperm count or if his little guys have problems with their shape or swimming capabilities, they may not make it for a full 48 hours. Due to these variables, it's best to have regular intercourse in the days surrounding your peak day. This does *not* mean you should have sex every day. In fact, for some, that can deplete sperm and aggravate your lady parts. Aim for every second day starting three to four days before you estimate ovulation will take place based on previous cycles and charting. The more months you chart, the more you should see a pattern and the better you will get at predicting the best days to have sex.

When Things Get "Funky"

Frequent, large amounts of creamy or egg-white consistency discharge in your luteal phase suggests you may have an excess of estrogen. This could be caused by a medical condition like fibroids or ovarian cysts. It could also be due to a diet rich in carbs and sugars that may cause bacterial and yeast imbalances in the vagina. Smelly discharge could mean you have bacterial vaginosis. A cottage cheese–like texture or irritation in your intimates suggests you have extra yeast. These are all symptoms you should track and mention to your practitioner. Many are easily addressed with dietary changes and herbs or supplements, and you may see even your most difficult symptoms pleasantly resolve after applying the tips presented in this book.

CERVICAL POSITION

Feeling around deep in your hoo-ha is awkward and uncomfortable for most women, but your cervical position is actually the most accurate of the three fertility signs. You can rely on your cervix because it always changes according to the phases of your cycle. During your period, your cervix is low and slightly open to allow the menstrual blood to exit your body. During the follicular phase, it closes almost entirely. That's why you barely see any goo in your panties right after your period. However, when it's time to ovulate, your cervix rises and opens up. This significant change is very noticeable if you're checking on your cervix daily. When you have to reach farther to find your cervix and you feel that softer, wider opening, it's a sure sign that your egg will be released in the next few days.

Checking in on your cervix takes some practice, but it's worth the learning curve. You'll first need to master the right stance. Either sit on the toilet or squat down near your floor. No matter which method you choose, make sure you keep it consistent. An inconsistency in your body's position could make your cervix position feel different to you even though nothing has actually changed.

Once you're in position, stick one or two clean fingers inside your vagina and feel your cervix. It's best to start checking right after your period. Your cervix will be lower and easy to reach, so you can get used to detecting it. You'll then be more likely to notice the change later on when you enter your fertile window. When your cervix is closed, it will feel harder, like the tip of your nose, and you won't be able to stick your finger inside. During ovulation, your cervix will be a bit harder to reach, and when you touch it, it will feel softer, like your earlobe. You'll notice an opening, and there will likely be an abundance of cervical mucus present.

If your app doesn't have the ability to chart the position and feel of your cervix, don't sweat it. This one is the easiest to chart on paper. All you have to do is number the days of your cycle and then denote with single letters whether your cervix was high (H) or low (L), firm (F) or soft (S), and open (O) or closed (C) on that day.

Charting cervical position isn't a cakewalk for everyone. Some women struggle to ever find their cervix, and some find the process painful. In those cases, don't sweat it; tracking your mucus and your BBT can provide sufficient data. For everyone else, however, its accuracy is worth the effort, the reason being that it can make sense of erratic mucus or temperature readings caused by illness, sleep issues, or boozy behavior.

BBT

BBT charting maps the temperature changes associated with the hormonal fluctuations that mark transitions in your monthly cycle. Simply put, your BBT is the temperature of your body at rest. By mapping that temperature throughout the month, you'll see peaks and dips that indicate you're moving from one phase of the cycle to the next. To identify your fertile window, you'll look for a spike that indicates an LH surge and the consequent release of your egg. On your graph, the temperature change will look something like a lightning bolt, rising sharply within a day or two, plummeting again, and then creating a gradual, more sloped rise that indicates you've entered the luteal phase. That secondary slow rise is created by the hormonal shift that moves you from ovulation into the luteal phase. The increase in progesterone in the luteal phase makes your internal temperature rise. It could also be referred to as "incubation" since

> If your temperature takes several days to rise rather than shooting up suddenly, you may have slight deficiencies of your thyroid, adrenal, or lady hormones.

the body is trying to create an ideal nurturing environment for the embryo (fertilized egg). If conception is achieved, the increase in temperature will be maintained past the time when your period was meant to arrive, indicating pregnancy. If the egg is not fertilized, your temperature drops right before or at the onset of your period. Keep in mind that, unless you're sick, your internal temperature is going to change only in slight increments of 0.1°F or 0.2°F.

Charting your BBT daily during a span of two or three months will provide a comprehensive picture of your hormonal shifts. Using that picture, you can determine the regularity of your cycle, predict when you're most likely to ovulate next, and increase your chances of conception. BBT charting will also help you identify hormonal imbalances, such as high FSH or low progesterone, so that you can address them with your practitioner. My patient Jodi was using BBT charting simply as an extra tool for pinpointing the best days to have sex with her partner, but she discovered a discrepancy. I had explained what a typical chart should look like, and she noticed that her temperature didn't rise mid-cycle as it should. Her body was not producing enough progesterone, keeping her recorded temps low. Armed with that knowledge, we worked on mindfulness techniques to reduce stress and added a Chinese formula called You Gui Wan to her regime. The following month, her chart looked perfect, and she finally had a clear picture of her fertile window. Even better, her newly balanced progesterone levels helped her body create the perfect environment for "incubation," and she conceived shortly thereafter.

To begin tracking your own BBT, you'll need a reliable thermometer. Some practitioners recommend a BBT thermometer, suggesting they are more accurate. Personally, I think a regular digital thermometer works just fine. The choice is yours.

WHAT TO REMEMBER WHEN TAKING YOUR BBT

- There can be slight variations between thermometers, so use the same one each time. If your trusty thermometer breaks and you have to buy a new one, make a note on your chart.
- Take your temperature right when you wake up, before you do any sort of activity. It's best to leave your thermometer within reach so you can use it before you even get out of bed.
- Take your temperature at the same time every day or at least within the same hour. If you overslept, your temperature may have risen as the day progressed. Should you hit the snooze button too many times, note the discrepancy or don't put a number down at all and indicate why.

Step 1

Ideally, start making your chart on the first day of your period. This means the first day of full blood flow (i.e., not spotting). However, you can still gather good information no matter when you start, so if you are ready to get started, then go for it. Even starting mid-cycle is still a good use of time despite the fact that it won't provide a full picture. If you're going old school and forgoing the app, you can print a template off the internet. I'd personally recommend an app, however, as it's simple and clean and will create a clear graph of the inputted temperatures for you. I'm betting your phone is with you at all times anyway, and if you mess up, it's a heck of a lot easier to fix. Paper is still a fine option—whatever works best for you.

Ovulation Spotting

Hormone levels shift dramatically at ovulation and can sometimes be slow to transition into the next phase. In some cases, progesterone rises too slowly to keep the uterine lining fully intact. This can, at times, cause you to have mid-cycle spotting. Don't assume you've started your period unless you see steady blood flow. Otherwise, you might actually miss ovulation. If the spotting turns heavy or carries on for more than a few days, consult a practitioner, as your hormone levels might be hanging too low or behaving erratically.

Step 2

It's best to take your temperature consistently every day for a month. However, missing a day is not the end of the world. Enter your recordings into your app or chart. Note any unusual circumstances, such as sickness, lack of sleep, or a boozy evening, and discard those as abnormal readings. Make a similar note for any adjustments to your routine, like a trip, a new medication, or even an extra-stressful day.

> Alcohol can also raise your temperature. It's not great for fertility anyway, so it's best to avoid it altogether. Should you indulge, however, make a note so that you'll know the culprit behind a wonky temperature change.

Step 3

Look back at your chart when the month has ended (marked by the onset of your period). Mid-cycle, or around days 10 to 18, you should see a spike in your temperature, followed by a drop and then a slow rise of up to 1°F, or 0.6°C. It should remain at that level for about three days. Those were the days directly following your ovulation. Typically, pre-ovulation temperatures hover near 97.4°F and post-ovulation is around 98°F or slightly above.

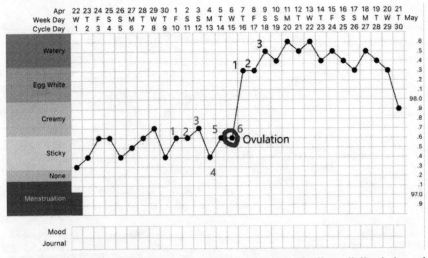

Figure 2.2. Basal body temperature chart demonstrating distinct rise of body temperature at time of LH surge and ovulation. *www.kindra.com*

Step 4

When you start next month's chart, make a note of which day your temperature first rose. If your temperature rose on the eleventh day of your cycle last month, this month, have sex on the ninth, the eleventh, and the thirteenth and keep an eye on your temperature to note the indicative spike and drop.

The Coverline Tool

Your charting app may have a function called the "coverline" to help you pinpoint your ovulation. Essentially, the coverline is a line placed between your pre-ovulatory and post-ovulatory temperatures on your chart. It's a visual tool to indicate you've entered the fertile window. Refer to figure 2.2 for an example of what that coverline will look like in your chart. In subsequent months of charting, insert your coverline in the same spot as the previous month. When your reading breaches the coverline, it means ovulation is in effect. Three consecutive days of temperatures recorded above your coverline means you are no longer fertile.

Atypical Cycles

Did your temperature spike unusually late in the month? Did you not see a rise at all? You could have experienced an atypical cycle. There are two types: a stress cycle and an anovulatory cycle.

A stress cycle is exactly what it sounds like. Extreme stress can essentially "short-circuit" your hypothalamic–pituitary–ovarian (HPO) axis, which can cause a hormonal imbalance that may signal your body to delay ovulation until the stress is eliminated. This kind of cycle is also common when you have been traveling or have experienced other drastic changes to your routine. We'll talk more about the physical effects of stress in chapter 6.

An anovulatory cycle means you didn't ovulate. Your estrogen may not have climbed high enough to mature an egg and trigger a surge in LH. Most women have one or two anovulatory cycles each year, and they are nothing to worry about. This may be the reason behind "faulty" ovulation predictor sticks that never show a positive no matter how frequently you test. Charting alongside or in place of predictor sticks is super helpful under these circumstances. An extended pattern of anovulatory cycles could indicate conditions like PCOS, hypothyroidism, or perimenopause (more on those in chapter 3). If you want double confirmation that you are, in fact, experiencing anovulatory cycles, there are tests your doctor can run.

Not everyone experiences steady rises in BBT. You could fall into a smaller category of women who experience a less obvious rise that makes detecting the prime three days more difficult. Other women experience erratic rises and falls right before and/or after ovulation, making identifying the true rise difficult. Eastern and natural medicine practitioners have multiple explanations for why this is occurring—ranging from hormone imbalance to stress to dietary factors. Regardless of cause, charting all three fertility signs and enlisting occasional help from an OPK can clear up the confusion with a more complete picture. Your fertile window can vary month to month, and having the extra data helps you pinpoint the true rise by matching one of your temperature peaks with the days you had fertile mucus or the days your cervix felt more open. Without all three indicators, you may get inaccurate readings.

If all this sounds stressful and unappealing, you are not alone. A better route for you might be to book an appointment with your gynecologist or a fertility specialist and request they "monitor" your cycle. Typically, this involves going to the clinic every few days to do a blood test and an ultrasound to monitor your estrogen rise and the growth of your egg so they can pinpoint when you're most likely to ovulate. They can also give you a "trigger shot" to release the egg once it has matured.

OTHER SIGNS OF OVULATION

There are a number of other ovulation signs and symptoms that are a little less obvious and measurable, primarily because they often mimic PMS. This typically makes it harder to identify them as true ovulation signs. However, your more solid data points for cervical mucus, cervical position, and BBT already tell you roughly when you should ovulate. Thus, these smaller signals become extra check marks on your list, not to mention indicators that you may have a hormonal imbalance.

As if menstrual cramps weren't annoying enough, it's also fairly common to experience pain in your ovaries during ovulation. This pain can manifest in your lower back or abdominal/pelvic area, just like period cramps, but some women feel this pain only when standing or sitting up. It will be slightly different for everyone. A smaller amount of women experience rectal pressure and some constipation. Jot down a note in your chart on days you're cramping but not experiencing bleeding. See if those days align with spikes in your BBT or the presence of fertile mucus. If so, you're likely ovulating. Experiencing cramping along with menstrual blood in what should be your fertile window is a different matter. In that case, you may be experiencing an abnormally short cycle, and you should inform your practitioner. This can be treated holistically or by using medications such as Clomid.

The Menstrual Cycle Experts

Consider seeing an alternative medicine practitioner to discuss cycle irregularities. Conventional doctors aren't as concerned with nuances in your cycle. Their primary focus is on larger issues that can be treated with medications and IVF, and there aren't great medical protocols for subtler imbalances. Alternative medicine specialists, on the other hand, are laser focused on your hormones, using them as clues to diagnose subtle imbalances in the body and develop a treatment plan involving lifestyle changes and natural medicine.

Feel like you inexplicably wake up in a fat suit mid-cycle? You're probably bloated and gassy as a result of ovulation. Oh joy. The mid-cycle munchies don't help either. The radical hormone shifts moving into the ovulatory phase make you crave salt, candy, ice cream, pasta, bread, and anything else generally unhealthy. You may also be subjected to bouts of irrational emotion. The resulting signs of ovulation may include but are not limited to crying over songs and movies, lashing out at your partner with sudden rage, or finding it hard to concentrate on simple tasks.

Knowing the subtle signs that indicate you've passed your fertile window is also helpful for rounding out your chart. Right after you ovulate, your breasts may feel tighter, fuller, and a little more tender as your hormones prepare to move you into the luteal phase. Skin breakouts and that oh-so-attractive water weight are other signals that you've just passed the ovulation mark. If you experience any of these less typical ovulatory symptoms, you may benefit from taking the hormone quiz on my website (https://naturnalife.com) to pinpoint a potential underlying condition.

Let's Get Busy

Now that you know all the signs of ovulation, you can easily predict the days your egg will be in the prime position. The next step is making the most of those days. Timing intercourse sounds cut-and-dry (get busy during ovulation, right?), but there are some subtle nuances that can

If you're downright randy, you're probably ovulating. Increased libido is your body saying, "It's time! Grab him!" Less interest could signify a hormonal imbalance or excess stress or indicate that the "window" has passed.

make all the difference if you are really trying to "nail" it, so to speak.

Whoa, Nelly!

Too much of a good thing can be detrimental. You may not want to have sex every single day leading up to ovulation. Why not? Sounds like it would boost your odds. Well, for some, it takes time to replenish sperm count after a good romp, especially if he's over 40 or has any sperm count/quality issues. Even if you've got yourself a prime specimen, having too much sex can make you sore and inflamed down there (and potentially more acidic, and acid kills sperm). Every other day leading up and two consecutive days at peak fertility is a safer bet. Line up your romps with your charted peak day and don't overdo it!

You might also ask your man to go lighter on the self-pleasing in the days leading up to your fertile window. You may think this is obvious, but he may not. You want that sperm to pack a punch, and if he exhausts his resources "practicing" right before you ovulate, you may have a problem.

On the other hand, you also don't want to make him "save up" for weeks ahead of time. That could mean there are a bunch of stagnant little guys who aren't as strong and can't swim as fast because they've been cooped up too long. Whether he gets his weekly "session" on his own or the good old-fashioned way is entirely up to you.

Been There, Done That?

The glaringly obvious hole in modern-day body education means that women must hunt down the answers to basic questions about their hormones. Internet searches are great, but they're also a breeding ground for misinformation. In your personal quest for answers, you've likely already heard of fertility charting and have previously researched the best days to have sex, but now you have the why, the how, and a concrete plan. Mastery of body basics is the foundation for all the fertility strategies to come.

Now that we have the lay of the land, we can move into what happens when the basics aren't matching your personal experience. You may be encountering issues such as a lack of fertile mucus, irregular periods, or a medical condition like PCOS or endometriosis. Maybe you can't even pinpoint a possible reason why you're struggling to conceive. The following chapters are designed to help you find answers beyond the basics for issues that persist no matter how perfectly you chart.

So, without further ado, let's meet all the culprits.

CHAPTER 3

Infertility in a Nutshell

Many of you reading this book may already have a name for your fertility foe. Many more, however, are wondering what unseen, unfelt issues are underlying your fertility challenges. You may already have an inkling that your struggles run deeper than an improperly predicted fertile window, but you aren't quite sure what to do next. Whether you've been at it for a while or just now embarking on your quest for a baby, its best to get the scoop on conditions that could act as barriers to conception. This chapter is designed to help you learn the ins and outs of the various disorders that could be playing a role in your fertility challenges.

The culprits responsible are varied, numerous, and sneaky. A doctor's visit is often the most logical step to identify a cause, but, unfortunately, it can be difficult to get a "diagnosis." Many fertility challenges are actually caused by a combination of several subtle factors that don't pop up on lab tests. As things stand, a (non)diagnosis of idiopathic (aka unknown cause) infertility is rampant. Reasons for this abound. Among them is that doctors are incredibly cautious about labeling a condition unless there is ample evidence to confirm it. Generally, this stems from their "evidence-based" training and the reliance on lab tests rather than observation. In some cases, it also sadly boils down to the fact that they have very limited time to spend with individual patients. If their schedules allowed for lengthier discussion, more information could potentially be gleaned, and a clear diagnosis and treatment direction might result. What I aim to do in this chapter is to help you begin to uncover some clues on your own that can give you some direction as to how to take action. Perhaps it also gives you the opportunity to bring up talking points with your practitioner so they may offer some guidance.

The root of your infertility could be a preexisting medical condition, a dietary issue, a lifestyle issue, an environmental issue, or any combination of these. Reading the details of such a condition may clue you in that you have a secondary, undiscovered diagnosis. That said, having a name for your problem doesn't automatically mean you know how to tackle it. *However*, giving the issue an identity can provide a firm foundation from which to start taking action.

Let's dive into "naming" our foe or, at the very least, getting in touch with possibilities of where to start.

Getting to Know Your Foe

Have you been told you have one or more of the following conditions? If so, feel free to skip to the relevant sections to learn a little more about your diagnosed foe(s). Each section discusses how the condition affects your fertility and what lifestyle factors might be influencing it. I do suggest, however, giving the whole chapter a thorough read. You may discover things that you never previously clued into.

If you haven't yet been tested for a preexisting condition, I would encourage you to read through the symptoms of each section to see if any match up with your experiences. The knowledge you glean will empower you to take action. If you think you might have one or more of these conditions, I encourage you to talk with your practitioner about getting tested.

About Your Eggs

Eggs are a hot topic in the world of fertility because egg quality is often blamed for many cases of idiopathic infertility. The major challenge with this diagnosis is that no one knows exactly what causes egg issues (other than age), and no one agrees whether there are any effective treatment options. Poor egg quality has been linked to metabolic issues, immune issues, toxin exposure, genetics, age, and more. Women over 35 are typically the first to get this diagnosis, as ovarian aging is probably the most frequently cited barrier to producing quality eggs that I've seen clinically. However, in my opinion, it pops up concurrently with other, subtler issues. Read on to get the full scoop on eggs.

LOW EGG RESERVE

Not every biological clock keeps perfect time. Some of our clocks are ticking faster than others. About 10 percent of women are affected by what's known as premature ovarian aging (POA). Your egg reserve declines naturally as you age, but POA implies that your egg reserve does not match your age. Your ovaries are essentially older than you. Often, this is a genetic gift, but I've noticed that many of my patients with diminished reserves are highly stressed-out ladies who are very hard on themselves. Other causes I've observed are chemotherapy, toxin exposure, certain medications, or immune confusion (discussed later in this chapter). I have a low ovarian reserve on top of my PCOS, which is an odd combination. PCOS usually involves an overabundance of eggs—just goes to show that none of us fit perfectly under any one label. POA often shows little to no symptoms, so it isn't commonly diagnosed unless you specifically request that your practitioner test your antral follicle count (AFC) and anti-Müllerian hormone (AMH) levels. Your results will be compared to the standard levels of women your age.

You Have Options!

Conventional Treatment: None according to many doctors, though some recommend dehydroepiandrosterone (DHEA) or CoQ10 supplementation
Holistic Treatment: Herbs (tonics) and supplements (CoQ10, DHEA), lifestyle (reduce stress, get good quality rest), detoxification

Request a Test

AMH tests are used to determine an egg reserve (i.e., how many eggs you are still working with). If your AMH level is low (registering under a 1 in an AMH test), it may indicate that your reserve is low. This might be a clue that you'll be less likely to have success with an IVF treatment, which is designed to stimulate your ovaries into producing *more* eggs than you would in a natural cycle. If there isn't an abundance of eggs, you won't have luck trying to stimulate them. A very high AMH test isn't necessarily ideal either. If your levels register above a 3, it may be an indicator of PCOS amenorrhea. You'll get a lot of eggs but may encounter an issue with the quality and end up with low fertilization rates or poor-quality embryos. I'm told the fertility sweet spot is between 1.5 and 2.5, but doctors would still rather see a high number over a low one.

AFC tests are the other, perhaps more accurate way to assess your egg reserve. Your fertility center will do an ultrasound on day 2 of your period. If they see an abundance of follicles (at least a few on each ovary), they'll give the go-ahead to start the cycle. In truth, these tests aren't 100 percent accurate indicators of your fertility or how an IVF cycle will play out. If your numbers aren't ideal, don't be discouraged. Follow the fertility-enhancing guidance in this book, and keep the faith.

POF OR EARLY MENOPAUSE

POF, also known as premature ovarian failure, means your ovaries stop responding properly to the pituitary gland's signals to make an egg (or eggs) grow. Essentially, your ovaries are no longer responding to the FSH hormone.

Common symptoms are the following:

- Irregular periods or no period
- Hot flashes
- Vaginal dryness
- Poor response to IVF, canceled cycles
- Irregular periods and ovulation

Like POA, this happens naturally as you age, but in some women, it is accelerated. POF can manifest as early as the teen years, and it can come on very suddenly. The main difference between POA and POF is that FSH is generally elevated in POF because your pituitary gland pumps out an excess trying (unsuccessfully) to get your ovaries to respond. The combination of low reserve and elevated FSH makes for a trickier, more advanced condition. The high levels of FSH mean that your ovaries won't respond to the stimulation from IVF medications. They may, in fact, go on strike. IVF cycles of POF patients are often canceled because their eggs either don't grow at all or produce only one or two, making the cycle more trouble than it's worth. However, hope remains. There are holistic methods to lower FSH levels through complementary medicine and lifestyle adjustments, which will be covered in this book.

Keep in mind that if your infertility has been linked to poor egg quality but your symptoms aren't aligning with those of the previously mentioned conditions, then carry on through this chapter. The upcoming sections, with the exception of "Structural Stuff," can affect your egg quality. It's a broad topic, so to get the clearest picture, it's best to understand how all types of hormonal and immune conditions can impact the health of your egg cells as they develop.

You Have Options!

Conventional Treatment: Mini IVF, IVF with donor eggs
Holistic Treatment: Diet (healthy fats, low acid), supplements (antioxidants), herbs (tonics), acupuncture, lifestyle (detox, stress reduction)

Request a Test

FSH tests are administered on day 2 of your period. If your levels are above 10, it may be an indicator that your ovaries are a tad on the fritz. A high FSH may indicate issues with egg quality and suggest a poor prognosis with assisted reproductive technology (i.e., IVF).

LH is the hormone that indicates that ovulation is occurring. LH levels should be high only when you are "surging" to release an egg. High LH early in the cycle can indicate that the signals between your brain and ovaries are a tad off balance and/or issues with egg quality. High LH numbers are characteristic of PCOS or POF.

Hormone Hell

In their natural, harmonious state, your hormones improve your skin, boost your mood, keep you focused, and help your uterus nourish a life. When some factor of your lifestyle, diet, or environment knocks them out of equilibrium, you can feel bloated, antsy, and volatile. Hormones play such an integral role in your basic bodily functions that a prolonged imbalance can create and feed various disorders that then hamper your fertility. The best way to prevent and combat these conditions is to learn how to harmonize your hormones.

PCOS

Of all the hormonal conditions that one could name, PCOS might be one of the most common misfits. Nearly 70 percent of all female infertility issues are attributed to PCOS, some of my own included. It's a complex metabolic condition that is hard to diagnose because it can manifest in multiple ways. Two women with PCOS could have widely different body types and manifestations. This is because it's a so-called spectrum disorder, meaning that you can have only a few or all of the symptoms (see list of symptoms below). Doctors hesitate to diagnose it because your symptoms can manifest differently at any given time. So, while one physician may say you have it based on one or two strong symptoms, another might assess the same symptoms on a different day and say you are unlikely to have it. I wasn't diagnosed until I was in my late twenties, though, when looking back, I was demonstrating textbook symptoms on the "spectrum"!

Thin women are typically not diagnosed with PCOS because it is thought that only overweight women qualify. Not true! I can't tell you how many skinny PCOS ladies I see. The difference is that skinny women with PCOS are generally gathering fat in their "viscera" (organs). They look trim, but they still have a tendency for high cholesterol and issues with ovulation. It goes unnoticed and untreated because doctors take one look at the patient's waistline and dismiss PCOS as a possibility.

For a clear diagnosis, your ovaries have to be enlarged and contain fluid-filled cysts. "Poly" means "many," and most women with PCOS have multiple cysts in their ovaries surrounding the eggs. They often look like rings of pearls on an ultrasound. Sounds interesting—unless you have it. These cysts affect your cycle, impede egg production and release, and scramble hormonal messaging between your brain and ovaries. However, some women don't experience multiple cysts at a time. PCOS can be diagnosed as mild, moderate, or severe, which is why the symptoms are so varied.

Common symptoms are the following:

- Irregular periods
- No period
- Difficulty losing weight
- Inflammation (feeling "puffy")
- Acne
- Excess body hair
- High blood pressure
- High cholesterol (or low HDL, aka "good," cholesterol)
- Pain in the ovaries
- Dark creases in areas where the skin naturally folds (arm pits, groin, and so on)

PCOS encompasses a plethora of hormonal issues. The exact imbalance and resulting symptoms will vary widely from woman to woman thanks to the spectrum nature of the condition. In some, it may cause high insulin, which can lead to many other metabolic issues, such as high cholesterol, heart disease, and type 2 diabetes. In others, the cysts may cause excess estrogen and awful PMS.

Request a Test

One determinant of PCOS is an LH:FSH ratio test. You want a 1:1 ratio, but if the LH levels become higher, such as 2:1, it may indicate PCOS.

My hormonal hell began as soon as I reached puberty. My emotions and energy levels fluctuated wildly, and I suffered with insomnia, making me even more moody and tired. Then acne struck with a vengeance and continued into my twenties. Once I started working, I felt drained and sick all the time. My weight could rise dramatically if I stopped my athletics for even a couple weeks.

At age 27, my period stopped altogether, and I became chronically constipated and puffy. Finally, I was diagnosed with PCOS, which connected all the dots: the mood problems, missed periods, weight gain, fatigue, and acne.

Sometimes I was a textbook case, and sometimes people didn't believe I had it. When I was finally diagnosed, I had not had a period in six months, had cysts all over my ovaries, and was having trouble controlling my weight. When I was an athletic teen, I had acne and a couple cysts here and there. The exercise was controlling the symptoms.

Over the years I've learned to adapt my lifestyle to force the PCOS into submission. I want to help you do the same.

What can you do to lessen your symptoms?

Due to PCOS's close ties to insulin excess and insulin resistance, the biggest changes you can make are diet and lifestyle related. The most problematic things for insulin resistance are dietary, specifically processed foods, alcohol, and sugar. Thus, your food intake can determine the severity of your PCOS and influence how symptoms come and go. If you are eating like crap (carbs, booze, sugar, dairy, and fried, greasy, gluten bombs everywhere) and not exercising, then you will likely feel as crappy as the quality of your food choices. If you are eating clean and exercising regularly, then you will feel relatively normal. I literally watched my cysts come and go according to my behavior. Pizza and candy made them appear. Interval training and a paleo-centric diet made them disappear. Giving up your guilty pleasure foods doesn't sound fun, but the payoff is significant and doesn't require conventional treatment or medication. PCOS is highly treatable through lifestyle adjustments alone! You'll reverse your symptoms and remove an obstacle to your fertility, and that's worth saying good-bye to even the most tempting treat.

You Have Options!

Conventional Treatment: Clomifene (encourages ovulation) and metformin (reduces insulin and blood sugar levels)

Holistic Treatment: Low-inflammation diet, interval training, acupuncture, herbs (Wen Jing Tang, Fu Zi Li Zhong Wan, Liu Wei Di Huang Wan, maca), supplements (myo-inositol, N-acetylcysteine [NAC], vitamin B6, probiotics, fish oil)

INSULIN RESISTANCE

While insulin is associated with obesity and diabetes in most people's minds, you don't have to be overweight to experience insulin imbalance. The disruption of this hormone's normal function can affect your fertility as much as your weight. Insulin is produced in your pancreas, and its primary function is to control your blood sugar levels. In the modern age of highly processed foods full of simple carbs and refined sugars, women of all shapes and sizes develop a resistance to insulin. That means that

> Spotting before your period? It could be an insulin or progesterone issue—or both! Many conditions come in pairs.

no matter how much insulin they produce, the blood sugar is not broken down and properly processed. The body keeps trying, though, and the excess insulin eventually throws metabolic and hormonal processes out of whack.

Clinically, I see insulin and blood sugar imbalance as a leading cause of "sub-fertility," meaning it's taking longer than average to conceive but hasn't yet been a year of unsuccessful trying. It is also often the underlying issue for many of the women diagnosed with the incredibly frustrating idiopathic infertility.

Common symptoms are the following:

- Easily puffy
- Craving sugar or carbs
- Craving sugar after eating
- Mood issues
- Difficulty controlling weight
- PCOS
- Brain fog
- Low energy

You Have Options!

Conventional Treatment: Metformin
Holistic Treatment: Low-glycemic, low-carb diet; acupuncture; supplements

Insulin resistance blocks fertility by suppressing ovulation and inhibiting proper blood flow to the endometrial lining in your uterus. It thereby affects both the growth and the implantation potential of an egg. Higher insulin and blood sugar levels can also increase free radical damage on the egg, lowering the quality. Should your insulin imbalance feed into PCOS, as it often does,

Request a Test

Fasting glucose, A1c, pricking finger at home (see chapter 5 for more information).

that can lead to a harder shell developing on the egg, making it more difficult for the sperm to penetrate.

OVULATORY DYSFUNCTION

Most ladies with this issue will have very long cycles, no period, or late ovulation (if at all). It's worth mentioning that a predictable 28-day cycle doesn't necessarily mean you're ovulating. A percentage of women who appear to menstruate normally are not actually releasing an egg. Most often, this is because their follicles are not actually fully maturing, although at times, the eggs don't actually break through the ovarian wall (i.e., escape to make the journey down the fallopian tube). To discover if this is the culprit behind your struggle to conceive, you can start with BBT charting. If your temperature never really goes up mid-cycle (or at any point), I encourage you to book an appointment with your doctor to get your egg development and hormone levels "monitored" through blood tests and ultrasounds. Through imaging and tests, your practitioner can confirm whether your eggs are maturing and releasing from the follicles during ovulation.

Request a Test

Ultrasounds and blood tests together can provide a full picture of your follicle (egg) development. Ultrasounds measure the size and growth of follicles. Blood tests provide snapshots of your estradiol (E2) and LH hormone levels, which allow the practitioner to assess the growth and maturation of your eggs. It's best to begin E2 testing early in your follicular phase (between days 2 and 6), drawing blood every few days until you ovulate. However, you can start as late as day 10 if you tend to have longer cycles.

LOW PROGESTERONE

Progesterone rises after ovulation occurs, fluffing the uterine lining, where your little one will embed and grow throughout the pregnancy. Progesterone is produced by the corpus luteum: a sac left over by the empty follicle when the egg is released. As such, a healthy ovulation must take place to produce adequate progesterone levels.

Without adequate progesterone, you can't maintain an endometrial lining, and thus the egg may either not implant or easily miscarry shortly after implantation. Low progesterone is common in hormonal conditions, such as PCOS, and in "hormonal transitions," such as perimenopause. In some cases, it can result from excess stress, overexertion, and/or too much caffeine. It has even been linked to immunological factors on occasion.

Common symptoms are the following:

- Bad PMS
- Bloating before your period
- Anxiety or insomnia before your period
- Spotting after ovulation before your period
- Early miscarriage
- Weight gain
- Infertility
- Swollen/painful breasts
- Water retention
- Heavy or painful period

Low progesterone can lead to a short luteal phase. Ideally, a luteal phase should last 10 days or more. If you notice on your chart that you seem to jump rather quickly from ovulation signs to your period, it's an easier diagnosis. However, sometimes a woman's chart looks perfectly normal up until after the temperature spikes at ovulation. If the chart doesn't show a sustained increase in temperature and/or you start bleeding soon after a temperature spike, it's likely you are not producing the right levels of progesterone during the luteal phase—a condition called LPD.

Request a Test

Ask your practitioner to evaluate your progesterone levels about a week after ovulation in what's known as a day 21 progesterone test. The timing of this test is important because certain hormones are active only during specific times in your cycle. You may remember that progesterone is dominant in the luteal phase (between ovulation and menses), so it's best to test at the midpoint. Seven to 10 days after ovulation, you want to see healthy enough levels to maintain a pregnancy (definitely above 10 but better above 20).

You Have Options!

Conventional Treatment: Progesterone supplements (topical, oral, or suppository), Clomid

Holistic Treatment: Stress reduction techniques, cut out caffeine, chasteberry, maca, acupuncture, Chinese herbs, dietary modification

Estrogen Dominance

Estrogen, one of the two primary female sex hormones, is not only produced in our bodies but also found in our food and environment. Estrogen increases feelings of wellness, maintains a youthful appearance, and promotes fertility. The downside is that, in certain cases, the body might have an estrogen overload that causes symptoms like water retention, mood swings, weight gain, migraines, and terrible periods. The culprits of this imbalance may be internal. Fibroids, excess fat, endometriosis, cysts, and polyps create an imbalance. The issues could also be external. Eating foods with phytoestrogens, like soy, or exposure to xenoestrogens in plastic, pesticides, conventional meat, and dairy products can also cause estrogen excess. The liver and guts are responsible for ridding these substances from our bodies. If our body's cleansing systems are backed up (most people's are), we end up with excess estrogens.

Common symptoms are the following:

- Puffiness/water retention and weight gain (hips and butt)
- Mood swings
- Anxiety/depression
- Insomnia
- Flushed face
- Weepiness
- Cervical dysplasia
- Breasts enlarged and/or tenderness
- Fibroids
- Endometriosis
- Heavy bleeding
- Painful period
- Migraine headaches
- Brain fog
- Gallbladder problems

THYROID IRREGULARITIES

Your thyroid gland looks like a delicate butterfly perched at the base of your neck, but it's actually more like a supercomputer that assists in the regulation of your entire body, including fundamentals like breathing and heart rate. For all you ladies dreaming of a baby bump, its most important functions are regulating your menstrual cycle, your temperature, and your cholesterol.

It does this by turning iodine in your food into two hormones: triiodothyronine (T3) and thyroxine (T4). T3 and T4 work together inside your blood cells to determine how fast your cells and metabolism function, which is why the thyroid can affect so many aspects of your body's day-to-day processes. A healthy ratio is also important for maintaining pregnancy. Thyroid levels are routinely checked for all women undergoing infertility treatment. Irregularities create major hormonal roadblocks and unpleasant symptoms.

Common symptoms are the following:

- Dry skin
- Anxiety
- Sleep issues
- Slow bowels
- Hair loss
- Brain fog
- Light period
- Long cycles
- Late ovulation or no ovulation

I had a patient named Sarah who had noticed a shift in her mood. She was tired and grouchy more often than not. Her sleep and bowel movements were inconsistent. Add constant bloat and a chill that wouldn't dissipate no matter how many layers she piled on, and you have a miserable situation. After a routine test, we discovered Sarah had hypothyroidism, a deficiency in her production and use of thyroid hormones. Essentially, Sarah's brain was trying to trigger the production of T3 and T4 using thyroid-stimulating hormone (TSH), but her thyroid wasn't receiving the signal correctly or perhaps just wasn't responding. Most women with thyroid issues suffer from a lack of hormone production, referred to as "hypothyroidism." Symptoms are commonly fatigue, chills, poor digestion, abnormal cycles, and infertility. However, some women suffer from an excess of thyroid hormones, in a condition referred to as "hyperthyroidism." Common symptoms for hyperthyroidism are hot flashes and slightly bulging eyes. An excess of these hormones may also cause a dizzying, manic feeling, like you're constantly running a mile a minute. Hyperthyroidism can actually

Some thyroid irregularity symptoms can mimic PCOS. Similar to those ladies with PCOS, women with thyroid issues often have weight problems, cysts, puffiness, constipation, and menstrual irregularities. Thyroid issues are often overdiagnosed, and insulin resistance (associated with PCOS and idiopathic infertility) is often underdiagnosed. Both conditions, however, can be present simultaneously.

be life threatening if left untreated. In some rarer cases, such as in Hashimoto's disease (autoimmune thyroiditis), the thyroid can fluctuate between hyper and hypo until it finally tires out and becomes permanently hypo.

> ## Request a Test
>
> If you think your thyroid might be acting out, ask your practitioner for a full thyroid panel, including T3, T4, and thyroid peroxidase (TPO) antibodies in addition to the standard TSH test.

The effects of unbalanced thyroid hormones manifest physically in a variety of ways. It's unclear the *exact* role that thyroid health plays in fertility and reproduction, but there is no denying it has a profound effect. Thyroid irregularities alter the feedback loops between all your hormone-producing glands: the hypothalamus, pituitary, ovaries, and adrenals. Your thyroid might underproduce or over-produce reproductive hormones important to fetal growth and development. Underproduction is associated with increased risk of miscarriage and poor development of the fetus.

Behind the scenes, your thyroid hormone is responsible for metabolizing cells, allowing for new cell turnover. Without proper cell metabolism, you can have lower BBT, lower egg quality, a suboptimal uterine lining, and irregular or inconsistent cycles, which makes pinpointing your fertile window a serious hassle. Thyroid imbalance

> ## You Have Options!
>
> **Conventional Treatment:** Synthroid, Nature-Throid, Armour Thyroid
> **Holistic Treatment:** Animal glandulars, gluten-free diet, low-inflammatory foods, herbs, acupuncture, stress management, detox

is also implicated in premature ovarian insufficiency and repeated IVF failures. The effects are pervasive.

Treat the Person, Not the Test Results

Lab tests don't always tell the whole story. I've seen women who show all the symptoms of hypothyroidism, but their labs come back negative for the condition. If this happens to you, don't give up on your hunch. Thyroid levels can fluctuate week to week. Try testing again in a different lab and aim to test during your luteal phase, when the thyroid levels tend to dip more. Another thing to keep in mind is that what you are experiencing might be early signs of a developing thyroid condition. If that's the case, then lean into nutrition, lifestyle, and natural medicine to address it before it has the chance to fully manifest.

Immune Confusion

The concept of immunological conditions, wherein your own cells react improperly to the embryo, is not widely accepted in the medical community. However, from my experience and observation of patients' journeys over the years, I believe they are worth mentioning. There are many unseen factors that affect fertility, and some experts point to malfunctions in the behavior of the immune system. Autoimmune conditions are pervasive, and they manifest in many different ways. Most of the rhetoric surrounding reproductive immunology deals with its links to miscarriage and recurrent pregnancy loss. That's not the whole picture. The effects can actually be far more varied. Common by-products of immune confusion are inflammation and free radical damage that attack eggs, sperm, ovaries, the uterus, or the embryo itself. Free radical damage may also trigger premature aging of the ovaries. The damage is far reaching.

Ask an Expert

I asked Dr. Eric Forman from Columbia University Fertility Center about what causes miscarriage. Here are his two cents: "Age is still the primary causal factor in miscarriages due to chromosomally abnormal embryos, but there may be other factors involved, such as structural/uterine issues (septum, polyps, fibroids), genetic issues (balanced translocation), autoimmune troubles (e.g., Hashimoto's thyroiditis, antiphospholipid antibody syndrome), or medical factors (e.g., insulin resistance/prediabetes). Lifestyle factors like excess weight or smoking can also increase your miscarriage risk." You may not have control over all of these factors, but you certainly have influence over a few of them.

Personal communication with author (2022)   •

An embryo contains only 50 percent of your DNA and tissue. The other half is the father's. To protect itself, your body's immune system may attack foreign tissues in your body just as it attacks viruses. When a fertilized egg implants in your uterus, your immune cells are sent out like defending soldiers to check out the situation. When they reach the egg, something changes those soldiers' primary directive, telling them to protect the embryo rather than attack it. The exact cause is still unclear, but some experts believe substances in your partner's sperm signal to your immune cells that the embryo is not harmful. Others believe that the father's half of the tissue in the embryo is what gives the signal thanks to a protein called antigen G.

Unfortunately, this mysterious signal sometimes gets mixed up. The mother's body does not properly recognize the embryo's tissue and attacks it with the natural killer cells that are meant to battle tumors or virus-ridden cells. Some experts believe this aggressive response occurs only in women with a natural overabundance of those killer cells.

Interestingly, new theories on the issue indicate that this attack response may not be the immune system target-ing a foreign tissue but rather a lack of the protective response that keeps the embryo safe through pregnancy. This occurs when the man's and woman's genetic makeups are too similar. Thus, when the immune cells examine the embryo, they can't distinguish the fa-ther's tissue from the mother's. With-out that distinction, the cells don't recognize that there's a pregnancy, so the mother's body never turns on the special protective response that shields the embryo from immune cell attack.

> ## You Have Options!
>
> **Conventional Treatment:** Immu-nosuppressive drugs (i.e., pred-nisone and Neupogen)
> **Holistic Treatment:** Low-allergen/low-inflammation diet and sup-plements; acupuncture; herbs

Another potential cause is the presence of antinuclear antibodies (ANAs), which are a more recent discovery. These antibodies destroy cell nuclei, the cen-tral and most vital part of all cells. These antibodies are usually present only in women with autoimmune disorders like lupus or rheumatoid arthritis.

Having a thorough assessment of thyroid health is also important since "antithyroid antibodies" can also cause miscarriage. This is typically linked to hypothyroidism and a deficiency of thyroid hormones.

> ## Request a Test
>
> An immunophenotyping test can assess your levels of natural killer cells. If you have an autoimmune disorder or have experienced past miscarriages, ask for an ANA test to check for antinuclear antibodies. Your doctor may have already issued one, as this is a somewhat standard test for those with former pregnancy losses.

BLOOD CLOTTING AND THROMBOPHILIAS

In the heavily debated field of immunology, thrombophilias make up yet another condition that falls under the umbrella of "Is it relevant?" medicine. Some stud-ies profess they don't affect IVF/assisted reproductive technology (ART) out-comes, while others state these abnormal blood coagulations are more prevalent in infertile women and miscarriages. Despite the wide range of research results, blood clotting due to thrombophilias is recognized by an increasing number of practitioners as an underlying cause of miscarriage. Thrombophilias block blood flow to the fetus via clotting, or they can even cause clotting around the embryo that unhitches it from your lining. There are two types: hereditary and acquired. If your family has a history of heart issues like high blood pressure, heart attack, or stroke, you could have the hereditary type. Doctors typically test for these thrombophilias automatically for women with a history of miscarriage, but if you fall outside those circumstances, you'll likely have to request such testing. Acquired thrombophilias are more commonly called antiphospholipid antibodies (APAs). You can acquire APAs through conditions like endometriosis, lupus, or Lyme disease, but only select laboratories in the United States are equipped to test for them. If you think you could have thrombophilias, speak with your doctor. The sooner, the better, as their presence automatically makes your pregnancy high risk, and your practitioner will need to move forward as such.

HEREDITARY THROMBOPHILIAS (GENETIC MUTATIONS)

A genetic tendency for thrombophilias has been more widely implicated in pregnancy losses, but other consequences less talked about are implantation failure and unexplained infertility. I see patterns of conception difficulties in women who have high toxin levels and issues with blood circulation, but these patterns would be considered subtle and perhaps imperceptible by conventional lab testing. It's via Eastern medicine's diagnosis of the tongue and pulse that the effects and patterns are made clearer. I've observed a tendency for patients with these mutations to suffer from more food sensitivities or mood problems. If you have similar symptoms, requesting a test may provide you with answers.

MTHFR

MTHFR is a commonly inherited gene mutation that makes it difficult to process synthetic folic acid into its natural form, folate. Around 25 percent of the population has a serious defect in this gene, meaning that they can't metabolize and properly absorb the folic acid found in prenatal vitamins. The natural form of this vitamin, folate (vitamin B9), is important before and after conception to decrease the chance of the embryo developing neural tube defects like spina bifida or anencephaly. Supplementing methyl-folate combined with vitamins B6 and B12 for optimal absorption can assist in this scenario.

If the MTHFR gene is not working properly, you also cannot convert the amino acid homocysteine to methionine. If homocysteine isn't converted, it sticks around in increasingly high levels, creating inflammation and free radical damage. When there are elevated levels of homocysteine, our bodies cannot properly break down folic acid to folate, eventually leading to a deficiency in folate. Women with a positive MTHFR gene mutation may have an increased risk of complications like miscarriages, preeclampsia (high blood pressure during pregnancy), and the inability to conceive, particularly when having two copies of the variant C677T or one copy of C677T and one A1298C.

Because this mutation is genetic, you cannot cure MTHFR, but there are ways to significantly reduce your symptoms and thus the risk to your fertility and pregnancy. The biggest changes you can make are dietary. Cut out foods with synthetic folic acid, like processed breads, pastas, and white rice, and instead consume natural sources of folate, like leafy greens, avocados, and dried beans. You'll also want to choose your prenatals with more care, looking for labels that list folate rather than folic acid.

> **You Have Options!**
>
> **Conventional Treatment:** None available
> **Holistic Treatment:** Dietary adjustments (anti-inflammatory, folate rich), detox

THE LEIDEN MUTATION

A recently discovered mutation in the blood protein, this genetic thrombophilia has been linked to 20 to 60 percent of deep vein thrombosis cases (abnormal blood clots, usually in the legs or lungs). Disruptions to circulation caused by this mutation have been proven to cause implantation and fertility issues. A study of the Leiden mutation revealed an increased risk of miscarriage and infertility in carriers of the gene. Women with this mutation were two and a half times more likely to have at least two miscarriages or infertility issues—a statistically significant increase.

> **You Have Options!**
>
> **Conventional Treatment:** Blood thinners such as Levonox and aspirin
> **Holistic Treatment:** Dietary adjustments (anti-inflammatory), herbal medicine, acupuncture, supplements (vitamin E, omegas)

PROTHROMBIN "FACTOR 2" MUTATION

The prothrombin mutation could potentially be the culprit behind your "unexplained infertility" diagnosis. Prothrombin is a naturally occurring protein in your blood plasma that helps the blood coagulate when needed, but in people with this genetic mutation, prothrombin doesn't function properly and can instead cause abnormal blood clots. A predisposition for abnormal coagulation and clotting affects blood flow to the whole body, including the uterus. So it's not too surprising that this mutation is far more commonly found in women with infertility issues than in women who are fertile. Testing for this mutation can give you a leg up in your quest for baby. If you know you're predisposed to poor blood flow, you can implement holistic methods that improve your circulation, such as acupuncture.

Request a Test

Genetic blood testing that isolates your DNA strand can determine if you have this mutation.

You Have Options!

Conventional Treatment: Steroids, dexamethasone or IVIG, intralipids, heparin or baby aspirin (for thrombophilia-related causes)

Holistic Treatment: Low-inflammation, low-allergen diet, detox, vitamins (C, E, N-acetyl cysteine [NAC], probiotics, omega-3), herbs, acupuncture

Miscarriage and Recurrent Miscarriage

If you have experienced one or more miscarriages, my heart goes out to you, and I am deeply sorry for your loss. I understand your pain because I have felt it. I hope you are able to find some additional solace here in better understanding some of the common causes and how you might combat them going into your next pregnancy. While about 50 percent of all miscarriages are caused by a chromosomal abnormality, the remaining 50 percent can usually be associated with one or more of the conditions listed in this chapter, such as insulin resistance, low progesterone, thyroid irregularities, structural issues, clotting factors, toxin exposure, infection, and autoimmune conditions.

ENDOMETRIOSIS

Arguably the most ferocious and painful autoimmune disorder, endometriosis produces excess and abnormal tissue growth in and around your uterus and ovaries. In fact, it can spread throughout your entire abdominal cavity. The growth has no distinct shape and doesn't form in predictable patterns. It's just extra tissue, but as it proliferates, this silent aggressor damages your uterus, fallopian tubes, and ovaries. Your body's immune system flares up to confront the perceived invader, creating inflammation throughout your reproductive system that further damages cells and creates hardened scarring. You may not be able to see the scars, but you may well feel them. Although most women with endometriosis often have painful periods and ovulation discomfort, for others it's completely silent. Some even feel the pain throughout the month. Relief is possible, but it requires some changes to your lifestyle. The ladies who complete my program often eliminate their pain entirely.

Common symptoms are the following:

- Pelvic pain (outside of regular period cramps)
- Bloating and severe cramping
- Bowel discomfort and difficulty: pain when pooping, bladder issues
- Painful periods
- Heavy periods
- Painful ovulation

The pain of endometriosis is thanks to white blood cells attacking the foreign scar tissue. The cells release substances that cause inflammation in an attempt to shield and heal the injury. The problem with endometriosis is that inflammation lingers too long, causing painful periods and internal chaos. Free radicals then swarm unchecked, attacking reproductive function at a cellular level. The scarring complicates conception from start to finish. It may prevent follicles from growing, resulting in no egg or a damaged egg that can't become a healthy embryo. Should your egg drop, the excess tissue could potentially block your fallopian tubes so that the sperm can't meet the egg. In some instances, partially blocked fallopian tubes may even lead to an ectopic pregnancy. If your egg travels successfully through the fallopian tubes and is properly fertilized, the scars can then make it difficult for the embryo to implant or lead to miscarriage.

Tubal Setbacks

Scarring and inflammation in and around your uterus and ovaries could predispose you to an ectopic pregnancy, wherein the embryo implants in your tube rather than your uterus. This can be life threatening if the tube grows too large and bursts. Most of the time, it's caught early enough, but it's a huge setback in your fertility efforts. The miscarriage drags out and often involves a drug called methotrexate to help it "resolve." This drug is a chemo agent and toxic to a developing fetus. So, if you've had this shot to resolve an ectopic, you'll have a three-month minimum wait time until you get a pass to try again. The wait time is closer to one to two menstrual cycles when you have the fetus removed surgically. Regardless, it's devastating and scary. When possible, preemptive action to reduce the swelling and scarring is always best.

Endometriosis is triggered by autoimmune issues and estrogens (yes, we have more than one kind) and is heavily influenced by our lifestyle: diet, stress levels, and so on. The exact cause behind endometriosis as a condition is still unclear. Interestingly, in my conversations with endometriosis specialists, many of them noted that most of their clients are type A workaholic personalities. One told me, "It's always the high-power, high-stress attorneys in New York City." However, the strongest links are to immune deficiency and the accumulation of toxic industrial chemicals, like polychlorinated biphenyls (PCBs) and dioxins, in the body.

In short, endometriosis is mean and sneaky. It spreads quietly and then causes all sorts of drama. This is why some specialists believe it is likely to be implicated in many cases of undiagnosed infertility.

Toxin Exposure

Toxins can build up in your body and nudge your natural internal processes off course, causing a plethora of issues (endometriosis not the least among them). Environmental toxins can be breathed in or ingested, and you'll find them in high concentrations not only in big cities and industrialized places but also on your average grocery store produce. Personal choices, such as smoking, alcohol, or drugs, can also expose you to harmful chemicals. The effects will vary based on your body and the specific toxins you are exposed to, but this is a pertinent factor that is often overlooked. Cut back where you can and see chapter 7 for specifics that will help you create your ideal regimen.

You Have Options!

Conventional Treatment: Laparoscopic surgery wherein the surgeon ventures into your pelvic cavity to look for tissue growth and scarring (highly invasive)

Holistic Treatment: Anti-inflammatory/alkaline diet, stress reduction techniques, eliminating plastics and other pollutants in your daily routine, acupuncture, herbs (raspberry leaf, Xue Fu Zhu Yu Tang), supplements (pycnogenol, melatonin, resveratrol)

Structural Stuff

If you're not exhibiting any concrete symptoms for any of the other conditions listed here, it may be that you have structural anomalies that are affecting your fertility. I once had a patient who had numerous IVF cycles only to find out later that she had a septate uterus, meaning she had a membrane dividing her uterus down the middle. She had it surgically corrected and was able to conceive successfully afterward. Generally, a septate uterus would be discovered in the early stages of testing by a reproductive specialist. However, further exploration is sometimes required.

Another fairly common uterine malformation is a bicorniate uterus, which means the uterus is split at the top into a heart-like shape, forming two conjoined cavities instead of one. Treatment for this structural issue is a bit more complex and is highly debated in medical circles.

In general, uterine malformations are associated more with pregnancy loss than inability to conceive. That still presents a roadblock to pregnancy and is still considered a fertility issue.

An "incompetent cervix" is an even more common structural issue that occurs during pregnancy whereby your cervix may shorten prematurely, causing miscarriage or pregnancy loss. Causes include infections, hormonal imbalance, or previous procedures that would have affected the cervix, such as a loop electrosurgical excision procedure (LEEP) (done when there is abnormal pap smear) or perhaps an abortion or other internal procedure.

You Have Options!

Conventional Treatment: Metroplasty (surgery to remove extra uterine membrane), cervical cerclage (procedure in which the cervix is stitched closed during pregnancy)

Holistic Treatment: Bed rest, acupuncture, herbs, manual manipulation

FALLOPIAN TUBE TROUBLE

Blocked fallopian tubes are a routinely tested structural issue. Your tubes can be blocked off by some extraneous growth or swollen tissue. Obstructions could be scarring as a result of a condition like endometriosis, appendicitis, or pelvic inflammatory disease. Growths in the uterus, such as fibroids, could also be to blame.

You Have Options!

Conventional Treatment: Corrective surgery
Holistic Treatment: Herbal medicine, acupuncture, castor oil, or cleansing but only in cases where the blockage is attributed to mucus or inflammation (if extensive scarring is blocking the tubes, neither surgery nor holistic methods will be of much use)

Request a Test

A hysterosalpingogram (HSG), or dye test x-ray, assesses whehter your tubes are open. If the dye introduced to your uterus doesn't flow through the fallopian tubes, it's a sure sign there's an obstruction. A TPP test, which gauges the function of your fimbria, isn't a commonly performed procedure, so you would have to request it. It's likely you may need to see a specialist, as access to this test isn't abundant.

ADENOMYOSIS, POLYPS, AND FIBROIDS

Adenomyosis, polyps, and fibroids are benign growths in the uterus. Adenomyosis is a benign mass of cells that grows within the uterine wall and makes it thicken. The distinction is that fibroids are defined masses that protrude from the wall of the uterus. Polyps are tiny growths that dangle off the surface layer of your uterus lining. Fibroids, endometriosis, and adenomyosis can significantly affect inflammation and blood flow in the uterus and are often treated today with Lupron. This unpleasant treatment can last up to two months and cause you to have migraines, mood swings, insomnia, and more. Polyps, on the other hand, are more easily removed with a "scraping" of the uterus, known as a hysteroscopy. Acupuncture, dietary changes, and traditional herbal medicine are natural approaches that can be used in many cases to assist conception in lieu of more invasive options.

Fertility challenges arise when these growths get in the way of an egg that's trying to implant. If you have a large fibroid or a cluster of little polyps blocking all the prime locations, your fertilized egg may dissolve before it can latch on. This is

Request a Test

Saline sonograms check the lining and contour of your uterus to determine whether there are any abnormal growths. Hysteroscopies explore the contour of your uterine wall while simultaneously scraping the polyps and small adhesions (scarring) from the surface. Hysteroscopies are a common method to "freshen" the lining before implantation, so they act as both diagnostic and treatment.

definitely a bigger problem with fibroids because their size is more substantial, but polyps can pose an issue. These growths, especially fibroids, can cause pregnancy difficulties even after implantation because they weaken the blood flow to the growing fetus. If substantial, they can even cause pregnancy loss.

Common symptoms are the following:

- Irregular bleeding/spotting
- Heavy periods
- Painful periods
- Severe PMS

A Holistic Viewpoint

Dr. Rebecca Sagan is a naturopathic doctor who is a master at understanding how lady hormones interact with thyroid function. She says that when it comes to hypothyroidism, simple hormone replacement may be the answer for some, but more often these imbalances are not so black and white. Signs of a thyroid disorder can often be missed with basic thyroid blood tests unless we dig deeper and look for the root cause of the hormone imbalances. Thorough testing includes not only the basic TSH test, but also testing the hormones from the thyroid gland (free T4 and free T3), along with both thyroid antibodies (thyroid peroxidase antibodies and thyroglobulin antibodies) and the protein from the thyroid gland, thyroglobulin. Antibody testing can indicate an underlying autoimmune issue like Hashimoto's. These tests will also let us see if you have a conversion problem with your thyroid hormones or subclinical thyroid issues, or if nutrient deficiencies may be contributing to your fertility issues.

The thyroid is part of the symphony of glands that secrete hormones, and the interplay between these glands determines how well our body works. High estrogen levels will interfere with our thyroid function and make the thyroid underactive. Cortisol, our stress response hormone, will also interfere with thyroid hormones. It is also essential to have great liver function and bile flow to ensure that we can break down, bind, and move hormones through our bodies. Without proper clearance of estrogen and cortisol, we cannot have a balanced thyroid.

Personal communication with author (2022)

Fibroids and polyps are also associated with hormonal imbalances—specifically estrogen excesses and, at times, deficiency of progesterone. Not only do they grow as a result of excess estrogen in your system, but they also produce and emit estrogen. The imbalanced ratio of these hormones is associated with inflammation and free radical damage. Furthermore, it can upset the timing of ovulation, affect egg quality, prevent implantation, and will likely cause painful and heavy periods.

How can you get rid of them?

Well, if you want to fully remove them, it requires surgery. This option is more common with fibroids, as polyps are considered to be a lesser issue. Although surgery is your only option for removal, there are some simple dietary and medicinal changes you can make to help slow their progression (growth).

You Have Options!

Conventional Treatment: Fully invasive surgery (fibroids), hysteroscopy (polyps) to scrape the uterus of mild adhesions (scarring) to freshen up the lining

Holistic Treatment: Avoid excess sugar, buy organic produce, swap estrogen-based medicines for alternatives, avoid dairy, eat more plant-based foods, try supplementing with diindolylmethane (DIM) or calcium D-glucarate (custom Chinese herb formulas, such as Gui Zhi Fu Ling Wan, shrink masses and inhibit inflammation)

What Do You Mean, "You Don't Know"?!

Undiagnosed infertility is easily the most frustrating condition of all. Sometimes, after running the standard panel of tests, your doctor's only answer for your struggles is, "We just can't determine the cause for certain." The uncertainty could be linked to an undiagnosed condition that is not tested for in a standard panel. Your symptoms may fluctuate or may not check all of the basic boxes, so your doctor has never seen a need to test for an underlying condition. For example, I see many women with a few symptoms of PCOS (aka "mild" on the spectrum) but not enough to get several doctors to agree. The same goes for endometriosis. Likely culprits for a "we can't be certain" diagnosis are PCOS, endometriosis, autoimmune disorders, structural problems, egg quality, nutritional deficiencies, or hormonal imbalance (i.e., everything I've laid out in this chapter). Most often, the "unknown" brand of infertility stems from a subtle interplay of lifestyle and environmental factors that have yet to be identified, making pinpointing a singular root cause difficult.

It's incredibly disheartening to be left without answers. So, if your symptoms aren't lining up well with any of what was covered in this chapter, then the next four chapters are for you.

Male Factor Infertility

Last but not least is the elephant in the room. The man's involvement in infertility is rarely discussed, even when their sperm quality is suboptimal. Sperm issues constitute around 30 percent of fertility challenges, yet very little attention is given to the topic. Why? One reason may be that fertility specialists are trained as obstetricians and gynecologists, so their specialty is highly focused on the female side. That said, the bigger influence is that IVF developed a neat little procedure called intracytoplasmic sperm injection (ICSI), which can select a decent-looking sperm and inject it right into the egg. It removes the need for the sperm to be strong enough to penetrate the egg and thus can improve fertilization rates for couples where the male side is somewhat (or significantly) lacking. There are, unfortunately, downsides to using this method. Albeit rarely, ICSI is associated with an increased risk of congenital defects and epigenetic syndromes. The risk may be due to the use of poor-quality sperm to fertilize an egg, but the jury is still out on the topic, and ICSI remains common practice in IVF.

Although I believe ICSI to be an amazing tool, my core belief is that if your man has less-than-ideal sperm parameters, then it would be best to address lifestyle factors to improve the quality and quantity of sperm, thereby improving pregnancy outcomes *and* mitigating risk.

A comprehensive review of sperm analysis is beyond the scope of this book, but to give you the basic breakdown, we are looking at the following:

1. Concentration: The amount of sperm your guy produces per ejaculate (e.g., quantity of sperm)
2. Motility: Their swimming capabilities (e.g., can they make it to your egg?)
3. Morphology: Their shape (e.g., are their tails crooked and unable to swim, or is the head malformed so that it can't penetrate the egg?)

Improving sperm quality is much like improving egg quality. Preferably, your man should set aside at least three months for applying the regimen before you try again (though improvements can be accomplished in less time). Much of it has to do with free radical damage, so reducing inflammation and stress, balancing insulin and blood sugar, and implementing a detox are all big players. It's also important not to "cook" his testicles—no hot baths, no hot tubs, keep the cell phone out of his pocket, and keep the laptop off his lap. Tight undies and long bike rides are also not recommended. Beware also of high fevers, as this can damage sperm for several months. Given the many cases of poor embryo quality and failed IVF attempts, it makes sense to give some attention to the other side of the equation.

> ### Request a Test
>
> A urologist or fertility center conducts a sperm analysis. As a follow-up, a deeper dive can be done through a DNA fragmentation test, though this test's validity is controversial.

There are some great vitamins and minerals to improve the trio above, all of which will be outlined in chapter 11.

> ### You Have Options!
>
> **Conventional:** Varicocele surgery
> **Holistic:** Vitamins and minerals such as zinc, selenium, vitamins C and D, and many more! Low-acid/low-inflammatory diet, herbs, mindfulness, acupuncture, moxibustion

> ### DNA Fragmentation
>
> This is a test used to identify damaged genetic material within the sperm that may influence the fertilization and progression of an embryo. Proponents of this test believe that high levels of DNA fragmentation lead to poor-quality embryos, implantation failure, miscarriage, and unexplained fertility. The medical community is divided on the validity of the test, so you may find that your doctor is not in support of recommending it. I find it valuable to point to the amount of oxidative stress in the male so that we can apply nutritional, lifestyle, and vitamin strategies to improve the situation. The upside: get him healthier and potentially with better quality sperm. The downside: not a whole lot.

The Big Four Fertility Foes

In my 18 years of clinical practice, four culprits continually cropped up in the daily lives of my fertility patients. These fertility foes are not preexisting conditions, but, in many cases, they exacerbate the symptoms of PCOS, endometriosis, POF, and so on. Other times, these four culprits are all present in varying degrees, creating numerous unseen, unfelt obstacles between you and that positive pregnancy test. I call them the Big Four, and they run rampant in the lives of modern women. Their presence isn't often acknowledged, but they're more prevalent than any preexisting medical condition. You're exposed to the Big Four every day, and if you're not aware of them, they can wreak havoc on your fertility, unchecked and unnoticed.

So what are the Big Four?

1. Inflammation
2. Insulin
3. Stress
4. Toxicity

You may find you aren't that surprised at this list, as all four of those words have cropped up elsewhere in this book already. They are by-products of modern living. Inflammation can be triggered by lifestyle factors as mundane as our food choices and sleep habits. Insulin takes over your bloodstream via those ever-so-convenient, fast, processed foods. Stress is the day-to-day norm of the modern woman everywhere, whether a high-powered lawyer or a woman of leisure. Toxins enter your system via the air, your food, and your everyday household products. More troublesome still, each of the Big Four has the potential to trigger the other three. They are interconnected, and they can all weaken your ability to conceive.

Liz, a 38-year-old corporate attorney, was under attack from all of the Big Four at once, locked in a vicious cycle that brought her to my office sobbing. After yet another month of painful fertility drug shots and high hopes, she had just gotten her period. On top of the crushing disappointment, the stress of the treatment was affecting her relationship with her husband and causing her to withdraw from family and friends. To add insult to injury, she had gained 10 pounds from the medications and was still without answers.

Before coming to me, multiple fertility doctors told Liz the same thing: "It's an egg quality issue." Unfortunately, the verdict wasn't followed with any kind of advice for how to improve her "egg quality."

Liz was left with even more questions. Why was it not good? How does this happen? What can I do?

As you now know, there are many reasons why a woman's ovaries aren't producing quality eggs, and Liz was affected by more than one. She'd been labeled with the stamp of "advanced maternal age," and she had endometriosis. However, her lifestyle was actually her biggest problem because it was worsening her medical condition.

Liz was constantly stressed and overworked. She was a partner at her firm and worked 80-hour weeks. She drank a lot of coffee to keep up the pace and used wine in the evening to wind herself down, not to mention the use of sleeping pills and antianxiety meds here and there.

Her diet also wasn't great. She skipped breakfast and ate out pretty much every meal. If she was on a time crunch at work, she would just munch on cookies in the afternoon and eat a big dinner at 9 p.m. before diving back into work until midnight. Her routine was putting her body through the wringer.

The more aggravated her lifestyle and the crappier she ate, the more her endometriosis created free radical damage and inflammation in her reproductive system. The path to baby required calming her mind and cleansing her body of junk and inflammation. The best way to do that was to address various aspects of her lifestyle in a treatment regimen designed specifically for her using my method.

I recommended Liz do a three-week elimination diet to cut out inflammatory and acidic foods such as sugar and booze. I gave her fish oil and magnesium supplements to reduce inflammation, balance stress, and improve sleep. She came for acupuncture two or three times per week to increase circulation to her ovaries and help detoxify her system. I also added specific dosages of coenzyme Q10 (CoQ10) and acai to improve her egg quality. I taught her basic meditation techniques and recommended some recorded fertility meditations to listen to on her commute. We dissected her work and home life and came up with a more manageable routine. Liz also started eating two of her three meals per day at home after learning some new (simple and quick) recipes. For the third meal, I taught her how to pick "safe" things from restaurant menus. Liz underwent this program for six months. Yes, it can take that long. While some women need less time, Liz needed an overhaul.

After the six-month program, Liz decided to start prepping for her next IVF cycle as she was waiting for her period to come around. She came to me in a state of exasperation because her period was late.

"What's wrong now? I can't catch a break!" she said.

I suggested she take a pregnancy test before we started troubleshooting a late period. At last, there it was, the long-awaited positive. She went on to have a healthy baby. Liz is now under my care prepping for baby number two!

Did it take a long time? Sure, but she did it without more painful shots or the expense of another IVF cycle, and she made changes that would serve her and her family in the long term. I'd say the wait was worth it.

Although Liz's age and her endometriosis were big factors in her fertility struggle, she didn't get pregnant by stepping into a time machine or by miraculously curing her endometriosis. Liz became pregnant by reducing the impact of the Big Four and her hectic lifestyle.

Many preexisting conditions are genetic, and making lifestyle changes isn't going to make them disappear, but creating a personalized treatment regimen using my method will be a significant aid in dealing with your condition. That's why you will notice that beside each condition, I noted the future chapter that will be most helpful for you and your needs. Feel free to skip there and read that chapter first after you've completed this one if you want.

Untangling the web of the Big Four is the core of my method. That's why, in the following chapters, I'll be laying down effective strategies to combat these four fertility foes in order to manage and improve the conditions listed in this chapter. We'll tackle them one by one so that you can begin to understand which areas of your life they're sneaking into, how they affect your fertility, and how to combat them.

It's not a quick fix. I am proposing a total lifestyle transformation to help you reach and *maintain* your fertility and overall health goals. It *does* get you results. Many of my patients have literally tried everything else, only for simple dietary and lifestyle changes to be the big ticket. The answer is not in pill form and will not provide miraculous benefits overnight. Commitment is key in overcoming your condition(s) and seeing the changes you want.

So without further ado, let's commit to a deep dive into the first of the Big Four.

CHAPTER 4

A Fire Inside

The first of the Big Four is stealthy. While it often manifests as pain or swelling, much of the damage it does flies under the radar, making it hard to peg. Meet *inflammation*. The word comes from the Latin *inflammatio*, meaning "setting on fire"—fairly appropriate for an immune response characterized by heat and redness. When you twist your ankle or bump your knee on that damn coffee table again, you put an ice pack on the injury for it to subside. But this Big Four champ isn't just external lumps and bumps from sports or clumsiness. When inflammation is present deeper inside the body, we tack on the suffix "itis." For example, "arthr" means joint, so arth*ritis* is joint inflammation. Sinusitis? Inflammation of the sinuses. Endometritis? Yep, inflammation of the lining of the uterus.

Inflammation can be a localized response due to an injury, but it can also be a reaction to toxins, infection, autoimmunity, or allergens. In essence, it's a beneficial, natural response involving immune cells swarming to rid the body of an offender. Inflammation is also your body's immune system gathering around the injured area to provide the necessary resources for healing.

Unfortunately, when this natural reaction goes haywire, it has the power to wreak havoc at a cellular level. Egg and sperm quality issues, for example, can be a side effect of chronic (and often silent) inflammation. And the damage doesn't stop there. The upside is that if you take control of your daily habits, this foe will be no match for you.

For the most part, we associate inflammation with pain. Generally, the discomfort is caused by "inflammatory mediators," such as bradykinin and histamine, flooding an area and irritating the surrounding nerves. Any pain in the body indicates inflammation, even if you can't see the swelling. Period pain, ovulatory pain, and those god-awful sensitive pimples that won't come all the way to the surface? Inflammation. The pain is our body cuing us to pay attention.

Although pain is a good clue that inflammation is present, sometimes the manifestations are much more subtle. You may not have a clue that it is happening at all. As a result, many women never realize that inflammation is playing a role in their fertility troubles, and it goes untreated for far too long. When inflammation lingers for long periods of time, effectively becoming "chronic," it can start to damage healthy tissues and cells and may even cause scarring. DNA damage and cellular changes don't bode well for egg or sperm quality or for implantation.

Conditions like endometriosis or fibroids are characterized by inflammation in the reproductive organs. Despite the near-constant unrest down there, many sufferers don't experience any pain. Instead, they might have low energy, look puffy, have difficulty losing weight, or have interrupted sleep. If you are having trouble getting pregnant, then consider that inflammatory processes gone awry may be at play.

> Inflammation disruptive to fertility can result from internal (endogenous) or external (exogenous) sources. Internal examples are an autoimmune condition, psychological stress, genetic predispositions, or poor gut health. External sources might be drugs (including medications), a polluted environment, exposure to toxins, or surgery.

Does this sound like you?

- I have painful periods.
- I have back pain or other persistent body pain.
- I have stubborn excess weight and/or fluid retention.
- I have migraines.
- I have allergies.
- I've been diagnosed with irritable bowel syndrome.
- I frequently have constipation.
- I have had a miscarriage(s).
- I have been diagnosed with endometriosis.
- I suffer from frequent infections.
- I have acid reflux.
- I am always tired.
- I have insomnia.

Did you check five or more of these boxes? Read on for more information about the root causes of inflammation and it role in hampering fertility.

Too Much of a Good Thing

Inflammation is supposed to be a helpful healing response, and it actually plays a natural role in many reproductive processes. It is a by-product of egg development, ovulation, and the formation of your lining. For example, you experience acute inflammation in your ovaries each time you ovulate. As the egg "bursts" out of the follicle, it causes a mini trauma, so inflammation occurs to heal the damage. An abundance of inflammation, however, may cause that familiar sudden twinge or sharp pain in your ovaries when your egg drops out of the follicle. Inflammation is a favorite tool of your immune system, which plays a crucial role in ovarian follicle (i.e., egg) growth. Your immune system regulates which tissues are allowed to grow and how much of that tissue is allowed to grow. It also decides which tissues to protect and preserve. This means it regulates the frequency of follicle renewal. This ability degenerates naturally with age, but if other issues speed up that degeneration, you can diminish your follicle (i.e., egg) count prematurely (Bukovsky and Caudle 2012). Persistent, long-lasting inflammation is one of those accelerating issues. It can cause cellular changes, affect DNA, and lead to low-quality eggs and poor development of embryos (Boots and Jungheim 2015). Fluid pockets in the uterus or fallopian tubes are also a common side effect of inflammation, which can pose challenges for implantation.

Inflammation is powerful. It has the ability to damage structures and lead to the development of scarring. Conditions like endometriosis and pelvic inflammatory disease (PID) are linked to chronic inflammation and scarring and pose serious fertility challenges (Weiss et al. 2009).

Antioxidants to the Rescue!

While inflammation is the inciting incident, it's actually the by-products of inflammation that are associated with reproductive damage on a cellular level. These reactive oxygens are also secreted by the select follicle that releases the egg during ovulation. They're natural, but the trouble for some people is that too many of these suckers are floating around in their systems. They don't have enough antioxidants in their body to "scavenge" the reactive oxygens. There is talk in the fertility community about supplementing antioxidants as a means of improving fertility. It's well documented that you can improve sperm quality with antioxidants, but there's less evidence associated with improvement of women's egg quality. We'll get there later, but I recommend adjusting your lifestyle to reduce the production of free radicals (reactive oxygen species) to stop the issue before it starts. In some cases, supplementation of antioxidants such as melatonin, resveratrol, NAC, acai, or CoQ10 might be helpful.

The (Auto)Immune Connection

If you've been diagnosed with an autoimmune condition, your immune system may be triggering "attack mode" without the presence of a true threat. It acts much like a loyal but misguided guard dog barking at innocent passersby. Victims of the assault may include anything from your partner's sperm to a fertilized egg (embryo) trying to nestle into your uterus.

There is mounting evidence that autoimmune issues can negatively impact both male and female fertility. It's one reason for the rising buzz surrounding topics such as natural killer cells, lupus, and silent endometriosis in the field of reproductive medicine.

Malfunctioning antibodies that attack your own cells are called *autoantibodies*. Research suggests that regardless of whether you've been diagnosed with an overt autoimmune disease, you can have autoantibodies that can affect the function of your reproductive system. There are many kinds of autoantibodies that have been linked to repeated IVF failure and infertility (Carp, Selmi, and Shoenfeld 2012). They assault your hormones and egg cells, causing premature ovarian failure or the widely loathed "poor egg quality" diagnosis (Haller-Kikkatalo, Salumets, and Uibo 2011). However, this connection hasn't been fully accepted by those in the medical field due to inconsistent findings between studies. Still, the topic keeps reappearing and is worth some attention. The solution doesn't necessarily have to involve aggressive immune therapy, but rather practicing an anti-inflammatory lifestyle when trying to conceive.

There are two well-known representations of immune dysfunction affecting the reproductive system that are far less disputed in the medical field: endometriosis and Hashimoto's disease. A hot topic in the fertility community is the concept of silent endometriosis. This condition is now classified as an autoimmune syndrome that attacks the tissues of the reproductive system. The strongest link experts have

Ask an Expert

Autoantibodies attack your eggs at all stages of their development. The chromosomal damage they cause leads to complications in egg growth, fertilization, and implantation. Should a chromosomally defective egg survive all that and manage to embed in your lining, the unfortunate likely scenario is a miscarriage.

One of the ways that modern medicine has sought to circumvent such miscarriages is the introduction of PGT-A testing during an IVF cycle. This test is performed after your eggs are taken out and before they're placed back in your uterus.

Dr. Forman from Columbia Med is an expert in this area. Here are his two cents:

"As many as 60 to 80 percent of miscarriages are caused by chromosomal abnormalities. Preimplantation genetic testing for aneuploidies (PGT-A) testing offers us a way to test the embryos in advance of the IVF transfer to lessen the likelihood of placing an embryo that may result in miscarriage. Prior to the advent of this testing, a common practice was to transfer several embryos in hopes of one 'taking.' The complication with this method was the higher likelihood of twins and triplets and the risks that come with such pregnancies. PGT-A testing's ability to select chromosomally normal embryos, on the other hand, results in 60 to 70 percent live birth success rates. As long as you are able to produce some chromosomally sound embryos, this could be a more direct and speedy route to a baby."

Personal communication with author (2022)

made in regard to the actual cause of endometriosis is immune system dysfunction. You have naturally occurring compounds called prostaglandins in almost all of your tissues. They have an array of hormone-like effects, one of them being inflammation. If your immune system is weakened or has a genetic abnormality, you can produce an excess of inflammatory prostaglandins in your lady parts. The chronic presence of this inflammation can result in abnormal tissue growth and scarring characteristic of endometriosis. Endometriosis, along with other autoimmune conditions like lupus, is associated with an abundance of antiphospholipid antibodies. These can cause complications through swelling and clotting, cutting off blood supply to an embryo or hindering implantation (Scher and Dix 2005).

Testing Your Uterine Lining

If you've experienced a previous unexplained miscarriage or suspect you may have silent endometriosis, it's possible you have inflammation and scarring that's preventing an embryo from nestling into your uterus. There is a way to determine whether your lining is currently in an adequate state to accept an embryo so that you can take preemptive action before trying to conceive again. To get answers, you can have a biopsy of the uterus called an endometrial receptivity test or endometritis test. They cut out a little piece of the uterine lining and test it for inflammation. It's thought that inflammation of the uterine lining is caused by bacterial infections, so conventional doctors often treat it with antibiotics. Unfortunately, I usually see the inflammation return in full force due to the antibiotics imbalancing the bacteria in the gut and reproductive system. The most effective method for banishing endometritis is a clean diet and good probiotics.

Hashimoto's thyroiditis is an autoimmune disorder involving autoantibodies that attack the thyroid and severely alter its function. An autoimmune thyroid condition is very dangerous and, in some cases, can be life threatening. Treating Hashimoto's can be difficult because the thyroid is reacting to any number of inflammatory triggers and can switch between hyper (overactive) and hypo (underactive). Medicating any autoimmune condition poses difficulties because the effects are "systemic," meaning many bodily systems are involved.

> For a full list of tests to assess autoimmune fertility challenges, see appendix F.

Hashimoto's disease can cause complications with anything from ovulation to implantation. Digestive conditions like irritable bowel syndrome (IBS) and leaky gut syndrome tend to exacerbate Hashimoto's disease. The upside is that this strong connection to the gut allows us a starting point. We can improve thyroid health and many other immunological and inflammatory issues by managing our digestive health. The catch? You gotta do the work!

Your Microbiome and Infertility

We know that inflammation can occur via genetic predispositions, toxin exposure, stress, drugs, injuries, and so on. But what we haven't yet discussed is how your gut bacteria could cause, perpetuate, or prevent healing of said inflammatory reactions.

The collection of microorganisms in our gut is known as our "microbiome." Unfettered, this army of good bacteria helps to fend off invaders, break down food to release energy, and produce vitamins such as B12. It plays a pivotal role in immunity and nutrition. But when microbiomes leak out into places they're not supposed to, they trigger inflammatory processes that wreak all sorts of havoc (Hakansson and Molin 2011).

Since about 70 percent of your immune system is located in your digestive tract, it is the hot seat of immune reactivity (Aleksic, n.d.). Your digestive and respiratory systems interface with the outside world via a mucosal layer that runs the length of your torso. This protective barrier is packed with immune cells and bacteria that attack and neutralize foreign substances such as germs and microbes.

Sometimes, however, the immune response can be altered due to damage of the mucosal layer and "dysbiosis," an imbalance of the healthy gut bacteria that usually inhabit our digestive system. Bacterial "endotoxins" can leak through a damaged mucosal layer into our circulation. This is a very common problem. In fact, studies have shown that a third of the molecules in most people's bloodstream are unhealthy gut bacteria (Pizzorno 2014). The weaker and more permeable your mucosal barrier, the more endotoxins are circulating. They damage cells and tissues of vital organs (Pizzorno 2014), including those involved in getting you pregnant! Endotoxins are implicated in POF, recurrent pregnancy loss (RPL), and repeated IVF failures. In my practice, I've found that, in most cases, gut health is the key to achieving pregnancy when implantation fails for unknown reasons.

> Endometritis (inflammation of the uterine lining), though controversial, is frequently caused by bacterial imbalances and is thus treated with antibiotics. This may help some women get pregnant, but for others, it poses harm to their efforts.

The Leaky Gut Connection

Some people have a genetically weaker mucosal barrier, but most of us unknowingly weaken our barrier through lifestyle and dietary choices. Overeating, eating too fast, overuse of medications, high stress, and unhealthy foods can assault the delicate internal lining of your gut. Over time, tiny perforations or "cuts" appear. Bacteria, food particles, and toxins can leak through those perforations into the bloodstream in a condition known as "leaky gut syndrome." Your lymphatic system scrambles to clean up the leak and calls on your liver to pitch in, acting as a filter for the gunk. A weakened gut becomes a systemic issue, causing a heightened level of inflammation and firing of immune and stress responses. According to a recent study conducted in Turkey, gut perforations and excessive gut permeability markers are one of the possible reasons why women with PCOS tend to inflame easier and have issues with egg quality and implantation.

A weakened mucosal barrier also leads to estrogen imbalances because your gut stops producing enough of an enzyme called beta-glucuronidase. This enzyme filters and recirculates active estrogen back into your system. As if all that wasn't problematic enough, a leaky gut is associated with anxiety and depression. Yikes.

Anik Ilhan and Yildizhan (2018)

INFLAMMATION MAKES YOU FAT

Sadly, I'm not kidding. An imbalance of your microbiome can lead to weight gain and obesity (Harakeh et al. 2016). Increased weight results in higher levels of inflammation. As our weight goes up, our fat cells swell beyond their threshold and start to leak. Once the leaked gunk hits our circulation, the lymphatic system, which transports your healing white blood cells, tries to clean up. Ever feel puffy? That's usually the result of a backup in your lymphatic system. It fills with liquid to try to dilute the junk it's filtering. Lymphatic health and gut health are intertwined. But it isn't just fluid weight that starts to accumulate. Inflammation messes with our blood sugar metabolism, blocking insulin from fulfilling its usual functions and leading to weight gain (more on that in the next chapter). If you feel yourself getting fatter for no particular reason or you're really struggling to shed weight, silent inflammation could be playing a significant role.

Ways to Test for Inflammation

If you suspect inflammation could be playing a part in your infertility but you aren't experiencing all of the symptoms, you can ask your doctor for the following tests to determine whether inflammation is present in your system:

1. *Immunoglobulin tests (IgA, IgG)*. Immunoglobulins are the antibodies your body uses to fight infections and foreign substances. The two most common are IgA, which are located in the mucus around your lungs and intestines, and IgG, which are in all of your bodily fluids and are meant to fight viruses. If your test results come back and your levels of either of these immunoglobulins are high, it indicates that your body is reacting to something and that inflammation is present. There are functional medicine tests that dive deep into this type of testing. Labs such as Genova offer this option.

2. *Alcat test*. This is one of the most well-known food and environmental sensitivity tests. It helps determine what factors of your lifestyle might be causing inflammatory reactions. You can choose cheaper à la carte options to test solely for food, environmental toxins, molds, and so on. If it's within your budget, however, I suggest doing the whole package and testing for everything. The Alcat test is available through Naturna Institute's website (https://naturnalife.com) or my personal website (www.christinaburns.com).

The Skinny on Probiotics

One strategy to rebalance your gut, improve digestion, and strengthen your immune system is with probiotics. Your gut is full of both good and bad bacteria. Probiotics help to balance those levels for optimal health and fertility. Research conducted on women undergoing IVF proved that the right strains of good bacteria (*Lactobacillus acidophilus*) have the potential to improve pregnancy rates (Moreno et al. 2016).

You already have probiotics in your digestive tract lining naturally. Actually, they are 10 times more numerous than actual cells in your gut, at least when your gut is healthy. But things like sugar, toxins, parasites, and genetically modified organisms (GMOs) feed the bad bacteria, leading to "dysbiosis": an imbalance of gut bacteria in favor of the bad guys. Dysbiosis has been linked to infertility, while good strains of probiotics have been linked to IVF success (Pelzer et al. 2013). Antibiotics can certainly help dysbiosis as well, but they kill off the good bacteria along with the bad. So, after using antibiotics, it is essential to eat a clean diet and take probiotics to repopulate the gut with good bacteria. Otherwise, you could have rebound infections worse than the one you treated.

I've had many patients with bacterial infections who took dose after dose of antibiotics only to have the inflammation return soon after. When those probiotic levels are reduced, it can throw off your entire gut balance and consequently your immune system, digestion, mood, and fertility.

Signs of dysbiosis include the following:

• Allergies
• Constipation
• Skin disorders
• Anxiety/depression
• Malnutrition
• Exhaustion
• Autoimmune disease
• Attention deficit disorder (ADD)/attention-deficit/hyperactivity disorder (ADHD)
• Infertility (obviously)
• Hormonal dysfunction
• Food sensitivities

Increasing your probiotic levels naturally means mixing up your diet a little. Sour foods like apple cider vinegar, kimchi, kombucha, sauerkraut, or any fermented veggies are all rich in probiotics. The caution with dietary probiotic sources is that they sometimes exacerbate candida (an overgrowth of yeast) when you first start taking them. A more controlled way to repopulate your gut is to use human strain probiotics from a reputable company. The best scenario is to see a licensed practitioner who can prescribe you an appropriate combination of probiotic strains (fun fact: the prescription will vary depending on your digestive, immune, mental, and vaginal health). In lieu of that, choose one of the items mentioned in appendix E.

Prebiotics are a nice add-on to probiotics, but they, too, have their downsides. I find them most helpful when there are issues with elimination because they help you poop more regularly. However, I've noticed that, for some, the fermentable fiber sources that naturally

> Prebiotics reinforce the effects of probiotics by giving them "food" to thrive. Many prebiotics are also combined with glutamine, which helps to heal a damaged gut lining.

contain probiotics—chia seeds, flaxseeds, asparagus, and apples—are in some cases quite bloating for those with an imbalanced gut.

As much as I'd like to tell you to get everything you need from food, I've observed clinically that some people do better to start with controlled doses of pre- and probiotic supplements while they clean up their diet. Studies have shown that probiotics make your intestinal wall stronger by increasing adhesion proteins in the tissue (Uusitalo et al. 2016). A stronger gut means less leakage, a lower inflammatory response, and thus less oxidative stress. Once the gut is in a healthier (and less reactive) state, supplements can be weaned, and foods can take the main stage.

> ### Did You Know?
>
> Probiotics help combat insulin resistance and the inflammation it brings.

I posit that balancing your gut bacteria, healing your gut wall, and maintaining a healthy microbiome are crucial factors in regulating immune health and controlling inflammation.

> ## Inflammation and Insatiable Hunger
>
> Hunger means that you need more food, right? Not necessarily. It could be inflammation messing around with two major hormones that control appetite: insulin and leptin. While insulin balance can indirectly affect appetite and cravings, leptin is literally your appetite-regulating hormone. It is secreted by your fat cells, and it tells your brain that you're full. But if that signal is disrupted by inflammation, you might keep eating past your normal capacity.

Cool Down

Maybe you don't think this chapter applies to you. However, I have yet to meet a woman or couple who didn't have some sign of inflammation in their body. You may not experience pain in your lady parts or the indirectly related symptoms like IBS or food sensitivities. That doesn't mean inflammation isn't underlying some of the fertility challenges you are facing, as there are many sneaky symptoms that indicate inflammation without pain.

If you prefer to have tangible data points to confirm an overactive immune response, you can request an IgA or IgG immunoglobulin test to see if you have an excess of antibodies that might indicate the degree of inflammation present in your body. Other tests that can pinpoint indicators for immunological issues more directly related to infertility are antiphospholipid, antinuclear, antithyroid, and antisperm antibodies. The caveat is that, by and large, fertility specialists do not support immunological testing as it pertains to fertility. There haven't been enough studies conducted and data collected for it to become standard procedure. That said, many IVF clinics are now routinely prescribing immunosuppressant drugs such as steroids or antibiotics in conjunction with fertility treatments. Theoretically, this means that a number of clinics are adopting practices to stamp out the immune response. While it's great that modern medicine is looking closer at more subtle fertility foes, the dilemma is that the common treatment involves pumping women full of drugs. This approach is physically, financially, and mentally taxing and will inevitably bring about harsh side effects. It's best to try cooling things down naturally before grabbing the big guns. If you've been diagnosed with "poor egg quality" or another vague, inconclusive diagnosis, I highly recommend following the directions laid out in this chapter.

Since your immune system is so closely tied to your gut health, some of the biggest changes you can make are dietary. Refined foods have been shown in numerous studies to adversely affect fertility, perhaps at least in part due to the effect they have on overgrowth of bad bacteria. No matter the exact source of the overgrowth, the inflammation that results from dysbiosis prevents you from properly absorbing nutrients. You can become deficient in nutrients such as vitamin D (Noventa et al. 2015), zinc (Spann et al. 2015), and selenium (Razavi et al. 2015) that are vital for fertility.

To rebalance your nutrient levels, reduce inflammation and reverse immune confusion, stick to the following basic dietary principles.

Avoid processed meat, pork, and grain-fed beef. Red meats are known to increase inflammatory biomarkers because they are full of saturated fats stuffed with endotoxins (Greger 2012; Ley et al. 2014). Your immune system reacts to endotoxins like foreign bacteria, flooding your bloodstream with inflammatory attack cells. Researchers at the University of California San Diego School of Medicine found that red meat contains a molecule that humans don't naturally produce called *Neu5Gc*. After ingesting this compound, the body develops anti-Neu5Gc antibodies and an immune response that triggers chronic inflammatory response (Tangvoranuntakul et al. 2003). Fish, poultry, and plant proteins should take the main stage when it comes to protein. If eating meat, choose "grass-fed and finished" since animals fed soy and corn tend to have higher percentages of bad fats.

Benefits and Detriments of Bone Broth

Many sources purport that drinking bone broth helps with both gut health and inflammation. It is mineral dense and contains collagen that is thought to help the lining of the gut. However, there's a pretty significant caveat. Bone broth also contains high levels of histamine, which produces an immune reaction in a lot of people. Bone broth has a lot of health advantages; if you feel inflammation may be a major factor in your infertility, it may be best to drink it in moderation or avoid it altogether.

Choose healthier oils when cooking. Common vegetable cooking oils are highly inflammatory. Because of the high levels of omega-6 fatty acids and low omega-3 fats in corn, sunflower, safflower, peanut, grape seed, and soybean oils, they are metabolized into hormone-like compounds that promote an inflammatory response. Instead, when you sauté veggies or bake fish, use macadamia oil, extra virgin olive oil, or coconut oil. These oils have a more equal ratio of omega-3s to omega-6s, meaning fewer inflammatory omega-6s. The only caveat is that you can't let these healthy oils "smoke." When they get too hot, they will turn carcinogenic and cause free radical damage. Oxidative damage from free radicals accelerates aging throughout the body, including your precious eggs. Fast and furious aging is, in essence, the death of fertility. Note that trans fats found in deep-fried foods, fast foods, commercial baked goods, and those prepared with partially hydrogenated oil, margarine, and vegetable shortening have also been found to promote inflammation, cardio-vascular diseases, and resistance to insulin, laying the ground for degenerative illnesses (Mazidi and Vatanparast 2017).

Try Water Sautéing!

Try using a bit of oil to first coat and sauté your protein and veggies, then add water to cook them through. If you're cooking protein, I recommend using the oil to brown it, then adding the water along with any veggies. Of course, there's always the option to just steam it all with water and avoid the risk of smoking oil altogether.

Avoid sweets, booze, and processed foods. These all equate to sugar in your blood. The entire next chapter is dedicated to this topic, so I'll keep it brief here. High-glycemic foods and drinks (i.e., those that spike your blood glucose and insulin levels) set off a chain of inflammatory responses in your body. The biggest culprits are refined sugars and grains, such as corn syrup, white sugar, and flour-based wheat or corn products. Excessive sugar intake, no matter the source, is linked to increased risks of obesity, inflammation, and chronic diseases like metabolic

Did You Know?

Binge drinking induces insulin resistance and may even leave you feeling down and less motivated to follow through with healthier diet habits.

syndrome and type 2 diabetes (Delli Bovi et al. 2017). Reducing grain intake can be very beneficial for gut health. In particular, a gluten-free diet has been shown to reduce inflammation, insulin resistance, and body fat (Soares et al. 2012).

The Progesterone Factor

A study done on pregnant women demonstrated that healthy progesterone levels seem to prevent inflammation and preterm labor. Maintaining healthy progesterone levels helps reduce inflammation and gut permeability by strengthening the bond between proteins in the gut, thereby fortifying the mucosal barrier. In order to optimize your progesterone levels, try seed cycling (see chapter 9 for details) and avoid excessive exercise and stress. Vitamin B6 or herbs such as chasteberry and maca may also be helpful.

Milk is for babies. You're probably not going to be very happy with me, but this must be said. Most people have some level of dairy intolerance. More than 60 percent of the population cannot properly digest milk. If you're in that percentile—and there's a big chance you are—your gut and mucosal lining can be negatively impacted. An allergy, even a mild one, triggers an immune response that results in inflammation. It's wise to suspect dairy as the culprit when experiencing pimples, painful periods, allergies, weight issues, hypothyroidism, cysts, PCOS, yeasty issues, or digestive complaints. Interestingly, a childhood fraught with ear infections is also an indicator. If you suspect inflammation is interfering with your fertility or if you have endometriosis or any sort of autoimmune condition, cut out dairy altogether. That means anything made from milk, including cheese and yogurt. I realize this is a big ask, but we have so many good replacements. Since dairy is a comfort food, I often suggest substituting healthier fatty foods, such as nut or seed butters, avocado, nut cheese, or coconut yogurt. If you absolutely must keep the dairy, then go for smarter choices that are more easily digested and contain little to no lactose. Your best options are unsweetened whole-fat goat or sheep yogurt or feta cheese. Somewhat surprisingly, you should avoid low-fat dairy altogether. A large study of 18,000 nurses linked the consumption of low-fat dairy to higher risk of anovulatory cycles and infertility (Chavarro et al. 2007c). The "fat-free" trend is toxic to our hormones and is basically just an excuse to overeat. It's much wiser to eat good-quality fats sparingly than chow down on anything with a "low-fat" label.

Worried that you won't be getting enough calcium? Seeds, nuts, and greens like broccoli and collards are packed with this important mineral.

ADDITIONAL STRATEGIES

Your food choices may be the most essential part of reducing inflammation, but lifestyle changes also matter. Excessive or inadequate weight, rigorous exercise, smoking, drugs, psychological stress, and toxin-heavy environments can all lead to oxidative stress that harms eggs, sperm, and uterine receptivity (Gupta et al. 2013). Making small changes to your daily routine is the key to successfully integrating healthy new habits.

Hydrate like it's nobody's business. One of the simplest habits you can introduce to cool your system is upping your water intake. Water cleanses our elimination systems and, by relation, *everything* else in the body. Without enough water, your cells are malnourished. Your metabolism then slows down and retains toxins, leading to more inflammation. The exact amount of water you need per day will vary based on your sex, your size, and how much you're exercising, but the basic rule of thumb is eight eight-ounce glasses a day, or roughly half a gallon/two liters. If you want to get super exact, the National Academies of Sciences, Engineering, and Medicine says that a woman should drink 2.7 liters a day. Hitting anywhere around that number is beneficial (Mayo Clinic Staff 2020).

Practice sleeping deeply. Studies have shown that people suffering from sleep deprivation have higher levels of inflammatory cytokines. Your sleep deprivation doesn't have to be extreme either. Sporadically interrupted sleep or just falling a few hours short of the eight hour mark will have the same inflammatory results. You must achieve at least four to five cycles of that deep rapid-eye-movement (REM) sleep to get adequate rest. It's during this restorative sleep that your body cleanses, heals, and cools itself. I know through personal experience that sleep is not easily attainable for everyone. I am a self-professed crappy sleeper. That said, I have noticed that practicing good "sleep hygiene" helps me rest much better. Here's what I've learned. Power down all screens (including phones and Netflix) by 8 p.m. at the latest. Next up, eat early. Before 7 p.m. is best, and avoid a massive hunk of meat or carbs as your last meal. As the old Chinese saying goes, "The digestive energy sets with the sun," so eat lighter in the evening. Booze of any kind pretty much slaughters sleep. It prevents you from attaining the REM state. You may think it's curative, but I assure you that you'll sleep better than ever without that evening cup of vino. Caffeine is obvious, particularly when consumed after noon. If you are a poor sleeper, then explore knocking it out altogether. Pause yourself entirely for five to 10 minutes in the afternoon so that you aren't super wired when you come out of your workday. You must allow your nervous system to wind down so that you don't enter the evening hours with your brain on fire. If you still can't sleep, then try valerian root. It's a great herbal sedative and doesn't have side effects. Chinese herbs also work wonders for sleep. Some of my faves are Gui Pi Tang, Suan Zao Ren Tang, and Tian Wan Bu Xin Dan. The tricky thing with herbal remedies is that the formulas are very precise and personal. If you try to create your own herbal concoction, you may actually make yourself feel worse. Seek out a qualified Chinese medicine doctor or herbalist or get a custom prescription through https://junkjuicemagic.com or by contacting the Naturna Institute (https://naturnalife.com).

Don't overdo the exercise. Exercise helps you cleanse your system and feel elated, but it can be inflammatory if overdone. A hard workout breaks down muscle fibers, which then heal stronger, building and toning muscle. The trouble is that this is essentially a mini trauma, and the healing process requires some level of inflammation. You'll recognize it as the burn you feel the day after a good session. The balance is different for everyone, but you'll see an outline of recommendations if you jump to chapter 10. As a general rule, go for nonimpact exercises like yoga, walking, swimming, and dancing. Why nonimpact? Impact causes stress on joints and tissues, resulting in inflammation. Avoid cross fit, boot camps, and running like the plague.

Try acupuncture. There are now many studies to support the use of acupuncture in regulating inflammation and immunomodulation. A skilled acupuncturist can target inflammation using techniques to calm swelling and pain, correct immune imbalance, and restore digestive health (Zijlstra et al. 2003). Scheduling an appointment couldn't hurt and may do worlds of good.

> Famous Chinese herbal formulas have been used to effectively treat inflammation. Shao Fu Zhu Yu Tang has been found to be efficacious in treatment of endometriosis, and Xue Fu Zhu Yu Tang is one of my favorite go-tos.

Vitamin C supplementation. One natural way to foster immune balance and reduce inflammation is as simple as taking vitamin C supplements regularly. When an inflammatory response occurs in your body, it triggers the production of a protein called C-reactive protein (CRP) in your bloodstream. An analysis of data on CRP levels in 14,519 U.S. adults showed a correlation between higher vitamin C intake and lower levels of CRP in the blood (Ford et al. 2003). A controlled trial study found that taking 1,000 mg of vitamin C a day for two months resulted in a 16.7 percent decrease in CRP levels compared to an 8.6 percent increase that was seen in the placebo group (Block et al. 2009). In another study, daily vitamin C supplements were shown to significantly increase the presence of an anti-inflammatory cytokine in the bloodstream of marathon runners (Peters et al. 2001). They also increased the circulation of cortisol in the bloodstream. Cortisol is an anti-inflammatory hormone that regulates your fluid levels. Whenever you exert yourself, cortisol is pumped into your system, but if your levels are too low, you can experience inflammation after strenuous activities. Vitamin C can help reverse that by helping your body better distribute cortisol where it's needed.

Omega-3 supplementation. Omega-3 comes from fish, such as salmon and sardines, as well as plant sources, such as flax and walnuts. This potent anti-inflammatory agent halts or tempers the effects of substances such as cytokines. As such, it's incredible for soothing and fortifying the nervous system, circulatory system, and immune system. It's one of the first recommendations I offer when a patient mentions pain or any type of "itis." One study showed that omega-3 is a great alternative to nonsteroidal anti-inflammatory drugs (NSAIDs) (medications like ibuprofen and aspirin) for a variety of pain conditions, ranging from neck pain to ulcers to heart attack (Maroon and Bost 2006). In terms of fertility, it's a huge aid for anyone with pro-inflammatory conditions like endometriosis and PCOS. Its anticlotting properties can help to thin blood and improve circulation in women whose infertility is tied to immune and blood-clotting factors. An animal study in 2012 showed that a diet rich in omega-3 can possibly even prolong fertility into advanced age (past 35 years old). The women who ate a diet rich in this magical fat had better egg quality than the control group. The authors thereby determined that omega-3 might be a way to slow the biological clock and improve fertility in advanced ages (Nehra et al. 2012). It even helps baby, boosting brain health in the womb.

The Truth about Turmeric and Other Spices

One of the most common herb recommendations for inflammation that you'll find in online searches is a yellow root called turmeric. This bitter herb *is* great for inflammation, as it actually blocks inflammatory cytokines, but it doesn't necessarily have any direct correlation to enhanced fertility. Excess amounts can even suppress both follicle development and the growth of the uterine lining. I prescribe it to patients who have pain, arthritis, and certain autoimmune conditions, but it is not one of my go-tos for women trying to conceive.

A lot of blogs will recommend you add "hot" herbs and spices to your meals, such as cayenne pepper. It seems counterintuitive to add "hot" spices to your food in order to "cool" inflammation, but it's true that they have anti-inflammatory properties. Unfortunately, peppers can actually irritate the lining of the gut in sensitive individuals (ahem, 60 million Americans). They also fall into the nightshade family of vegetables and are inflammatory for those with autoimmune conditions.

THE PAYOFF

Given that we often can't see or feel inflammation and may not have identified its source, a multifaceted approach may be the way to go. In my experience, tackling it from several angles improves the chances of achieving your desired results in a timely manner. Apply these techniques over just a short period, and you will notice systemic benefits such as improved mood, digestion, energy, sleep, and appearance. You may even find yourself knocked up. Take my patient, Paula, for example.

Paula was a 39-year-old and had worked in finance since her early twenties. She got into the office at 6:30 a.m. and didn't emerge until 6:30 p.m. most evenings. She ate at her desk because she was glued to her multi-screen workstation. As a day trader, she didn't have a lot of time to take her finger off the "go" button. Her evenings often involved dinners with clients at upscale New York restaurants. Steakhouses and other American fare were constants, as were the wine and cocktails that went along with the evening's festivities. Even when not out entertaining, she liked rich foods. Filet mignon, lobster, and fried indulgences were on her plate at least a few times per week. During her brief breaks, she also scarfed down the sugary crap that was easily available from her office vending machine, not to mention the coffee in the break room. Red wine was making an appearance nightly as a way to relax. Paula essentially ate like most of her mid-fifties male coworkers, and she was beginning to look like them, too. Her skin was reddish and blotchy, her midsection wide, her whole body puffy.

Paula had been trying to get pregnant with donor sperm (sans partner) for three years. She had done eight IVF cycles to no avail. She had a high egg count but was having trouble getting good-quality embryos. A few times, she managed to produce better embryos, but then they failed to implant. When Paula came to see me, she was preparing for her ninth transfer. As we chatted in my office, she began to slump in her seat as she detailed her struggles, weighed down by them. She seemed cynical and hopeless that anything would improve her odds. She met my eye and confessed that the only reason that she came to me was that her doctor had recommended that she do so.

I explained to Paula that I believed inflammation was her issue and recommended that she do some additional testing regarding her gut and immune system. Paula's results showed that her immune system was overactive. It was potentially attacking the embryos so that they couldn't implant and thrive. I immediately put her on an anti-inflammatory diet that involved cutting out beef, gluten, shellfish, fried foods, booze, and sugar and replacing them with vegetables, small amounts of game meats and fish, herbal teas, and clean, filtered water. I suggested she stay on the program for a minimum of three weeks before her next transfer. Paula also came to me for acupuncture two or three times per week to help calm her immune system, improve blood circulation, and reduce inflammation. As a final touch, I added a few supplements to hasten results: vitamin C, omega-3s, probiotics, magnesium, and Chinese herbs. Over the course of three weeks, she lost 10 pounds of water weight. She deflated as we cooled her immune system. Her bowel movements regulated, she slept soundly, and she remained energetic throughout her day. I also saw her demeanor change, becoming much more hopeful about the upcoming transfer. Paula stuck to the regime throughout the implantation period of 10 days following the transfer. Her human chorionic gonadotropin (HCG) hormone came back positive, and she went on to have a healthy pregnancy and delivery.

Preconception Planning

At least 21 days before renewing your efforts to get pregnant, begin making as many of the following "cooling" lifestyle adjustments as possible:

- Cut out red meat, pork, dairy, vegetable cooking oils, and sugar.
- Begin a nonimpact exercise routine.
- Purchase a reusable water bottle and set a goal to drink two liters a day.

The Beauty of Informed Action

No matter the source of your inflammation—whether it be genetics, gut health, immune dysfunction, or toxins—you have a level of agency. With the tools provided in this chapter, you can take action. The causes of your inflammation are unique to you. However, there are commonalities between all scenarios (e.g., free radical damage) that provide a general guideline for treatment. Follow the ground rules in this chapter, and you can create a calmer, more receptive environment to make a baby. It may seem basic, but attending to sleep quality, stress reduction, and smart food choices are the best strategies you can employ. It's the small, everyday changes that will coax your immune system back into balance.

The Big Four rarely exist independently; in fact, they play off each other. In the next chapter, you'll be swayed to think twice before indulging in that sweet something. This temptress impacts your hormones on many levels and is also likely to set up an inflammatory cascade. While it may seem complex at first, as you familiarize yourself with these concepts, you'll likely notice there are commonalities among these culprits, the benefit of which is that one positive change will be likely to reduce the impact of several of the Big Four all at once.

CHAPTER 5

Sweet Tooth

The second member of the Big Four gang may be associated with having a sweet tooth, but there's nothing sweet about the effects of an insulin overload. Diabetes runs rampant in America, so most of us are familiar with the terms "high blood sugar" and "insulin." The threats that diabetes poses to our health are fairly common knowledge, but we typically don't pay much mind unless we receive a diagnosis. We have enough on our plates without worrying over things that don't directly affect us. There is, however, a lesser-known offender in the blood sugar game. It's called insulin resistance, and it could be your number one fertility foe regardless of whether or not you have diabetes.

Insulin resistance affects 34 percent of the American population and is a growing area of research among reproductive specialists. It's a subtle and insidious hormonal imbalance that is hard to peg, yet it influences everything from our fertility and energy levels to our mood and appearance. It's even a determinant of how well we process alcohol! A staggering 84 million people in the United States alone are insulin resistant. It's fair to assume that you might be, too.

Due to modern-day food trends, processed foods and sweet snacks are everywhere. We are taking in more refined, sugary foods than our sedentary bodies can handle. The abundance of easily accessible "fast carbs" and the lack of discussion on the subject has allowed the prevalence of insulin resistance to rise unchecked. This chapter's aim is to shed some light on this widely impactful topic in hopes that you acquire the knowledge to make its influence obsolete.

Once you have the know-how, you will have significantly more control over whether insulin resistance can affect your fertility. Because it's so tightly intertwined with diet and daily habits, you can reverse most of its negative influences with simple changes to your routine. This chapter will assist you in crafting an effective plan to beat down insulin resistance, but first let's dig into "why" before arriving at "how."

Metabolic Nuts and Bolts

Most of us know that eating too much sugar is bad, but understanding why is a far rarer tidbit of knowledge. Insulin is a hormone that comes from your pancreas and is indirectly but very powerfully linked to your reproductive health. It influences blood flow to your lady parts as well as hormone production, egg development, ovulation, implantation, and more!

Whenever you eat, your blood sugar rises to some degree. More sugar in your food means a higher level, of course, but most foods will cause a rise. When your blood sugar goes up, insulin is released. Insulin's main job is to make your cells open, gobble up that glucose (aka sugar), and then divert it out of the bloodstream and into different tissues, like organs and muscles, to use as fuel. Once all of the glucose is rerouted, your insulin levels drop, and you are returned to a state of homeostasis, or equilibrium. Your hormones are in balance.

Frequently bombarding your body with processed foods and sugar and overeating create frequent blood sugar highs. This forces your pancreas to secrete high levels of insulin. Over time, your cells grow weary, and they become desensitized to its effects. Essentially, insulin keeps pumping, but your cells ignore the cue to take in the glucose to use as energy. Eventually, it will take higher and higher levels to push the same amount of sugar out of your blood and into your muscles, organs, and fat cells.

Many people have a genetic predisposition to insulin resistance—think parents or grandparents with diabetes or heart disease. Insulin resistance does not equal diabetes, but it is a precursor to type 2 diabetes and leads to all kinds of metabolic and reproductive complications. While anyone can experience pancreatic "burnout," if you have a genetic predisposition, you are likely to get there faster.

Hungrier before Your Period?

Research has shown us that women with type 1 diabetes have more insulin requirements in the luteal phase. That means they had to inject more insulin to bring their levels back into check. If you experience intense cravings in the week or so leading to your period, it's likely because insulin and blood sugar imbalances have gotten out of hand. Since insulin resistance plays a role in failed implantation and miscarriage, it's best to curb consumption of sugary, refined foods; excess fruits; juice; or alcoholic beverages.

Trout et al. (2007)

Am I Insulin Resistant?

Most sufferers don't realize they have an issue, and a deep dive into genetic and physiological markers for insulin resistance is not standard protocol for most doctors. Typically, hemoglobin A1c (HgA1c) is the most common test that is used to assess whether you have an issue, though I've met a lot of insulin-resistant women whose A1c is normal. To conduct more thorough lab tests, you'll want to contact an endocrinologist. In lieu of having a good one in your area, you might try getting a home glucose monitor and testing your sugar levels first thing in the morning and two hours after you eat. If you have notable spikes in your sugar (e.g., over 100 fasting and 140 or higher after food), then you might consider exploring further by reaching out to a professional and following the recommendations laid out in this chapter.

Request a Test

Assessing your insulin and blood sugar is important. The standard HgA1c test only measures the average of your blood glucose levels over the past three months. Dr. Zev Williams, director at Columbia Fertility in New York City, can best explain why you should explore further test options:

"HgA1c is a good indicator of the average glucose levels. However, what we've found is that it is actually elevated insulin, not glucose, that is toxic to the cells of the early placenta. With insulin resistance, you can experience extremely elevated insulin levels in response to a glucose/carb load, but the pancreas is able to make sufficient insulin to keep glucose levels within normal limits. So the HgA1c would be normal, but the insulin would actually be high.

"I have patients do a 75-gram glucose tolerance test (they can do it at Quest or Labcorp). We check a fasting and two-hour glucose and insulin. The critical value I look at is the two-hour insulin."

Personal communication with author (2022)

Lab tests are amazing modern medical assets, but I'm also a proponent of exploring things symptomatically, meaning that if it walks like a duck and quacks like a duck (you know how it goes).

Does this sound like you?

- I struggle with my weight.
- My body reacts poorly to alcohol.
- I am plagued with frequent colds and infections.
- I have heart palpitations.

- I am frequently fatigued without a clear reason.
- My small cuts and bruises take an unusually long time to heal.
- When I'm nervous, my palms and feet sweat.
- I crave sweets.
- I crave salt.
- I'm always thirsty.
- I get dizzy when I stand up.
- I feel weak and shaky a lot.
- I have irregular, "masculine" body hair.
- My bowel movements are difficult and/or infrequent.
- I pee frequently.
- My pee is dark and smells strongly.
- I have PCOS.
- I have had one or more miscarriages.
- I have trouble building an adequate uterine lining.
- I have infertility of no known cause.
- I have infrequent or no periods
- I have a high AMH (over 2.5).
- I tend to easily get belly fat.
- I have a very strong appetite.
- I crave sweets after meals.
- I have high cholesterol.
- I have a fatty liver.
- I often feel puffy or bloated.

If you checked off five or more of these, there's a good possibility you are insulin resistant. Let's take a deep dive into why these symptoms occur.

"Hangry"

Insulin resistance makes you hungry, even downright "hangry" at times. You might crave sweets after a meal or still be hungry despite having just eaten. What's at play is an interaction between insulin and the hormone called leptin.

> Balanced insulin is the key to balanced weight. Feeling a little soft around the midsection? Focus on your blood sugar and insulin, and the weight will fly off.

What's leptin, you ask? Leptin comes from the Greek *leptos*, which means "thin." This is a hormone we all want to have around. It tells your body when you've had enough to eat. Whenever you eat a meal or snack, your fat cells swell and dump leptin into the bloodstream, which makes you feel full and stop eating. Should insulin disrupt leptin's signals, your hunger may go awry. Take my patient, Jaclyn's story, for example.

> Abnormally high levels of insulin suppress leptin.

Jaclyn confessed she craved something sweet after every meal no matter how much she'd already eaten. When you're not properly absorbing the glucose in your blood, your cells aren't being fed. So they ask for more, meaning you start craving the sugary foods and fast carbs that are causing the issues in the first place. All Jaclyn knew was she really wanted a donut; she had no idea she actually had an excess of sugar already floating around in her blood causing problems. The more she ate, the worse her cravings became. Hello unwanted weight. The added pounds reduced her insulin sensitivity further, and the vicious cycle continued. We often think that if

> A sugar high crashes into a sugar low, which equals more sugar cravings. Those lows can even affect your mood and mental health, sometimes going so far as to cause feelings of depression.

we crave something, it's what our body wants or needs. This couldn't be further from the truth in many cases. In Jaclyn's case, excess insulin had not only disrupted her leptin signals but also made it harder for her body to ovulate by suppressing the function of her reproductive hormones.

It's Your Insulin

When insulin metabolism is out of balance, many body systems are deprived of energy. This can consequently impair many bodily processes involved in reproduction. Circulation becomes weak in the ovaries and uterus, and hormonal feedback systems break down.

The hormonal hell caused by insulin dysregulation can cause problems producing eggs and triggering ovulation. Another side effect is that low hormone production can cause your uterine lining to remain thin. As

> Do you crave a nightly glass of wine? Well, unfortunately, that's just another face that fast carbs wear. It's sugar on a rocket ship called ethanol. Avoiding dessert and opting for wine won't help insulin resistance.

a result, insulin resistance is implicated in many cases of failed implantation, miscarriage, and recurrent pregnancy loss, but until recently, there was little understanding as to *why* it caused these issues. Enter Dr. Zev Williams, director at

---

The Low-Down on Carbs

Carbs get a bad rap, and it's only half deserved. Healthy whole foods like vegetables and fruits have carbs, but the difference is the type of carb it contains. Carbs are made up of carbon, hydrogen, and oxygen. There are two main types:

1. Simple, or "fast," carbs are monosaccharides like glucose and fructose or disaccharides like maltose, sucrose, and lactose. "Mono," or "single," sugars are naturally found in fruits, but candy and other sugary foods are jam-packed with processed versions like high-fructose corn syrup. "Di," or "two-sugar," carbs are found in beer, liquor, fruits, veggies, milk, and sweeteners like honey and maple syrup. Both types of simple carbs are likely to cause a spike in blood sugar that will inevitably result in a crash thereafter.
2. The good guys are the complex carbs, or polysaccharides, like starch, glycogen, and fiber. Starch and glycogen are the storage form of carbs for plants and animals, while fiber forms the structural walls of plants. They are found in root veggies, nuts, seeds, leafy greens, and legumes. Fiber is useful in balancing blood sugar because it is built to withstand digestion and passes largely unchanged through the small intestine, assisting healthy bowel movements. It breaks down and absorbs slowly, which keeps your blood sugar and insulin levels relatively stable.

Columbia Fertility in New York City, who has spent countless hours researching the topic. He and his team conducted a study that revealed that high levels of insulin were actually toxic to placental cells, making it impossible for the fetus to get nourishment and thrive (Vega, Mauro, and Williams 2019).

THE CHAIN EFFECT

Insulin resistance is often connected to other members of the Big Four. Together they create chaos that's detrimental to fertility and overall wellness. Chapter 6 dives deeper into the effects of stress hormones on fertility, but for now, the important thing to understand is that cortisol (one of your main stress hormones) triggers a survival response designed to help you preserve fat (i.e., store food for later). This occurs when insulin resistance prevents you from taking energy into your cells, which can trick your body into thinking it's starving. While storing fat was historically a beneficial survival mechanism in times when food was scarce, today it's making us pack on pounds. Those extra fat cells produce their own inflammatory cytokines called adipokines. The combination of inflammation and oxidative stress leads to rapid premature aging. You lose muscle, gain fat, and become chronically inflamed, and your cells begin to deteriorate. Oh joy! This aging applies to your egg quality and supply, and if your partner is riding a similar roller coaster, it can affect his sperm quality.

Stress hormones also make it harder to sleep because your mind and body are on edge. Sleep deprivation increases your appetite and sugar cravings, and that means less willpower to make good decisions. The consequence? The potential to pack on more pounds. Your partner isn't immune to these effects either. In one study conducted on a group of men deprived of two days of sleep, the results showed an increase in ghrelin, the hunger hormone (Schmid et al. 2008). Their leptin (hormone of satiation) was decreased, and they craved fast carbs.

The "Skinny Fat" Factor

Don't think you have a blood sugar or insulin issue because you are thin? Around 12 percent of skinny people are insulin resistant. The fat that causes insulin resistance for these women is hiding in organs (called visceral fat) and can actually be more dangerous than the unsightly fat that you see on overweight people. Visceral fat has been linked to breast cancer, type 2 diabetes, and cardiovascular disease. This fat is essentially another organ. It can release hormones and cytokines, making it a hot seat for inflammation and metabolic havoc.

MAN-ISH

There are some cases where you begin to share more with your lover than you want! The more insulin resistant a woman becomes, the more she has the propensity to take on male characteristics. Chronic insulin spikes lead to androgen excess, and the major androgen in our bodies is testosterone.

When people think excess testosterone, they think of jacked macho men. It's sort of the male equivalent of estrogen in that it is thought of as exclusively a "male hormone" while estrogen is the "female hormone." However, women actually need small amounts of testosterone for a healthy balance just as men need a little estrogen. Testosterone in the correct amounts supports your libido, energy, and muscle tone. If you are doing intense workouts and not getting results, low testosterone might be at play.

High Insulin = Low Estrogen

Insulin resistance and estrogen levels are intertwined. This is most prominently seen in women in the perimenopausal and menopausal years because their estrogen is already naturally declining, leading to a rise in insulin and a higher likelihood for reduced sensitivity. So insulin resistance can contribute to premature perimenopause or be caused by it. Most women in this era of their lives complain of belly fat that suddenly appears without a change in their diet or exercise. Insulin resistance combined with low estrogen levels leads to weight gain, sugar cravings, and ovulation issues.

While low testosterone poses its own set of issues, high testosterone is a fairly significant roadblock to fertility. "High T" is associated with conditions like ovarian cysts, polycystic ovaries, high prolactin, and long cycles (late ovulation or anovulation). Symptoms generally include greasy skin, pimples, and abnormal hair growth like sideburns or nipple hair. Sexy. And don't forget thinning head hair and bad temper!

> Taking vitamin D? If not, you should be! Vitamin D is an essential fertility nutrient and is often found to be low in women with PCOS. Consider supplementing it, especially in the winter when days are shorter and sunlight is scarcer.
>
> Wallace et al. (2013)

Normally, a balanced body produces cells called sex hormone–binding globulins. These globulins act as chaperons for sex hormones (estrogen and testosterone), latching on and leading them where they're needed. In women, they bind stronger to testosterone so that they can better guide it to the few places it's needed in the female body, not allowing it to bring its influence elsewhere. Unfortunately, excess insulin suppresses the concentration levels of these globulins, leaving testosterone to float freely in your system, messing with hormonal signaling.

High T can attack ovulation by shutting down follicle growth or preventing the formation of a thick uterine lining, causing implantation failure. Abundant testosterone is a cause and/or component of complex conditions like PCOS. With PCOS, you may experience irregular cycles, challenges with ovulation and egg quality, uterine lining issues, and estrogen-emitting cysts that disrupt hormonal balance further.

Pro Tip

Chromium is a trace mineral that strengthens your insulin transduction pathways and reduces carb and sugar cravings. It's found in foods like broccoli, green beans, garlic, and basil.

If there's one lesson to take away from this book, it's that one out-of-whack hormone inevitably knocks another askew. Lucky for us, the solution is within reach.

Simple Changes, Big Impact

Since insulin resistance is so closely tied to our food choices, you will no doubt see the quickest and most effective impact by tending to your daily nutrition. The connections between excess glucose, stress, and inflammation make it imperative to cut simple sugars from your diet and focus on high-fiber foods as well as slow-burning macronutrients like protein and fat. These substitutions will help buffer the absorption of sugar into the bloodstream, calm your appetite, and stabilize blood sugar and insulin levels.

The Scoop on Gluten

Gluten is a protein found in grains like wheat, barley, and rye. Previously, gluten was a major problem only if you had an autoimmune reaction to it (i.e., celiac disease) or if you were part of a small group with a high sensitivity. Now the number of people with a sensitivity is rising along with the severity. Some speculate that this is due to the hybridization of wheat crops and the consequent increase in gluten content. If you are insulin resistant, have signs of inflammation, and/or have a damaged gut, gluten may trigger a systemic immune response. A study conducted on mice showed that animals put on a gluten-free diet achieved glucose homeostasis and a significant reduction of inflammation in comparison to those put on a gluten-heavy diet.

CONSCIOUS EATING

Let's start at the beginning—of your day, that is.

Quit skipping breakfast! I know you're busy and you have places to be, but just stop it. Take five minutes to sit down and eat a small, smart meal. If you skip breakfast to arrive at that morning meeting 10 minutes early (or maybe sneak in a spin class), you're setting yourself up for a desperate meal choice later. Your blood sugar will drop too low, and your stomach will start growling. You are likely pouring coffee into the rumbling belly, only worsening the situation with a spike in cortisol. When you finally free yourself to get some food, you grab one of the first things you see—maybe a bag of starchy potato chips or, worse, a donut from the staff room. Uh oh, you just dumped a bucket of sugar into your blood. Up goes the insulin, and down goes the leptin. When you finally manage to take your lunch break, your hunger is insatiable. You grab a sandwich and an iced coffee. Up goes the cortisol and insulin, and down goes your energy. By the time dinner rolls around and you actually take time to sit down, you aren't feeling so great. You're bloated, you've got to pee every 10 minutes, and you're falling asleep sitting up. Wine or a cocktail is your pick-me-up to go alongside the pasta you've ordered. Booze sends more sugar into your blood, and you feel great after the first glass. But by the end of the meal, you are feeling pretty woozy and worn out, and you've set yourself up for a crappy night's sleep.

> Free-range eggs with sautéed spinach make a great, fast, protein- and fiber-rich breakfast.
>
> Soares et al. (2012)

Start your day with protein and/or fat. Avoid the sugar crash by starting your day with protein or fat (i.e., nut butter, avocado, or protein shake). Have a little with each snack and meal. With this simple addition, you will feel more satisfied with less food and be able to prolong periods of (intermittent) fasting. "How much protein and fat?" you ask. It's tough to say without knowing your activity levels. A general rule of thumb is to try to eat seven grams per day for every 20 pounds of body weight.

> Bulk up a salad with beans, seeds, and nuts for lunch. Drop in some avocado or olive oil, and you've implemented additional healthy fats. Grilled chicken (organic pasture raised is best) or fatty fish (salmon, sardines, or Spanish mackerel) add more sustenance and great nutrition but remember to be mindful of portions.

Choose snacks wisely. Being prepared with healthy snacks will help make sure you aren't getting too hungry between meals. That's the most common reason slip-ups happen (besides skipping breakfast). Have something on hand for blood sugar dips that occur mid- to late afternoon (2:30 to 4 p.m.). Curb the temptation to reach for chocolate or something carby as a pick-me-up by keeping a smarter snack handy.

Fat Makes You Fatter

Excess weight causes low-grade inflammation throughout your body. The consistent low-grade inflammation caused by excess body fat can disrupt insulin's functions. If your body isn't properly reacting to insulin due to these disruptions, you become increasingly insulin resistant. The real kicker is that the more weight you gain, the higher your likelihood of worsening both the insulin resistance *and* inflammation in your body. If you have a body mass index (BMI) of over 25, losing a few pounds is a way to reduce inflammation and increase insulin sensitivity.

Slow down. Speedy eating leads to minimal chewing, and then you run into fermentation and bacterial growth from the undigested food. You also may overeat because your body hasn't had the time to register that it's been fed!

Mind your portions. Keep in mind that overeating even the healthiest of foods is still overeating. It strains your digestive system and can lead to fermentation of the food that hasn't digested properly (see chapter 4 for the nitty-gritty on gut health). Eating less actually gives you *more* energy since you are effectively reducing the load your body has to process. To best control your portions, practice more mindful eating. Avoid meals in front of the television or computer screen. Without distractions, you'll be able to pay more attention to chewing your food and better tune in to feelings of satiety. Smaller, smarter

> Omega-3s are healthy, polyunsaturated fatty acids you can incorporate into your meals fairly easily. Eat high-omega fish like salmon, sardines, or Spanish mackerel. If fish doesn't suit your fancy, then try walnuts and/or ground flaxseeds in porridge, a paleo muffin, or breakfast smoothie.

portions leave you looking and feeling light while providing you with the fertile nourishment that you need to get knocked up.

Up your healthy fats to keep you satiated. Just because something contains fat doesn't mean it's going to make you fat. It's true that saturated fat from red meat and palm oil in excess will raise bad cholesterol, inflammation, and the number on your scale. One study linked a diet heavy in red meat to negative, diabetes-like glucose metabolic indicators in women who didn't actually have diabetes (Ley et al. 2014). The study showed that swapping out red meat for other proteins (chicken, fish, and legumes) reduced both insulin and inflammation in the body. The trans fats in processed foods aren't any better than those in red meat since they spike your insulin and increase your chances of ovulation

> Fibrous foods such as brussels sprouts, kale, and artichokes make great dinner sides.

failure. However, mono- and polyunsaturated fats are good for you and can help you reduce your food portions by making you feel full. These are fats that are liquid at room temperature (like olive oil or avocado oil). They lower bad cholesterol and help your body burn fat, which helps control blood sugar, calm inflammation, and improve your chances of getting pregnant.

Add fiber-rich foods to your meals. These slow down the release of sugars into your blood. Fibrous foods take much longer to break down, and they absorb a lot of liquid. This means they expand and linger in your stomach, making you feel full and curbing overeating. When they do break down and leave your system, they sweep out toxins as they go (more on that in chapter 7).

Avoid refined and high-glycemic grain products. Refined/processed grains like white flour products (i.e., white bread, noodles, pasta, biscuits, and pastries) land high on the glycemic index, which means they are more likely to spike insulin. They are also devoid of fiber and B vitamins when compared to whole, unpolished grains. Seek out minimally processed/gluten-free grains like brown rice, buckwheat, quinoa, and millet as smarter fertility choices.

Drink water. Curb cravings by hydrating all day, every day. Many people's brains confuse hunger and thirst signals. When you get that "craving" feeling but you aren't sure what exactly you want, try drinking a glass of water before you reach for snacks. A lot of times, that mystery hankering will subside. To add a little more flavor to your hydration and add a nice, cozy ritual to your evenings, try herbal tea. It can be super effective in offsetting that snacky feeling.

Did You Know?

Binge drinking induces insulin resistance and may even leave you feeling down and less motivated to follow through with healthier diet habits.

Back Away from the Booze!

Alcohol is kryptonite for anyone hoping to heal insulin resistance. Due to its acidity and tendency to spike insulin, alcohol causes inflammation throughout the body, affecting digestive function and overburdening your pancreas and liver. Just ask Suzy, a young attorney and a patient of mine who told me she blacked out every time she drank alcohol. She couldn't understand why drinking the same amount as her friends affected her so differently. Suzy's body couldn't handle the booze because her pancreas would malfunction after the heavy influx of alcohol sugars (i.e., ethanol). Booze made her insulin spike so high that her body would just shut down to try to manage the assault. As an alternative to a boozy nightcap, try adding bitters, essential oils, or lemon to your water. Fertility-friendly teas such as raspberry leaf, nettle, hibiscus, mint, lavender, and red clover are also great options.

Eat clean. Certain toxins, now being called "diabetagens" by researchers, actually trigger the onset of autoimmune diabetes. Some poison insulin receptor sites and impair the ability of the pancreas to secrete enzymes and insulin. Others scramble the brain signals that control hunger, hamper your thyroid and liver function, slow your metabolism, and thus lead to weight gain. The best way to prevent these issues is to eat organic when you can.

Learn sugar's many aliases. Check food labels for the sneaky names that hide sugar in its many forms: corn syrup, invert syrup, dextrose, fructose, golden syrup, maltose, sorghum syrup, sucrose, cane sugar, and so on. Also be wary of any bottled, pasteurized fruit juices. Apple, orange, and pineapple juices contain concentrated fruit sugars, which can have a similar impact to refined sugars. Think Splenda is a good alternative? Think again! Fake sugars are a menace for your hormones. Studies show that synthetic sweeteners such as aspartame and Splenda actually increase your appetite and are associated with weight gain (Yang 2010). They may not spike your blood glucose, but they send your insulin through the roof.

A Conventional Option

If you want an extra helping hand in reducing your insulin troubles, the drug metformin has been shown to restore ovulation, assist implantation, and reduce the chances of miscarriage for some women. I've found dietary and lifestyle changes to be the most effective strategies, but I offer this tidbit for a well-rounded chapter of info. Note that metformin appears less ideal for already thin women, as it may result in being underweight, which brings with it another set of fertility challenges.

These are just a few diet substitutions to start thinking about, but for a full diet tailored to reversing the effects of insulin resistance and the other members of the Big Four, see chapter 8.

BEYOND FOOD

Your daily choices are your strongest ally in tackling insulin resistance. Outside of diet, insulin and blood sugar issues are also massively improved with stress reduction, regular exercise, and natural medicine.

Move your body. Physical activity is essential to increasing insulin sensitivity (i.e., helping your cells gobble up sugars). It also helps control appetite and mood and sleep. One study on women with PCOS showed that exercise significantly improved blood circulation and reduced insulin resistance. These women did aerobics like brisk walking, cycling, and jogging for at least 30 minutes, three days per week, for 16 weeks (Stener-Victorin et al. 2012). Simple and effective!

Try acupuncture. While regular old acupuncture effectively reduces inflammation and treats insulin resistance, the women in the previously mentioned study underwent electroacupuncture treatments for 16 weeks. This is acupuncture involving a small, low-frequency electronic pulse between two expertly placed acupuncture points in the abdomen and lower legs. They had 30-minute treatments twice a week for two weeks, once a week for six weeks, and once every other week for eight weeks, resulting in restored ovulation in most cases. Acupuncture has proved time and time again to be effective in improving insulin resistance when done in a series of treatments. In one study on 40 obese women who underwent ten separate 20-minute acupuncture sessions, the practice was shown to reduce excess insulin and promote weight loss (Güçel et al. 2012).

Sleep! When you are tired, you will crave quick carbs and sugars to give you quick energy. Your willpower will also decline with inadequate sleep. I notice for myself that if I don't get adequate rest, then I'm trying to sneak in some chocolate, gluten-free granola, or dried apricots. Yes, these sound like they aren't too bad, but they are still caffeine and sugar! Get those much-needed Zs to balance your appetite. Aim to get seven to eight hours per night to control cravings, lower inflammation, and set yourself up for success.

Tips and Tricks in the Supplement Category

The following supplements and herbs may help reverse insulin resistance, but when possible, schedule a visit with a qualified practitioner to ensure they're right for you:

- Omega-3s and probiotics indirectly treat insulin resistance by reducing the inflammation that blocks insulin receptor sites, restoring sensitivity.
- NAC improves insulin sensitivity in women with PCOS. I have also noted clinically that NAC is incredibly effective at reducing anxiety. Theoretically, this suggests it could effectively reduce the stress response (cortisol) that increases weight and insulin resistance.
- Magnesium levels are commonly low in women, and studies have suggested that supplementation to restore healthier levels can improve insulin sensitivity.
- Wen Jing Tang (Warm the Valley Decoction) is one of my favorite Chinese herbal formulas for women with insulin resistance and/or PCOS who aren't ovulating regularly or producing a thick lining.
- Vitamin D is an essential fertility nutrient often found to be deficient in women with PCOS.

SUPPLEMENTAL STRATEGIES

In terms of dietary supplementation, there is a fair amount of evidence to support the use of myoinositol to help regulate insulin and blood sugar. Myoinositol acts sort of like a vitamin form of metformin, reducing blood glucose and insulin levels to improve endocrine function and reduce fat accumulation. It's an insulin sensitizer that improves pregnancy rates because it can activate your insulin-signaling pathways (Bevilacqua

Having a period doesn't necessarily mean you are ovulating. BBT charting, OPKs, and monitoring your cycle with your doctor are ways to assess if your egg is dropping.

and Bizzarri 2018). My patients taking between 3,000 and 6,000 milligrams daily notice reduced cravings and appetite, less bloating, more balanced mood, clearer skin, and weight reduction in most cases. Another study showed an improvement in egg quality when combined with melatonin (Vitale et al. 2016).

MONICA'S STORY

A personalized schedule was exactly what my patient Monica needed to combat her insulin issues. Monica was a 32-year-old speech therapist who had been trying to conceive for two years unsuccessfully. She arrived in my office distraught and disheartened. She couldn't figure out why, at such a young age, she was having trouble conceiving. She and her husband had recently seen a fertility doctor who was recommending IVF. Based on her high egg count and young age, he believed she would be a great candidate. But Monica wasn't quite ready to go down this road, and she opted to see what she could do naturally first.

Monica explained that she got her period regularly and was quite sure she was ovulating. I asked her how often her period came and what she was doing to track her ovulation. She said that her period arrived every 35 to 42 days and that she had intercourse daily (often two times per day) from day 10 to day 16. Right off the bat, I explained to her that with her longer cycles, she could very well be missing her ovulation entirely, as she was almost definitely ovulating later than she thought, if at all.

Know Your Triggers

One of the best things this journey can offer is an opportunity to learn (besides having a baby, of course). Most people with elevated blood glucose or insulin are unaware of the internal goings on. Do you ever feel out of sorts but don't know why? Your blood sugar or insulin could be out of whack. It can manifest in such symptoms as anxiety, agitation, or wild fluctuations in energy and focus. A fun trick for figuring out how you are reacting to what you eat is to buy a home glucose monitor (nothing fancy; try a pharmacy or Amazon). Prick your finger first thing in the morning and then one or two hours after eating. If you have high morning sugars, look at the previous day. You could have had a heavy dinner, too much booze, not enough exercise or sleep, or too much refined food or meat (meat can spike glucose and insulin by way of an inflammatory reaction). You might be shocked by what sets it off. I had one patient whose insulin jumped to 160 after eating an apple. Another had high morning levels every time she ate meat for dinner the night before. Going through this exercise for just a week will make you better informed in making decisions based on your unique makeup.

I counseled her in BBT charting and cervical mucus observation and told her to use an OPK just for good measure. We needed to home in on the fertile window.

Next up was identifying the source of Monica's long cycles. She'd had long and slightly irregular cycles for as long as she could remember, and ovarian cysts came and went. She also had adolescent acne that was still present now to a lesser degree and was worsened by stress and certain foods. Monica was generally in good shape but said she had to watch her weight and often gained pudge in her midsection. She had a high-stress lifestyle and was prone to emotional eating. Carbs were her drug of choice, and a bottle of wine in one sitting wasn't far out of the ordinary either. Monica felt that, as a vegan, she was quite healthy, but I explained that vegans often crave more carbs to make up for the lack of protein. This diet is okay for some women but not always for those who are insulin resistant. Given Monica's long cycles and history of irregularities, cysts, and acne, I suspected she was insulin resistant and perhaps on the PCOS spectrum. I suggested protein first thing in the morning via a smoothie with hemp or collagen. She also agreed to eat fish and eggs a few times per week. These small changes naturally reduced her cravings for carbs, resulting in smaller portions and less frequent meals. Monica started a program of eating protein at each meal and selected whole foods over refined flour products. She went gluten free, and booze was limited to a vodka or tequila soda once per week. Myoinositol and

Preconception Planning

Whether you have one week or several months before your next "try," begin making as many of the following adjustments to your diet and lifestyle as possible.
   Starting points:

- Cut out fast carbs/simple sugars and saturated or trans fats.
- Increase intake of insulin-balancing proteins, fiber, and healthy fats.
- Have a slow-burning snack handy for desperate times. Think nuts, seeds, paleo muffins, a protein smoothie, or something of the like.
- Set a bedtime that allows seven to eight hours of sleep.
- Move your body daily and schedule in 20 to 30 minutes of exercise at least three days a week.
- Hydrate morning, noon, and night at least 30 minutes *before* a meal or one or more hours after.
- Eat organic as much as possible.
- Start your supplement regime.
- Consult with an acupuncturist to establish a customized treatment schedule.

Fulghesu (2002); Rodríguez-Morán and Guerrero-Romero (2003)

magnesium were implemented to improve ovarian function, manage stress, and sensitize her cells to insulin. Monica came for acupuncture two or three times per week to improve circulation, regulate her cycle, and calm stress hormones. At the end of the fourth cycle (we had cut them down to 32 days), she was pregnant naturally and went on to have a healthy baby.

Big Upside, Little Downside

Arguably, there are a ton of women who are insulin resistant and will never be diagnosed. Regardless of whether or not you fall into this category, it's undoubtedly beneficial to avoid an excess of refined foods and sugars. We know that sugar and refined carbs are inflammatory. We know that they cause oxidative stress. That should be enough to make us all pay serious attention!

Shifting your eating habits can be challenging, but minor shifts in daily habits may work wonders in the realm of your fertility. Make small but conscious changes every day and don't stress yourself out! Speaking of stress, the next chapter is dedicated to dissecting the mechanics of the fight-or-flight response. Get ready to learn all about how our mind-set can impact our journey to conception.

CHAPTER 6

Fight or Flight

Ever been told that simple relaxation will help you get pregnant? Maybe your doctor suggested you take a vacation. Maybe your best friend casually said, "Stop thinking about it, and it will happen. Remember Suzy did all that IVF, too, but she got pregnant only when she quit trying." Right. They mean well. How could they know that those words pierce your soul? Sure, it's easy for people to say, "Chill out. Relax. Take some *you* time." It's a lot harder for an alpha female to slow down. It's even harder to dull the deafening sound of your ticking biological clock. The wait is grueling, especially when you've laid a careful plan for your life. You're ready to say, "Baby, check. Next!"

Life is busier than ever because we are always plugged in. From the moment we wake to the moment our head hits the pillow, we're engaged, communicating, and absorbing information at lightning speed. Many of us have big goals and aspirations, and the majority of us place unnecessary pressure on ourselves to get it all done *now*. We may not realize how exhausting it is because we're high on stress hormones like cortisol and adrenaline. Stress is pretty much a daily occurrence and at fairly high levels, too. No big deal. Friday will come, and we can wind down, right?

What you may not realize is that the effects of frequent or chronic stress linger long after you get that rush of adrenaline. Yes, it's infuriating to be told that if you just chill out, a baby will land in your uterus. Sadly, there is some truth to this frustrating and often poorly delivered concept.

Type As like to push the limits, and there's nothing wrong with that—other than the somewhat deleterious effects it can have on our ability to conceive. One of my mentors told me, "Stress is waging an internal war." That has stuck with me for 20 years. In my practice, I've seen a direct correlation between higher stress levels and difficulty conceiving. As I write this chapter, I'm in quarantine amid the age of COVID-19. My in-box is now flooded with patients writing to announce that, after many failed IVFs, they are finally pregnant. It happened at home, the old-fashioned way. I have no doubt that less rushing and more rest-ing is to thank. In some cases, stress reduction alone can lead to enough internal change to create space for baby.

The Urgency Is All in Your Mind

We alpha-wired females spend the majority of our days in pursuit of productiv-ity and efficiency. This mind-set creates a tendency to take on too much at once. Because we are out there giving our all, patience can be quick to snap. Even small inconveniences become huge stress inducers because we've forgotten how to relax. Those little things build up, and we either lash out in anger or (arguably worse) fume in silence, keeping that negativity bottled up. If something doesn't turn out the way we envisioned, we can lose our cool even faster than we can let that f-bomb fly. So our glands fire out a mixture of cortisol, epinephrine, and adrenaline (to name a few), screaming at us to either get out of that stressful situ-ation or fight to resolve it. However, "fight or flight" is an antiquated response. We can't just jump up and flee our offices in the middle of the workday. So we stress eat and ruminate on stupid things instead of running. It puts you in a tizzy, often causing more stress.

The Type A Tizzy

We alpha-wired females more frequently exhaust our bodies as a consequence of un-relenting competitive drive, overachieving mentality, and constant sense of urgency. A type A woman feels guilty about watching TV after a 10-hour workday because she didn't quite finish her long list of tasks. So she pulls out her computer and answers email while she watches TV to try to ease that guilt and feel more productive. She schedules her meetings back to back, and if you get in her way on the route to her next engagement, duck and cover. But hyperefficiency in lieu of rest takes a major toll. The cardiologists who first defined type A personality actually linked it, via an eight-and-a-half-year study, to heart disease. Even when factors like smoking and other poor lifestyle habits were factored in, type A test subjects were twice as likely to develop heart disease than the more relaxed, type B test subjects.

Even if you don't identify as a hotheaded type A personality, you may tend toward perfectionism or chronic multitasking. As a result, you rarely give yourself a break. No break means you never fully wind down. The constant overstimulation inhibits the function of your reproductive organs and hormone-producing glands. Over time, stress essentially downgrades the function of your ovaries and the receptivity of your uterus. The correlation is cut and dried. It can't be ignored. So let's explore what's actually happening behind the scenes.

Ready, Set, *Go!*

Your nervous system is essentially your body's electrical wiring. You have nerves and specialized cells called neurons all throughout your body, and they transmit signals to each other to control both your conscious and your unconscious actions. Right now, your nervous system is telling your heart to beat and your lungs to breathe without your having to think about it. That subconscious part of your mind is called the autonomic nervous system. Each time you decide to turn a page of this book, you're activating your central nervous system, which is controlled by your conscious mind.

Your autonomic, or subconscious, nervous system is separated into two crucial parts. You have your sympathetic nervous system (SNS) and your parasympathetic nervous system (PNS). We'll call them Go Mode (SNS) and Chill Mode (PNS).

Go Mode governs your fight-or-flight response. It is activated when your brain signals to the body that you are in some sort of distress or danger. We don't typically have wild beasts stalking us anymore, but our fight-or-

> In Chinese medicine, your Chill Mode would be equated with yin: your feminine, quiet state. Your Go Mode would be associated with yang: your "masculine," active state. If yang takes over for extended periods, yin is depleted. The two need to be in balance for all systems to work efficiently, hence the yin–yang symbol that shows the two as interwoven equals.

flight response still lingers. Guess what sets it off these days. You got it: stress.

For the majority of your day, you want your Go Mode to be dormant while you operate in Chill Mode. Wikipedia refers to this more relaxed system as "rest and digest" and "feed and breed." It's the state in which your body's resources are geared toward conception. The Chill Mode system also controls all those vital tasks, like telling your heart how fast to beat, your intestines

> Noticing a thinning hairline or thin, brittle nails? Chronic stress could be the cause.

to digest food, your liver to filter junk, and so on. It even governs how fast your hair and nails grow.

If you've had a crazy week and you're neck deep in work or a family crisis, on top of your typical responsibilities, you're likely to trigger Go Mode. Stress has turned into distress whether you're aware of it or not. Stress is just your body's response to a change in your environment, thoughts, or body that requires you to adapt. Got a new assignment at work? Your mind must adjust to this task quickly, and that urgency triggers stress, which can manifest physically, mentally, or emotionally. Last-minute decisions, like where to eat lunch before your next meeting, can trigger a mild stress response. Even happy things can cause a stress response. If you get a big promotion, buy a house, or go on vacation, those things require major adaptations. They are positive changes, of course, but your mind and body must adjust to the new conditions. Running in Go Mode for a prolonged period can manifest a plethora of unpleasant physical symptoms. According to the American Psychological Association, stress is actually linked to the six leading causes of death: heart disease, cancer, lung ailments, accidents, cirrhosis of the liver, and suicide. It also directly impacts your fertility.

Does this sound like you?

- I have tension headaches.
- I feel nauseous in the middle of the workday.
- I have anxiety.
- I've been diagnosed with high blood pressure.
- I sometimes experience chest pains.
- I have been diagnosed with depression.
- I have a loss of appetite.
- I have insomnia.
- I have chronic muscle pains.
- I have frequent indigestion.

If you checked off five or more of these, there's a good possibility you have chronic stress.

The Brain-Gut-Inflammation Connection

It turns out that your gut has its own nervous system: the enteric nervous system (ENS). It covers your gastrointestinal (GI) tract from your esophagus to your rectum and is made up of "two thin layers of more than 100 million nerve cells." New research is showing that those cells are likely there so that your ENS (gut) can talk to your central nervous system (CNS) when things aren't quite right in there. Given this intimate connection between the gut and the nervous system, your digestive health can impact your mood. Ready for the real catch 22? If you already suffer from mood disorders such as chronic stress, anxiety, or depression, your digestive system is impacted by the resulting stress hormones that flood your circulation. So stress impacts your gut, and your gut then makes you more unhappy. An overactive nervous system can literally cause perforations (holes or gaps) to form in our intestinal wall (think leaky gut). Bacteria and toxins leak through the perforations and into your bloodstream. Your gut alerts your brain that foreign toxins are present, and your brain sends out cytokine soldiers. The result? A cascade of inflammation that could impact the development of your eggs or the receptivity of your uterus.

More Than a Feeling

How can a "feeling" cause so many issues? Well, stress isn't just a feeling. It's a state. Two walnut-sized glands above your kidneys called the adrenal glands produce up to 50 hormones, and a balance of all of them is required for a healthy body. One of their main influences is to help you react to stress through the production of stress hormones—two of the most prominent being adrenaline and cortisol. Adrenaline is the danger response. It gives you that sense of urgency that tells you to get the heck out of a bad, stressful situation. But if you don't get up and flee your car, office, or house, then your stress hormones just swirl around in your body creating oxidative damage. They need to be diffused. The need to reduce stress is what generally leads people to drink, smoke, do drugs, run, or yell.

The fight-or-flight response reroutes your body's resources to prioritize only the most vital organ functions so that you can survive a dangerous scenario.

Guess what isn't considered a vital bodily function? Reproduction. When your body hands the wheel over to Go Mode, your subconscious mind believes your life is in jeopardy. Your muscles and heart are given priority for blood circulation, oxygen, and nutrients so you can flee. Your reproductive organs are running a deficit and thus begin to tire and lose functionality. Yes, some women who are in real jeopardy and much more stressful environments than, say, a typical middle-class American still get pregnant, but many more do not. Your lady parts aren't the same as the woman next to you. Some women's fertility is more affected by stress than others.

You may think you're powering through a stressful week like a boss, but that's your central nervous system talking—your conscious brain. Stress, however, wreaks havoc via your unconscious mind, so you have no concept of how much your body is freaking out. All you know is that you've been diagnosed with "unexplained infertility," "poor egg quality," or the like.

Short Circuit

A lot of women are under the impression that stress simply causes a few headaches, some mood swings, and maybe some acne here and there. Not so. There is mounting evidence that stress makes your route to baby a grueling, lengthy journey.

Chronic or prolonged stress disrupts important signaling and feedback pathways of your hypothalamic–pituitary–adrenal (HPA) axis: the connection between your hypothalamus, pituitary gland, and adrenal gland. All three pieces play a role in controlling your hormone production and the functionality of your reproductive organs.

The HPA also regulates your hypothalamic–pituitary–ovarian (HPO) axis, which is the pathway to the gonadal glands, meaning your ovaries or your man's testes. A disruption to this connection, thanks to increased stress hormones, suppresses HPO function by limiting the production of LH and gonadotropin-releasing hormone (GnRH), which regulate the development of your eggs and trigger ovulation (see chapter 1). Essentially, chronic stress breaks up communication lines between your brain and your lady parts. The glands that produce your hormones then short-circuit, and the resulting hormonal imbalances make conceiving a baby highly unlikely.

Let's take a closer look at what's happening behind the scenes.

ADRENAL FATIGUE

At first, the adrenal glands are overworked, being repeatedly stimulated by stressful situations that cause a constant release of adrenaline and cortisol. The presence of adrenaline, the hormone released during stressful times, signals to your body that conditions are not ideal for conception. Adrenaline inhibits your body's use of progesterone, which is essential for fertility. It also causes the pituitary gland to release higher levels of prolactin, which may contribute to infertility. Research tells us that stress inhibits the body's release of GnRH, which governs the growth of eggs and ovulation because it stimulates the secretion of the main sex hormones like FSH and LH. This subsequently suppresses ovulation, sexual activity, and sperm count.

The longer chronic stress continues, the harder it becomes for the adrenals to keep up. Pumping out all that cortisol, epinephrine, and adrenaline leaves them weak and sluggish, reducing their hormone outputs. This is a condition known as "adrenal fatigue." You're probably thinking, "That means less stress hormones. Isn't that a good thing?" Unfortunately not. When your adrenals are fatigued, so are you. It can lead to lack of sleep, depression, muscle weakness, low immunity, foggy brain, and even bone mass loss. Your adrenal glands are also responsible for providing precursors for the production of reproductive hormones such as estrogen and progesterone. This may lead to hormonal imbalance. Not enough hormones are being produced or released. Other endocrine glands are not being signaled to release their hormones, and the entire chain of communication within the endocrine system is broken.

An Enzyme of Evidence

Chronic stress can make your HPA signal the release of the stress hormone epinephrine, which increases salivary alpha amylase. In heightened levels, alpha amylase is associated with a longer time to achieve pregnancy and higher infertility.

The breakdown in communication between the brain and ovaries is where things start to get sticky. You may experience long cycles (more than 35 days), decreased sex hormone production, suppression of ovulation, and poor IVF outcomes (fewer eggs retrieved, poor fertilization rates, and low pregnancy and live birth rates). Without estrogen, your ovaries don't produce eggs, and your uterine lining stays thin. If levels really dive, your cycle will stop altogether. I experienced this firsthand in grad school. I was so stressed by the smothering workload and several part-time jobs that I stopped having a period. I wasn't ovulating at all.

Women with PCOS, like myself, are more radically affected by high mental and emotional stress because we are already prone to under-producing "female" reproductive hormones. We already have excess androgens in our systems in many cases, and stress has the potential to increase testosterone secretion even further. Stress thus exacerbates PCOS symptoms and, in fact, has even been implicated in the *development* of PCOS. The catch is that PCOS worsens mood disorders and anxiety, creating a vicious cycle.

Frantic

You may recognize the symptoms of imbalanced progesterone and estrogen if you know anyone going through menopause. That's because menopause signals a slowing down of ovulation, eventually leading to no ovulation at all. If you don't ovulate, you don't produce progesterone because there is no follicle (corpus luteum) left over to secrete it. If there is too little progesterone to counterbalance estrogen, you can feel crazy. In proper levels, estrogen helps you feel energized, but when out of balance, it can actually make you frantic. Your anxiety is heightened, you can't think straight, and your mood is all over the place. You're essentially experiencing PMS 24/7. Many young women with low hormone levels (those with PCOS, chronic stress, and POF) may experience physical and emotional symptoms similar to their menopausal counterparts. Talk about stressful.

OXIDATIVE STRESS

The ties binding emotional wellness to fertility are surprisingly strong. As much as we talk about "feelings of the heart," emotions are actually created in the brain. When your mind is overwhelmed with an emotion, sad or happy, your body reacts by creating physical tears. Scientists and practitioners recognize the strength of this mind–body connection and take it into account in all clinical trials. Whenever a new method or medication is tested, a placebo is added because people's minds have the power to heal their bodies. If people believe a method or pill will help heal them, their bodies start to manifest that belief. In some cases, for some conditions, a placebo can produce up to 80 percent improvement. That's a huge number and cannot be dismissed as a fluke.

Emotions have consequences, good and bad. Although they may be fleeting, they can leave lasting traces.

Emotional stress causes oxidative stress. It's a word that gets thrown out a lot in antiaging product commercials along with "free radicals." Oxidative stress is an imbalance of your cell's production of oxygen and antioxidants. It causes cellular damage and can even alter DNA synthesis, which is destructive to growing eggs or a developing embryo. From damaged or poor cells come damaged or poor eggs, meaning less chance of conception. Stress can also cause failed implantation regardless of ovulation and egg quality. One study conducted on mice placed the subjects in a high-stress environment but gave them hormonal supplementation. Despite the boost in hormones levels, their uterine lining still showed poor receptivity to embryos. These more cryptic infertility struggles, like poor egg quality and failed implantation, often cause excess stress, leading to further fertility suppression, and the cycle continues.

Oxidative Stress and Your Mental Health

Your brain requires and absorbs lots of oxygen to function, but when you have an imbalance of reactive oxygen (oxidative stress), your brain is highly susceptible to a multitude of nasty cell degeneration effects. As a result, oxidative stress has been linked to mental health disorders ranging from anxiety and depression to schizophrenia and bipolar disorder. The emotional distress caused by these conditions only leads to more emotional imbalance, creating more stress and making breaking free of the loop more difficult.

Metabolic Mayhem

Worse for your fertility is that chronic stress makes your body enter a state called catabolism, which is destructive metabolism. This means your metabolism is breaking down complex molecules, like muscle proteins, into simpler molecules, such as amino acids, that help create more sugar to burn instead of fat. The excess blood sugar triggers your pancreas to release insulin. Excess insulin in the blood leads to more inflammation and oxidative damage. When your body is catabolic and your adrenals are fatigued, thyroid function is slowed down as a precaution. The thyroid is in charge of regulating many vital hormones, including those needed for reproduction, from ovulation to implantation and beyond.

Take Care of Your Thyroid

Your thyroid's effects on your reproductive system are somewhat indirect, but that doesn't mean you should neglect it. Thyroid health is just as important as ovarian health in many ways. Around 80 percent of my patients are put on thyroid medication by their fertility doctor. Both excess estrogen and excess cortisol can lead to hypothyroidism, which is a deficiency in thyroid hormones. Hypothyroidism is more common in the luteal phase due to the slowing down of your liver function at that time. The liver turns T4 (inactive thyroid hormone) into T3 (the active form). Fluctuating thyroid hormones in the luteal phase may play a role in premenstrual anxiety and insomnia. It can also cause a low basal body temperature, which means an unsatisfactory environment for a fertilized egg. Be conscious that IVF drugs, which are designed to stimulate estrogen production, can lower your thyroid hormone levels. Stress reduction techniques and an improved diet are simpler, long-term solutions.

Stress and Miscarriage

Stress doesn't just affect your ability to *get* pregnant. Studies have shown that psychological stress can cause spontaneous pregnancy loss early in gestation (fetal development). One meta-analysis on eight different miscarriage studies showed that women who reported a stressful negative life event during pregnancy or who had a history of psychological stress exposure were twice as likely to miscarry. Stress diverts so much energy away from your reproductive system that it's hard to maintain that delicate balance of hormones necessary for a healthy pregnancy.

My patient Carrie's miscarriages were a result of similar circumstances. Carrie was 36 and already a mother of two, but her attempts to conceive a third child had left her distraught and weary. She had conceived her two previous children without a hitch, but for some reason, this time around, she'd had one chemical pregnancy and a seven-week miscarriage. Her doctors said there was no issue and encouraged her to just keep trying. Unfortunately, the losses were causing Carrie a great deal of anxiety and stress. A friend told her that acupuncture could help with pregnancy, leading her to me. We discussed her daily routine, and she confessed that she never really had downtime. Her periods were few and far between. When it did appear, her flow was very light. It had gotten worse after the miscarriages, she said. Why was this one so much harder? We discussed her lifestyle and identified the lack of sleep and constant rushing as problem areas. I explained that this lack of rest could hinder adequate blood flow in her uterus and ovaries. We needed to calm her nervous system down and send the blood flow to her reproductive organs so that they could do their job properly. I prescribed CoQ10, omega fatty acids, magnesium, and herbs to calm her system and improve the function of her ovaries and uterus and then acupuncture two times per week in addition to a couple more hours of sleep and a lot less caffeine (dark chocolate and coffee were creeping in way too often). After three months on the program, Carrie again became pregnant, and this time, she carried all the way to term, healthy and happy.

The Daily Grind

Do you feel stressed and anxious without any real reason? A genetic predisposition could be at play, but more likely, chronic physical or emotional stress has depleted your happy hormones. Cortisol damages the receptor sites for neurotransmitters such as serotonin, dopamine, and gamma-aminobutyric acid (GABA). With low levels of these happy brain chemicals, you'll feel out of sorts even at the best of times. The slightest of annoyances will trigger severe stress because your brain chemistry has predisposed you to an inability to cope. The stress you feel only worsens the imbalances, perhaps causing you to indulge in substances that help you "escape." Alcohol, marijuana, benzodiazepines (such as Xanax), and sugar change your brain chemistry temporarily to give you a break. The issue is that the more you use them, the more they compound the imbalance. You may crave coffee to help you feel alert and motivated, or you may turn to "comfort foods" when you can't find the energy to be productive. Every fertility journey is packed with ever-changing emotions. They're unavoidable. How you react to them is what makes all the difference.

Stop Revving the Engine

If your typical morning starts with coffee or even caffeinated tea, pick a new pick-me-up beverage. Caffeine makes your heart race and kicks in your adrenaline, meaning your adrenal glands start firing shortly after you drink it. Go Mode switches on, and you've already started your day outside of the "rest and digest" mode. Worst of all, this coffee high is hard to come down from. This, along with the fact that coffee promotes gastric emptying, means food passes through you quickly and doesn't absorb very well. You are basically adding fuel to the fire or burning a gas tank that is already close to empty.

Stress Makes You Store Fat

Cortisol, remember, is a lingering hormone from more primal days in human history, and it tricks your body into thinking there isn't enough food in your environment. Your body has the choice to burn either fat or sugar for fuel. If you're in Go Mode, your body conserves fat because you might need it later, so it chooses to burn sugar instead, retaining fat and fluids.

Sugar is not an efficient source of fuel. When you burn sugar, you get a short burst of energy. In a dangerous situation, this would give you tons of energy all at once and allow you to fight hard or get the hell out. But you're not actually in danger. You're just stressed. You actually need the slow, steady release of energy that comes from burning fat. It's also better for your waistline. The bloating and inability to lose weight increase your stress, and the cycle begins anew. It's even harder to return to Chill Mode, which is ideal for digestion and fat burning. Toxins are lingering in that fat along with a bunch of excess estrogen. So you're overweight despite your workout routine, you feel frantic, your toxicity levels are through the roof, and your thyroid is being suppressed. A sleepy thyroid slows your metabolism, you retain more weight, and the hellish loop continues.

Instead of overloading your body with caffeinated, fatty, and sugary stressors, you can preempt and curb these cravings by implementing new, purposeful habits. Choose to add regular activities to your routine that ease you into a state of relaxation multiple times a day. Switch from Go Mode to Chill Mode consciously with preplanned "pauses" so that you can improve your fertility by nourishing your mind and body.

A typical day is full of obstacles that activate Go Mode. Traffic, deadlines, scheduling, relationships, and overwork all force your brain to problem solve all day long. There isn't anything wrong with an active lifestyle at its core, but you need to make sure you have a designated time each day to shut off your brain. Constant work forces your adrenals to fire in excess. Try to designate a "wind-down" time (or several). For example, maybe you take a walk during your lunch break or after work to stretch your muscles and get some vitamin D. Maybe you stop answering emails or doing anything work related after 6 p.m. Take time to make that rule a habit. Stick with it and remember to stop neglecting daily periods of personal enjoyment and relaxation.

Boost your nutrient intake and soothe stress with supplements. I recommend B vitamins such as B5 or brain balancers such as GABA. Herbal formulas like Gui Pi Tang are also helpful, but keep in mind that there isn't a one-size-fits-all when it comes to herbal remedies, so it's best to consult a professional.

Perhaps, in the past, you have used exercise as your escape from the daily grind. Exercise is great, but it comes with a large caveat. Say you've started a workout routine before or after work, and just like everything else in your life, you go big. You dedicate yourself fully to a high-intensity regime to burn that fat. Instead of being worn out, you're still hyped—high on the endorphins released during exercise. Thus, high-intensity workouts keep you in Go Mode. In general, working out is healthier for you than no exercise, but if you are constantly exerting yourself like this, you continue to drain your body and tire out your adrenals even more. If you're a workout-aholic, swap out a few SoulCycle or boot camp sessions for barre classes. You can get results without overdoing it, *and* there will be resources left over for your lady parts to do their job. Doing yoga or some other form of low-intensity, relaxing workout can not only help you stay in Chill Mode throughout the day but also help you get to sleep at night.

> Be kind to your digestive system, which can begin to falter when your body is weary and stressed out. Chew your food thoroughly. That little change makes a huge difference, helping your body draw nutrients from food. Choosing soup and smoothies for meals also prevents a buildup of large food particles that could ferment in your gut and cause inflammation.

Power Down

You can't power down if you never power off your devices. Stop staring at screens for a minimum of an hour before heading to bed. Your phone, computer, and TV emit blue light that tricks your brain into thinking it's still daytime, so your body's internal clock is confused when you lie down to sleep. If you can reduce your screen time throughout the whole day, even better. You can also find blue light–blocking glasses if your job requires you to sit at a computer all day.

As the final stage of your "unplugging" routine, schedule a set bedtime for yourself and stick to it. It may sound silly and childish, but there's a reason children are generally happier than adults. Make sure you're in bed at least eight hours before you need to wake up so you have time to settle in and get a full night's worth of REM sleep. If you don't experience a full REM cycle deep sleep, you'll wake up with your nervous system already in Go Mode.

> ### Small Steps to Better Sleep
>
> Try moving up your bedtime by 15 to 30 minutes per week to let yourself adjust. Ideally, you should aim to be asleep by 11 p.m. at the latest.

Sleep deprivation, even after just 48 hours, can make you feel a little crazy. Your hormones and energy levels go wildly awry, leading to more stress and further struggles with conception. Taking naps during the day but sleeping only a few hours at night doesn't cut it either. Aim for at least eight hours every night. If that means shutting down your Instagram a few hours earlier or resisting the temptation of the next Netflix episode, do it. Ask your partner to do the same. He needs equally good sleep habits in order for you both to make a baby. Without rest, he will severely diminish his sperm count.

Christina's Favorite Sleep Remedies

1. *GABA.* An essential neurotransmitter for sleep
2. *Suan Zao Ren Tang.* A simple Chinese herbal formula that helps reestablish sleep cycles
3. *Gui Pi Tang.* A Chinese herbal formula to treat anxiety and sleeplessness
4. *Magnesium.* A mineral that calms you and helps reestablish healthy sleep cycles
5. *Valerian.* An herbal sedative to calm your nervous system and help you nod off
6. *Bao He Wan.* A Chinese herbal formula that helps those whose sleep troubles are a result of overeating or eating too late

To all my alpha-wired females, please, stop trying to do *everything* in a single day! Instead, accept the notion of doing less and doing it well. If you want to go back to your hectic routine after having a baby, then have at it, but for now, consider prioritizing the quest for baby and what it entails. You may find you experience a lasting transformation that enhances your quality of life and better prepares you to be present for your child.

Preconception Planning

At least 21 days before renewing your efforts to get knocked up, begin making as many of the following adjustments to your lifestyle as possible:

- Select your "shutoff time" for work.
- Set a bedtime that allows eight hours of continuous sleep.
- Adjust your diet to reduce strain on the adrenals.
- Cut out caffeine.
- Treat your lunch break as a true break.
- Reduce screen time or purchase blue light–blocking glasses.
- Switch high-intensity workouts for a yoga or tai chi routine.
- Implement pranayama breathing techniques in your daily life.
- Meet with an acupuncturist if possible.

Learning to Pause

Stress has become ordinary in today's world. It doesn't always take the shape of major, traumatic events like the death of a loved one or losing your job. Triggers are widespread and can be as mundane as a tight work deadline, heavy traffic, missing keys, or a glitchy computer. The repercussions of daily, chronic stress are felt by your lady parts whether you're aware of it or not.

Pushing yourself to your absolute limits feels good in some ways, but sometimes that mentality is not exactly serving your quest for baby. Taking moments to pause, deliberately unplugging, and introducing daily mindfulness practices have the potential to transform your life. That trigger response that flooded your system with stress hormones will be replaced by a moment of reflection where you'll *decide* what reaction you'd like to embody. You'll start to view things differently and see opportunities rather than a series of grievances. Much like stress, positive emotions can send a strong vibration through all the cells of your body. It's best we tap into that energy and get off the stress high.

Now that you're aware of the havoc that stress can wreak on your fertility, it's time to discuss some other triggers that are invisible to the naked eye. They're called toxins, and their prevalence and connection to infertility is a major cause for concern. In the next chapter, we explore how they invade, how they hamper reproductive health, and what steps to take to reduce their impact. Let's get started.

CHAPTER 7

Our Toxic World

Arguably one of the most overlooked causes of infertility lurks in almost every aspect of the modern world. Chemical toxins are in the air you breathe, the water you drink, the products you use, and the food you eat. The average person isn't aware of their presence because they hide in unexpected places, and their effects on our fertility isn't a topic that typically crops up in casual conversation. While it's true that your body has an amazing ability to process and eliminate toxins, it's also true that a constant influx of them, especially when paired with poor lifestyle practices, will wear down your ability to detoxify.

From our mid-thirties and beyond, we are branded with the unpleasant label of "advanced maternal age." We know that our age greatly impacts our ability to make babies and are constantly reminded of the ticking clock. Alas, some women's clocks are ticking faster than others either through genetic predispositions *or* factors such as toxins. A study of more than 30,000 women based on data from the National Health and Nutrition Examination Survey (NHANES) discovered that those with high levels of 111 different endocrine-disrupting chemicals hit menopause 1.9 to 3.8 years earlier than their less exposed counterparts (Grindler et al. 2015). That is a big deal if you consider our fertile life span is already waning in our late thirties! Essentially, toxins cause accelerated aging—one of our biggest rivals in overcoming infertility.

A Toxic Cascade

On ingestion or exposure to toxins, stress hormones start firing to send out the alarm that something is awry. Your immune system activates defense mechanisms, causing an inflammatory response. Your organs then start working overtime to activate the detoxification pathways that process and eliminate the junk. In an attempt to "deactivate" the toxins, the body may also try to siphon them out of circulation and hide them away in organs or fatty tissues.

What does this have to do with baby making? Toxins are foreign substances that confuse and scramble communication between your brain and your hormone-secreting glands, such as the pituitary, ovaries, thyroid, and adrenals. By binding to the "receptors" on your cells where your natural hormones are meant to attach, chemicals can disrupt hormonal feedback systems, causing interruptions in body mechanics such as ovulation. Your body can then be tricked into thinking you have too much of a certain hormone and thus not produce the amount needed to grow eggs, ovulate, or fluff your uterine lining. When locked on to your receptor sites, they may also damage cell membranes, turning off your signaling capabilities so that your cells no longer respond to hormones like insulin, predisposing you to insulin resistance and diabetes. The disturbances don't stop there. Toxins also damage enzymes, which means you can't prevent free radical damage or produce hemoglobin. They can even hasten the rate at which your eggs are degenerating by damaging DNA. With such widespread damage and disruption, it's not too surprising that toxic exposure had been linked to diminished ovarian reserve, poor egg quality, endometriosis, and issues with ovulation (Vabre et al. 2017). In pregnancy, these endocrine (hormonal) disruptors have been linked to miscarriage and abnormal fetal growth (Krieg, Shahine, and Lathi 2016). Toxins may actually modify gene expression, which can span generations.

Does this sound like you?

- I have allergies/sinus problems.
- I have asthma.
- I am prone to bronchitis.
- I have frequent back pain.
- I regularly experience constipation.
- I suffer from depression and lack of motivation.
- I always seem to have a cold or the flu.
- I have frequent headaches.
- I have indigestion, gas, and bloating.
- I am frequently lethargic and fatigued.
- I am obese and struggle to lose weight.
- I have trouble concentrating.
- I have a skin or hair condition.

If you checked off five or more of these, there's a good possibility you have some level of toxic load. The liver is the hot seat of detoxification, separating good from bad and then pushing the bad out through elimination systems, such as poop, pee, and sweat. If overwhelmed by an excess of toxins, it can't flush you out properly, meaning that the more toxins you're exposed to, the more clogged your "filter" becomes and the harder it is to flush them out.

The strategy outlined in this chapter and the next is intended to reduce exposure and employ tactics to help our bodies detoxify. Let's jump into identifying where you'll find them so that you have the know-how to reduce their impact.

Wherever You Go, There They Are

Today, we use chemicals in the production and processing of just about everything. Toxins are also by-products of the conveniences we use day to day: car exhaust, cleaning products, and modern farming practices, to name a few. In most cases, toxins are man-made. But we also have a tendency to use naturally occurring toxins, like dioxins, at extreme, harmful levels. Their prevalence makes avoiding exposure a bit trickier but not impossible. The first step is to home in on where you're coming into contact with them in your daily routine.

THE TOXINS WE GOBBLE

It turns out that most toxins are ingested through the food we eat and the containers and bags that store our groceries and leftovers—think plastic bottles, food containers, and the like.

In most modern farming processes, massive quantities of pesticides and herbicides are sprayed by industrial-sized machines that scatter them over crops like a chemical rain. They keep bugs from destroying crops, and in some cases, they enhance growth. Sure, you can rinse away some of the chemicals on the surface, but no washing method can remove 100 percent of what lurks in these fruits and veggies, as they don't only sit on the surface. Chemical pesticides are also absorbed into the fruit or vegetable via an artery, such as the stems or root systems of plants. One farmer told me that squashes are some of the major offenders because the big leaves easily absorb the pesticides and carry them into the veggie itself!

The danger is that pesticides are essentially poison, designed to kill bugs. They aren't meant for consumption. A Harvard study in 2017 examined government recordings of average pesticide residue and then surveyed 325 women in the process of infertility treatments, asking them how many servings of pesticide-exposed fruit and vegetables they consumed per day. Women who consumed two servings were 18 percent less likely to become pregnant than women who had only one serving (Chiu et al. 2018).

GMOs

Some believe that GMOs have revolutionized mass farming practices by making crops more resilient to pests, weather, and so on. Others lament GM crops for destroying fertile land and annihilating small farms. Politics and environmentalism aside, our bodies may be reacting poorly to this new era of food. Many speculate that GMO foods may also underlie the pervasiveness of modern autoimmune issues, autism, asthma, and allergies. Perhaps making them more resilient to pests or weather also makes them tricky to digest. Eat non-GMO foods as much as possible.

The jury is still out on whether organic is in fact more nutritious than conventional, but there isn't much dispute over the fact that it's safer. However, many of my patients have concerns over the availability and cost of organic foods. Although it's ideal to eat organic, there are other tricks to find the "cleanest" options. Certain crops, such as strawberries, grapes, peppers, and spinach, are known to have a higher-than-average volume of pesticides. They are commonly found in the "Dirty Dozen"—a list available online that indexes the foods with the highest pesticide residue. Rather than avoid these fruits and veggies altogether, you can opt to buy organic *if* your budget allows. Farmers markets are another great source of clean produce. Not every local farmer opts to pay the fee required to have their produce certified organic, but you can ask them directly if they spray their crops. The "Clean 15," another online resource, catalogs foods that have lower pesticide levels, even when farmed conventionally. So if eating 100 percent organic doesn't fit the bill, refer to the previously mentioned lists to make smart choices.

Many toxins, including most pesticides, are endocrine (aka hormone) disruptors called xenoestrogens. *Xeno* is taken from a Greek word that means "foreign," "stranger," or "host." Xenoestrogens enter your system through your environment, food, and water and mimic and interfere with your natural estrogen and its processes.

> What's an endocrine disruptor? "Endocrine" refers to hormone-secreting glands like your ovaries. Endocrine disruptors are chemicals that mimic or interfere with your natural hormonal systems, usually causing a variety of imbalances.

These fakers can scramble the rhythm of your cycle and potentially disrupt many of the important roles that estrogen plays, from egg growth to the development of your uterine lining. Xenos can exacerbate conditions such as endometriosis and fibroids. Two of the most well-known xenos are bisphenol A (BPA) and dioxins, commonly ingested through foods and by-products of food and drink packaging.

BPA is used in the production of polycarbonate plastics and epoxy resins. It's *everywhere*—think plastic containers to beer cans to the receipts you collect at checkout. It's even used to make water pipes, meaning your tap water is potentially contaminated, too. Polycarbonate plastics are used to make water bottles, and epoxy resins coat the tops and seal the insides. Until very recently, even baby bottles were made out of this stuff.

In 2003–2004, the Centers for Disease Control and Prevention (CDC) conducted NHANES III. They took 2,517 urine samples from people ages six and up, and they found detectable levels of BPA in 93 percent of them. Unfortunately, BPA has been linked to low follicle counts, which presents major challenges in getting viable eggs either naturally or via IVF (La Merrill et al. 2020).

No More Beer Cans for Your Boo!

Drinking alcohol is already a sperm killer, but if your man loves knocking back his favorite brew in a can, his little swimmers are in even bigger trouble. Tin beer cans are lined top to bottom with BPA, and multiple studies have linked BPA exposure to lower sperm counts and reduced sperm quality. Swap his cans for a glass bottle and perhaps suggest cutting back if he is drinking more beer than water.

The resins that contain BPA break down and leach into liquids (i.e., water, beer, and so on) or come off the plastic packaging and soak into your food. This leakage can happen as the packaging ages, but primarily, BPAs get into your food if the packaging gets too warm. Never leave water bottles in your car or in direct sunlight. In fact, ditch plastic bottles and containers altogether. The plastic can even be overheated on the delivery truck before you even get your hands on the product. Invest in reusable drinkware instead.

Tips for Cutting Out BPA

Here are a few actions you can take to significantly reduce your BPA exposure:

1. Purchase glass, stainless-steel, or ceramic, containers instead of tin cans and plastic.
2. Any plastic containers you keep should be washed by hand instead of the dishwasher, which gets hot enough to cause that BPA leakage.
3. Never heat your food in a plastic container, even if it says it's microwave safe.
4. Receipt paper is coated in BPA. Opt for digital receipts when you can or take pictures of physical receipts rather than stuffing them in your purse.

Mínguez-Alarcón, Hauser, and Gaskins (2016); Cariati and D'Uonno (2019)

We spoke in chapter 4 about how certain toxins cause inflammation. It's actually dioxins, the second most prevalent endocrine disruptor, that are a major inflammatory trigger. They are directly linked to the prevalence and severity of endometriosis (Rier and Foster 2002). Dioxins are naturally produced by combustion, like wildfires. In the modern world, you can potentially be exposed to them by waste incinerators, paper, and chemical manufacturing plants and transformers or fluorescent light fixtures installed before 1977. However, the far more common means of exposure is food. Animals like cows and other livestock can inhale or ingest dioxins because the chemicals often leak into the soil that grows their food. The dioxins collect in the fatty tissues and can stay there up to 11 years. If you have endometriosis or another inflammatory disorder like PID, be very careful where you source your meats. Organic, grass-fed is your best bet or, even better, a farm-share program like a Community Supported Agriculture (CSA) system that makes local fare even more accessible.

Fish also frequently ingest harmful chemicals and metals due to the poor treatment of the lakes, streams, and oceans that serve as their homes. When you eat fish, there is a good chance you're ingesting chemicals like PCBs. These chemicals are released in landfills and dump sites, and when those facilities dump, spill, or leak into the water, the fish ingest them. Farmed fish, regardless of species, are often purposefully fed antibiotics and toxic food dyes.

High- versus Low-Mercury Fish

Fish are a great source of vitamin A and omega-3 fatty acids and are generally easier to digest than protein from land animals. However, large, deep-water fish like ahi tuna, swordfish, and Chilean sea bass contain potentially high concentrations of mercury. Take care when buying your fish and cross-check your selection with the FDA's list of mercury levels in commercial fish and shellfish (https://www.fda.gov/food/consumers/advice-about-eating-fish). Tuna and swordfish have some of the highest levels, while anchovies, catfish, clams, scallops, and sole are typically safer.

Sadly, it's not just food that's full of chemicals. Heavy metals like aluminum, cadmium, lead, and mercury can be found in your water supply. The levels and the types of metal will vary based on your location, but heavy metal runoff is common in public water systems. The deplorable state of the water in Flint, Michigan, has been in the news on a wide scale, but a USA Today study released in 2016 found 2,000 more lead-heavy water systems in the United States, many of them supplying schools and day care centers. To cut down your risk of exposure, buy a carbon water filter (I use the Berkey) or have a filtration system installed in your home. Note that a Brita or comparable brand will *not* cut it.

Get Rid of Heavy Metals

Chelation therapy is your best bet at flushing heavy metals from your body. Supplement your diet with chelating elements, meaning minerals like magnesium, zinc, copper, and manganese. They grip onto the heavy metals and pull them out as they pass through your system. It's best to use chelating elements in conjunction with fiber and other liver-supporting substances to ensure that the body eliminates them rather than reabsorbing them.

Here are some great food-sourced chelators:

- **Cilantro leaves:** A potent detoxifier of mercury
- **Garlic and broccoli:** Help to detoxify cadmium
- **Chlorophyll:** Great all-around heavy metal detoxifier (I used it for a detox years ago and got cystic acne from the junk it was pulling out. Many years later, I realized that I should have been using supporting agents such as NAC alongside it.)

A few additional supplements that support chelation are NAC, alpha-lipoic acid, glutathione, and selenium.

TOXINS IN YOUR BEAUTY ROUTINE

If you were handed a jar labeled "chemicals," I highly doubt you would rub it all over your face. However, you may already be doing this a few times a week or, more likely daily, each time you apply your moisturizer and/or makeup. Your skin is fairly resilient, but it is far from an impenetrable shield. It's actually your largest organ, loaded with pores that absorb whatever you put on and transport it to your bloodstream. Most conventional cosmetics and deodorants are loaded with heavy metals like aluminum, which can accumulate in your soft tissues and impair organ function. If enough junk piles up, you could be looking at anything from infertility to kidney damage or high blood pressure. Heavy metals, especially lead and mercury, have also been shown to contribute to miscarriage.

No Smoking Allowed

Tobacco has the potential to severely impact your fertility, accelerating the biological clock and diminishing your egg reserve. There is hope, however, for women willing to give up smoking. A study conducted by El-Nemr et al. (1998) to measure the effects of smoking on ovarian reserve showed that it was possible to reverse the damage within six months after quitting. The study's experts recommended "reducing oxidative stress through improved lifestyle, nutrition, or intake of antioxidants" for three to six months before undergoing any fertility treatments.

de Ziegler et al. (2013)

Parabens are another harmful type of chemical that show up consistently in cosmetics and hair products. They are used as a preservative and are found in just about all personal care products, from makeup to hair products to perfumes. You're likely putting them directly on your skin almost every day.

In 2013, a Harvard study on female rats that were orally given regular doses of parabens showed a reduction in ovarian weight, which means a depletion in egg reserve (Smith et al. 2013). In that same study, parabens were found to disrupt T4 hormone levels, potentially causing thyroid issues.

Luckily, we are seeing a plethora of "clean products" gracing the market, and even some of the big names are developing less toxic options. When shopping for personal care products, read labels. Parabens come in many forms, but they will always have "paraben" somewhere in the name, such as methylparaben and propylparaben, to name a few.

Ladies living in the United States may want to skip nail polish altogether. Another common cosmetic chemical called phthalates are found in abundance in nail, skin, and hair products. Studies have linked them to implantation failure, high blood sugar, and excess weight gain during pregnancy (Messerlian et al. 2016). You can check for "3-free" or "phthalate-free" labels on your cosmetics, including nail polish. Toluene has been banned in Europe because it's been linked to birth defects and organ damage, but here in the United States, it's found in gasoline, paint thinners—and your nail polish (Donald, Hooper, and Hopenhayn-Rich 1991). Inhaling this chemical can lead to issues with fetal development. Check your polish labels for the "toxic trio": formaldehyde, toluene, and phthalate. A few brands that exclude these are Zoya, Suncoat, Piggy Paint, Sheswai, Honeybee Gardens, and RGB. If you are frequenting the nail salon, you are also exposing yourself to harmful fumes. Look for organic/nontoxic nail salons in your area and opt for their services if available.

If you work in the beauty/nail industry and you're inhaling these fumes on a regular basis, consider getting an air purifier for your "zone of influence" in the salon and perhaps consider trying out some products that are lower in chemical residue.

Even the products you use to clean your face and body can contain phthalates—body wash, shampoo, hand soap, and anything else that lathers. Antibacterial labels usually mean the presence of triclosan, which is another hormone disruptor. You don't have to forgo your beauty routine, just be more conscious of the brands and products you choose. It will take some effort on the front end, checking ingredients on labels, but you'll end up with a safer makeup collection on hand. There are a lot of all-natural beauty brands cropping up in the market, and they're worth hunting down in the noble quest for a baby, not to mention keeping things clean for pregnancy.

HOUSEHOLD TOXINS

While you can certainly be exposed to toxins by polluted air outside or at your place of work, the place you need to be most conscious of toxin exposure is in your own home. In an enclosed space, any synthetic chemicals, such as volatile organic compounds (VOCs), that are released from items like particleboard furniture, paints, wood finishes, and even your home's foundational materials are points of exposure. They are trapped in the air you breathe in every room. Air filters can help, as long as you select a high-efficiency air particulate absorbing (HEPA) filter. You might also buy a few houseplants, as they're natural filters that produce clean oxygen for you.

The Scoop on Air Filters

Stick to HEPA filters since the non-HEPA versions can release ozone. In recent years, medical researchers have begun exploring the effects of ozone on fertility. In 2016, Patricia Silveyra, PhD, of the Pennsylvania State University College of Medicine and her research team discovered that exposure during ovulation significantly decreased the progesterone levels of mice and even reduced the number of eggs they ovulated (Mishra, DiAngelo, and Silveyra 2006).

Federation of American Societies for Experimental Biology (2015)

Now let's talk about the things you're spraying on your household surfaces. Phthalates don't just show up in cosmetics. These common xenoestrogens are also in many household cleaning products and anything vinyl. That's because, like BPA, they are "plasticizers." They are used to make plastics more flexible and durable. They also act as solvents and make fragrances last longer in products like air fresheners, laundry detergent, dish soap, and green-colored cleaning sprays. Even toilet papers, yoga mats, and shower curtains may contain

> Higher phthalates are associated with lower AMH (ovarian reserve) and hormonal imbalance.
>
> Dominguez (2019)

them. In 2000, the CDC tested 289 random people, and every single one of them had high levels of phthalates in their blood. Men are also at risk of negative effects. Phthalates disrupt testosterone production and can lower sperm swimming capabilities quite significantly.

Renovating?

If you're planning a home improvement project, take care in the materials you select. Common paints, glues, and flooring materials release toxic chemicals. "Antifungal" paints are some of the worst culprits, but also look out for paints that use formaldehyde as a preservative. It will typically show up as "methanal" on labels. Instead, look for Green Seal-11–certified and low-VOC stamps when shopping and consider milk paints, which are a healthier alternative to water-based latex or oil-based paints. Some trusted brands for home improvement products are Forest Stewardship Council (FSC), Global Organic Textile Standard (GOTS), Oeko-Tex, Standard 100, and Greenguard. Also be sure to leave all the windows open to release fumes and introduce a good air filter.

Phthalates aren't the only chemicals invading your cleaning routines. Avoiding ammonia-based products is equally important. Ammonia is a popular ingredient in cleaning liquids because it gets the job done. It is commonly found in glass/window cleaners, toilet bowl cleaners, polishing wax, oven cleaner, and drain cleaner. Regular exposure to the fumes can lead to reproductive issues in both men and women.

A 2018 study on male mice found that ammonia air pollutants reduce sperm quality in the exposed male and his male offspring (Zhang et al. 2018)! In another study, a scientist at Washington State University noticed that her female lab mice demonstrated a serious decline in fertility (Maher 2008). Only about 10 percent were able to get pregnant after mating, and many of those had serious (and in some cases fatal) difficulties in childbirth. Through the process of elimination, she and her team discovered that it was the ammonia-based cleaning products used in the lab and mice cages.

Beware of Electromagnetic Fields

Are you or your partner gadget junkies? If you're like most modern folks, you are probably addicted to your cell phone. Electronics of all sorts release electromagnetic fields (EMFs). A strong field or prolonged exposure can stimulate nerves and muscles and even affect biological processes. If you've seen a fertility doctor, it's likely he or she suggested your partner keep his cell phone out of his pocket and to avoid having his laptop directly on his lap for an extended period of time. According to a 2014 study, heat and EMFs cause DNA fragmentation in the sperm cell, causing it to grow abnormally (Wright, Milne, and Leeson 2014). EMFs can also interfere with the sperm's swimming trajectory. Although there isn't much in the way of research on it yet, if cell phone radiation can zap sperm, it may also negatively impact our eggs. Use airplane mode or turn it off as often as possible!

Gorpinchenko et al. (2014)

Now, are you a mouse? Obviously not, but if ammonia can have such a profound effect on the reproductive systems of mice, it can be assumed that exposure is probably not the best for any mammal. Strong ammonia-based cleaners are nice for disinfecting, especially in hospitals, but they might not be necessary in an average household, especially not at such a high personal cost.

Small Changes, Big Impacts

While most of us are aware that our air is polluted and that plastics are a big environmental problem, many still aren't tuned into the fact that minor everyday choices can affect our chances of getting pregnant. Yet in my personal and professional experience, equally small alterations to one's routine can deliver big payouts.

Carol was a 38-year-old celebrity hairstylist who worked at a prestigious hair salon in New York City. She spent three days per week in the salon and also freelanced on movie sets and fashion shoots. Carol always looked fabulous, and her eloquent French accent completed the package. On the outside, she had it all together, but Carol had been trying to get pregnant naturally for eight months to no avail, at which point she sought the advice of a fertility specialist. She dove into IVF, but after three rounds, she was back where she started. The eggs retrieved during her cycles were of such poor quality that they didn't survive long enough to make the "transfer" (the part of the IVF cycle when the embryo is placed into the uterus). Carol's doctor told her it was an "egg quality issue" and said there wasn't much that could be done. He suggested she come see me to assess whether any natural methods might help.

Carol and I sat down and did a thorough lifestyle intake. As I imagined, she ate mostly "on the fly" from plastic takeout containers. Organic was not easy to come by when ordering takeout, and tap water or plastic bottles were her source of hydration.

Carol's hair was full of product, her face perfectly made up. Suffice it to say, she was exposed to hefty amounts of parabens, phthalates, and even formaldehyde (yikes!).

At home, Carol was a clean freak and germophobe and had her apartment cleaned professionally every week. Her partner, Rob, worked from home and was getting a heavy dose of ammonia and phthalates—not great for his swimmers. In addition to New York City's polluted air, Carol was getting slammed by toxins daily.

Carol's fertility program was centered around reducing her toxin intake and gently cleansing her system. First up was swapping out all her toxin-heavy products and containers both at work and at home. I then placed Carol on a three-week detox diet with the addition of supplements to assist her body in cleaning out the built-up toxins. She felt horrible for the first week as her body unloaded the junk, but an energy boost soon followed. In fact, she felt so good that she agreed to stay on a modified version of the diet for another month. After a few weeks on the cleanse, I added some antioxidants and a custom herbal formula to reenergize her ovaries and enhance egg quality. The next IVF cycle was fruitful. She got more eggs this time, and five of them proceeded to the blastocyst stage (the most advanced stage of development for increased odds of success in an IVF cycle). They were sent off for testing, and two returned as good quality. She is now pregnant with one and has one on ice for baby number two.

Detox Your Life

Toxins may lurk everywhere in the modern world, but solutions are also abundant.

Start a dietary detox. Cleanses like the one I placed Carol on are an effective way to flush out pollutants and re-sync your cycle. A catered detox program is an amazing opportunity to reset your body and start fresh with healthier (fertility-friendly) habits. It also gets your head in the game for baby making by instilling an amazing sense of clarity and purpose.

Cleansing Vitamins and Herbs

- NAC is a potent antioxidant that assists your liver in processing toxic elements (more on this personal favorite in chapter 11).
- Milk thistle both cleanses and protects the liver from damage. Try drinking one to two cups daily during a detox regime (see chapter 8).

Shop produce according to the "Dirty Dozen" and "Clean 15" lists available online. Both are updated yearly to educate the public on how to avoid toxic exposure through food. While you're at it, peek at the Food and Drug Administration's (FDA's) list of mercury levels in commercial fish and shellfish and cut out those with the highest.

To get comprehensive lists of all products and produce that contain toxins, you can check out the Environmental Working Group's website (https://www.ewg.org). It's the "everything" guide to avoid toxins in your life. You can find even more resources in appendix A.

Take inventory of your day. Start by making small investments in items like glass food containers; a nylon, cotton, or polyester shower curtain; a yoga mat free of polyvinyl chloride (PVC); and a reusable steel water bottle. Then, as budgeting allows, add larger purchases like a HEPA air filter and a water filter capable of cutting out heavy metals.

Look for "green" beauty brands. These include OSEA, Ren, 100% Pure, and Juice Beauty for your shampoos and washes. To crowd out even more phthalates, replace your perfume with essential oils. You'll have the choice between an array of lovely scents like jasmine, geranium, and sandalwood and they come with therapeutic benefits! The sweet smell of stress relief, improved sleep, and antibacterial/antiviral properties.

Clean doesn't have to be toxic. Some of the worst toxin-laden offenders in the average household are air fresheners, aerosol sprays, laundry detergent, dishwashing liquid, wood floor polish, and carpet cleaners. Where you can, replace them for plant-based and nontoxic options from brands boasting labels like "biodegradable," "chlorine-free," "phosphate-free," "fragrance-free," and "no dyes."

> For do-it-yourself household cleaning products, use white vinegar, baking soda, lemon juice, or hydrogen peroxide as disinfectants. A mixture of diluted olive oil mixed with lemon juice can polish and shine furniture.

The information outlined in this chapter was designed to help you reduce the impact of toxins commonly found in your home and environment. In the next chapter, I guide you through a comprehensive nutritional overhaul to cleanse your body and optimize your fertility.

Preconception Planning

At least 21 days before renewing your efforts to conceive, begin making as many of the following adjustments to your lifestyle as possible:

- Buy glass or stainless-steel bottles and food containers.
- Clear your makeup collection of toxin-heavy products and opt for cleaner brands.
- Use all-natural cleaners in your home.
- Invest in quality water filters.
- Fill your home with plants or shop for a HEPA air filter.
- Be more selective in the produce aisle, choosing organic where you can.

CHAPTER 8

Cool, Calm, Cleanse, Balance

What you eat sustains you. It also has the potential to transform your life. The foods you choose are determining factors in the wellness of your body and mind, including your reproductive health. While I've provided snippets of information on this topic throughout the Big Four chapters, I'd now like to offer you a complete cleansing program as the first phase of your path-to-baby protocol.

The Big Four affect everyone differently, but their adverse effects boil down to pervasive "unrest" deep within your physiology. They aggravate, complicate, and hinder vital reproductive functions. This chapter's cleanse protocol is designed to calm your system as a whole, improving your fertility and overall health. It will also help you discover your own personal inflammatory foods or hidden allergies. It is a process to help you both diagnose and address your health challenges.

For three weeks, I'm going to ask you to remove certain foods and food categories from your diet and replace them with essential nutrients and botanicals that assist in cooling inflammation, calming the nervous system, cleansing your body of pent-up toxins, and balancing blood sugar and insulin (i.e., cool, calm,

As Old as Time

There's a good chance you've been on some sort of diet plan at one point in your life. However, this isn't a fad diet or a fleeting trend. This form of dietary plan has been at the center of holistic practice for millennia. Cleansing is a regular practice in countries such as India and in religious communities all over the world. Traditional cultures partake in cleansing and fasts according to the full moon and auspicious religious dates. You'll find cleanse retreats around the world that you can visit and reclaim your health, but for the purposes of convenience and ease, I have adapted traditional cleanse regimes to fit into your everyday life.

cleanse, balance). These modifications are carefully chosen to allow your body's detoxification systems, which may be overburdened or compromised, to function efficiently again. Think of it as a "reset" of sorts for your reproductive health.

In the pages to follow, you'll learn a wellness strategy that you can incorporate into your life for the long haul. Although aspects of the program may be challenging, this form of cleanse allows you to lead a somewhat normal routine while still achieving deep benefits. You don't have control over all aspects of your fertility journey, but you do have a great deal of control over what you put in your body.

The changes proposed in this program may be considerable for some. If you have a history of eating disorders or severe digestive complaints, taking this on might warrant some extra consideration. In such cases, you may consider consulting your health care practitioner to see if a modification is required. In lieu of doing the Conception Cleanse, you can home in on the nutritional tips in chapter 9.

Timing Your Detox

It's best to attempt to get pregnant *after* completing the cleanse and beginning a maintenance plan (see the next chapter). While you're cleansing, the body is pulling toxins out of their hiding places in order to process them for elimination. Those circulating toxins do not foster an ideal environment for conception and, in some cases, can be dangerous to a growing fetus.

Set time aside for cleansing so that you can best prepare yourself for this endeavor. It's not ideal to start this program if you have travel plans and many social engagements on the roster. You'll want to start out being close to home so you can be grounded

> The life cycle of eggs is around 90 days. It takes around three months for one egg to fully develop and be selected for ovulation. Sperm, too, has a life span averaging 80 to 90 days from early development to its "exit." If you are seeking to improve your egg quality, then it's most efficacious to start this process a few months in advance of trying to conceive.

and ready for the changes to come. It's a great idea to be fertility charting simultaneously (see chapter 2 for a refresher) so that you can log data and get in tune with your rhythms alongside the cleanse.

When Is Detox Appropriate?

There are some telltale signs that your body is overburdened. If you identify with the following list, you'd likely benefit from a cleanse, pronto.

Common symptoms of Big Four interference are the following:

- Allergies/sinus problems
- Bad PMS
- Heavy or painful periods
- Mood issues
- Asthma/bronchitis
- Back pain
- Constipation
- Depression/lack of motivation
- Frequent colds/flu
- Headaches
- Indigestion, gas, and bloating
- Lethargy/fatigue
- High BMI
- Poor concentration/foggy head
- Skin and hair conditions
- Diminished ovarian reserve
- Cysts
- POF/high FSH
- Endometriosis
- Fibroids
- Post-IVF or medicated IUI
- History of drug use
- Cessation of medications and pharmaceuticals

Post-IVF Detox

Going through IVF? Perhaps you've packed on a few pounds. Or maybe you are feeling foggy and not quite yourself. Consider detoxing after a cycle to help your body process all the excess estrogens and medications introduced during the process. Many women get thrown off physically and emotionally after IVF or even simply after a medicated IUI. A detox can help you get yourself back on track and improve the odds of success in your next round.

Is This Really Necessary?

On occasion (ahem, often), I get a bit of pushback from patients with regard to the detox concept. A comment that pops up repeatedly is "Why is it necessary to detox when people with severe addictions and poor physical health can still get pregnant?!" To be clear, the impact of toxicity and an imbalanced lifestyle may differ substantially from woman to woman. A clean lifestyle and detox program is more essential for some than others. For example, women with the MTHFR gene mutation typically retain more toxins because their natural detox systems are less efficient. Women with endometriosis and PCOS are highly prone to inflammation and more reactive to inflammatory and allergenic foods. Have a diminished ovarian reserve? Exposure to toxins accelerates the aging of your ovaries. Toxins and poor dietary choices aren't good for anyone, but they are definitely worse for some.

Conception Cleanse Principles

There are many detox programs out there. This one is specifically designed to tackle the Big Four in a gentle way. Liquid fasts and other extreme measures may be too harsh for the body when you are preparing for pregnancy. This Conception Cleanse is a modified "elimination" diet combined with detox principles to assist your body in calming inflammation, dispelling toxins, and balancing hormones. It is a fast track to rid the body of foods and food-based chemicals you may be allergic or sensitive to. The aim is to prevent and reverse premature aging of eggs and support your reproductive organs in functioning optimally.

This isn't just about giving you a list of foods you can't eat, though I will do that. I'm also going to tell you *why* they aren't recommended and provide lists of easy alternatives. Bonus recommendations include tips on other lifestyle strategies to support the cleansing process.

To further understand the "why," I've outlined three guiding principles to follow.

PRINCIPLE 1: ELIMINATE FOODS THAT IRRITATE AND INFLAME

Cleanse programs generally involve a certain amount of willpower to execute. This one is no exception. The premise involves an elimination of foods, drinks, and habits that overload your body with toxins, stimulants, and acidic substances. I'm talking about booze, caffeine, red meat, fried foods, dairy, refined carbs, sugar, and common food allergens.

You may be wondering what is left over after we cut these things out. Don't worry, we will get there. For the time being, try a shift in mind-set. Instead of looking at it as deprivation, see it as a delayed gratification. First, you'll get the satisfaction of knowing that you held out. Second, you're going to look and feel better from the inside

> Soy is used as a filler to "bulk up" many processed foods, but it acts as an endocrine disruptor because it is full of naturally occurring estrogens. It can also lower sperm count and sperm quality in your partner. Check package labels for soy before buying.

out. That "clean" feeling will make you wonder how you lived any other way.

Throughout the process, you will "crowd out" the junk by replacing it with nourishing foods, drinks, and activities. You'll become more aware of the foods that may not be serving you and experience the benefits of renewed health.

Bye for Now!

Throughout my years of practice, most of my patients have expressed their preference for "black-and-white" cleansing rules. They want to know the dos and don'ts, period, because it's easier for them to stick to clear-cut guidelines. This strategy will allow you to accomplish more in less time.

Say good-bye to the following:

- **Potentially toxic edibles:**

  ○ Conventionally farmed fruits and veggies (pesticides)
  ○ Deep-water or farmed fish (toxins and heavy metals)
  ○ Alcohol (by nature, a toxin)

- **Inflammatory/allergen foods:**

  ○ Common cooking oils
  ○ Gluten (wheat, farro, barley, and so on)
  ○ Conventionally raised meat and poultry (especially pork and beef)
  ○ Highly acidic foods (chocolate, coffee, and red meat)
  ○ Dairy
  ○ Sugar
  ○ Booze
  ○ Soy
  ○ Processed foods (e.g., chips, cookies, packaged sauces, and so on)
  ○ Artificial additives such as monosodium glutamate (MSG) and aspartame

Organic versus Conventional Poultry

Conventional poultry are full of a GMO- and pesticide-ridden diet just like cattle. When shopping for chicken, look for "free range" or "organic" labels.

The pH Scale

The cleanse diet is designed to replace acidic items with lots of alkaline options so as to create a "friendlier" environment where egg and sperm can meet. An overly acidic cervical fluid may actually kill the sperm before they can reach your egg. An acidic digestive system also cultivates bad bacteria and yeasts that trigger inflammation. While plants tend to be more alkaline than animal products, some plant foods, such as grains, legumes, and nuts, can lean more acidic. Aim for a diet rich in leafy green vegetables.

- **Foods and drinks linked to insulin and blood sugar dysregulation:**

  - Sugar and its many aliases
  - Wine, beer, and dark liquor
  - Gluten
  - Corn and corn derivatives
  - Refined foods (i.e., flour products)

- **Caffeine and other stimulants:**

  - Coffee
  - Energy drinks
  - Kombucha
  - Chocolate
  - Black, green, oolong tea (or any other caffeinated teas)

PRINCIPLE 2: REDUCE THE BURDEN

A cleanse works best when you take steps to reduce the burden on your digestive system. The easier it is for your body to process your food, the swifter the detox. One of the best ways to aid digestion is to eat, for the most part, alkaline, plant-based foods. Most animal products are more acid forming than their vegetable and fruit counterparts, and their proteins take much longer to break down and move through your system. The slower transit time means greater chances of fermentation and dysbiosis—think leaky gut and inflammation.

The other key dietary change is eating smaller meals with simpler ingredients. Your digestive system has to work hard to break down food, particularly if it's heavy or if you scarf and forget to chew. Periodically reducing your food intake can give your digestive system a rest period to rejuvenate itself and become more efficient. It's the same principle as taking a days' rest between strenuous workouts or taking the weekend off after a stressful workweek. You perform better when you're rested, and your digestive system is no different. The best way to give your gut a needed break is to cut portion sizes by one-third or one-half, focus on plant-based foods, cook everything, and potentially skip dinner in favor of a cup of tea, broth, or soup. If you are underweight or have a tendency to lose weight too easily, forgo cutting portions and instead focus on eating purees of vegetables and smoothies with healthy added fats.

> Make it a habit to drink room-temperature or warm drinks rather than cold, icy fluids. Drinking cold liquids, especially close to meals, weakens your production of digestive enzymes, slowing the digestive process.

Cooking Methods Ideal for Detox

The best ways to prepare your warm foods are with the following acid-reducing methods (in order of preference):

1. Steaming
2. Water sautéing
3. Boiling
4. Stewing
5. Baking

From an Eastern paradigm, these methods are energetically "neutral" and put the food in a state that's easy to digest. Overall, steaming is the best option, but there are select advantages to each. Water sautéing is perfect for greens, keeping the crunch. Boiling is best for root vegetables because it's most effective at softening them. Stewing is preferable for meat and bones so as to draw out more collagen and minerals. Baking is great for those nights you feel a chill but use it less if you have constipation or feel hot at night.

How you prepare your food matters, too. Foods warmed by thorough chewing or by cooking are easier to digest than raw foods. Whenever possible, cook your foods or reheat items that come out of the fridge. Eastern traditions have advocated for this choice for centuries, but if you think about it, even Western cultures have unconsciously adopted it. When you're sick, no one offers you salad. They offer you hot soup or hot tea with lemon. Many of my patients experiencing bloating or gas after meals rectified those issues by simply replacing salad with steamed veggies. If your body requires healing (reproductive or other), focusing on foods that require less energy to digest leaves more resources to do so.

Recall from chapter 6 that lifestyle habits are major influential factors on digestive and reproductive health. Staying alert, active, and busy keeps you from entering "rest-and-digest" mode. If your tendency is to function in a highly productive, rushed state, then for the duration of this program, consider simply sitting down when eating to foster healthy digestion.

Chew!

Digestion starts in the mouth, where the food is broken down by chewing and mixing with enzyme-rich saliva. If you scarf your food, you are swallowing whole chunks, leaving your digestive system to deal with the added burden. A famous doctor in China was known to take a look at patients' tongues to assess the state of their digestive systems. If he saw signs of digestive insufficiency, he would tell the patients to go home and chew their food. If they still had issues in a month, then they could return. Many never had to return.

It's not uncommon for busy women to put off eating a full meal until dinner. The evening, however, is not a great time to calorie load. Heavy meals and snacking at night put a blob of food in your gut when it doesn't have the abundance of enzymes to fully break it down, so that food lingers and ferments, contributing to a leaky gut. And since we tend to be more sedentary in the evening, the elevated blood sugar and insulin that occur as a by-product of digestion just swirls around in our bloodstream wreaking havoc.

Simpler Meal Ideas

Breakfast: Green plant protein smoothie
Lunch: Coconut chickpea and root vegetable curry *or* cooked broccoli and steamed pumpkin with salmon
Snack: Smoothie, nuts, paleo pumpkin muffin
Dinner: Vegetable soup, sliced avocado salad with olive oil and lemon juice

---

PRINCIPLE 3: FOSTER ELIMINATION AND AID DETOXIFICATION

You can't detoxify without showing the junk the exit. Your main means of elimination are breath, sweat, poop, and pee. Food, water, and exercise all facilitate elimination and are your allies in the cleansing process.

Water is essential to a detox because it provides the "ride out" via urine, sweat, and bowel movements. It's difficult to tell you exactly how much water to drink, as it varies according to the climate you live in as well as your activity level. As a general rule, seek to drink half your body weight in ounces or two to three liters daily.

High-*fiber*, plant-based foods work together with fluids to bind waste products and sweep them out of the body. In addition to helping you feel satisfied on the program, fibrous foods and water assist in the healthy disposal of excess estrogen metabolites. Fiber sources

> Increase your intake of fibrous veggies like broccoli, cauliflower, cabbage, and brussels sprouts. They contain indole-3-carbinol (I3C), which assists the liver's cleansing process.

include unpolished grains such as buckwheat and brown rice, fruits (pears are great for elimination), beans, squash, and dark leafy vegetables. Fresh ground flaxseed or chia seeds are wonderful insoluble fiber options that bind to toxins and flush them from your system.

If *exercise* isn't part of your weekly routine, it's time to step it up. Exercise enhances detoxification by increasing oxygen intake in all your organs and tissues; cleansing your liver, circulatory, and lymphatic systems; and helping your

Nutrients That Aid Detoxification

The first phase of detoxification begins in the liver. It has specialized enzymes that transform substances like caffeine, alcohol, pollutants, and medications into water-soluble molecules via chemical reactions. However, people with any intolerances to these substances may have issues with this transformation process, leading to a buildup in their organs and tissues.

Assist the cleansing process with herbal remedies like milk thistle, turmeric, green tea, and grape seed. They offer antioxidants and other nutrients that support liver function, making it more efficient at detoxification. For additional detox boosts, you can check out protein powder smoothies from companies like Thorne, Apex Energetics, and Metagenics. Their powders contain a slew of vitamins, enzymes, minerals, and herbs, such as B vitamins, magnesium, NAC, lipoic acid, and glutathione. All are powerful detoxifiers.

The second phase of detox occurs after your liver partially breaks down the toxins. Junk travels out through "exits," such as bowel movements and urine. You can boost your body's efficiency at this process by supplementing with nutrients like B and C vitamins, folic acid, glutathione, selenium, molybdenum, and zinc and, even better, if you can find supplements that also contain amino acids like glycine, cysteine, methionine, taurine, and glutamine. The smoothie powders and supporting supplement combos offered by the companies mentioned above contain all these nutrients. My team and I can also offer you catered detox packages via my website (christinaburns .com) or at https://naturnalife.com.

organs of elimination to drain. Moving your body essentially helps you circulate and eliminate toxins more efficiently.

Keep in mind that when undergoing detoxification, a gentle exercise routine is recommended so as not to overload your body, which is working overtime to rid you of a toxin buildup. If you're used to high-intensity workouts, give yourself a break and adopt a lower-intensity routine for the duration of the cleanse (see chapter 10 for more on exercise and fertility).

Too Much Too Fast

We want results now, but sometimes, it comes at a cost. Cleansing should be slow and steady to allow your organs of elimination to gently process and remove toxins. This is one of the main reasons why fasts (including juice or liquid fasts) should be done only under the guidance of a health care professional and *not* when seeking to get pregnant. Much of the fasting craze is doing damage to our already taxed systems by overloading them with waste too quickly. When trying to restore vitality to the reproductive system, we must be gentle with ourselves. Rapid weight loss (beyond just losing water weight) could shock your system and add strain. When on the quest for baby, there is no time for unnecessary setbacks. Don't jump the gun!

One of the most effective forms of exercise for detoxification is yoga. It is incredibly sophisticated, and many poses (asanas) are designed to "wring out" organs to help them remove waste more effectively. The gentle nature of yoga makes it perfect for detox programs. You may also end up finding salvation in this ancient practice, as regular yoga will help you feel more relaxed in body and mind.

Yoga Poses That Facilitate Detoxification

1. *Twists*, such as seated spinal twist, eagle pose, and revolved chair pose. The twisting movement of these poses wrings out the liver, kidneys, and digestive system. The pressure on these organs as you breathe deeply helps to mobilize toxins. As you release the pose, the toxins circulate through the liver and lymphatic systems and find their way out through the organs of elimination. Twists also help to improve digestion.
2. *Inverted poses*, such as headstand, handstand, and shoulder stand, use gravity to allow all fluids in the body to travel with ease through the heart and circulatory system. Fluids sometimes gather in the lower limbs and become stagnant. Inverting helps mobilize them through the circulatory and lymphatic systems for faster cleansing.
3. *Forward bends* give the internal organs a massage similar to twists but less intense. Forward folding also lengthens the spine, leading to a release of toxins in the back muscles and spinal column.
4. *Supine positions*, such as cobra pose and boat pose, cleanse the digestive and reproductive systems. The increased oxygen intake with each expansion of the lungs improves the cleansing process through the bowels and breath.

Committing 100 percent to a new diet or workout routine can be tough at first. Why not pamper yourself with cleanse-friendly spa activities to assist the process? Here are a few optional add-ons that can enhance detoxification.

Your Do-It-Yourself Detox Practices

Saunas help you work up a sweat by sitting back and letting the day's stresses melt away. Since your skin is the largest organ of elimination, you release toxins via sweat through your skin's pores. Infrared saunas are particularly helpful in assisting the liver and gallbladder to remove toxins and fatty gunk. The infrared rays penetrate deep into tissues and allow you to sweat longer at lower temperatures than traditional saunas.

The ever-popular practice of *cupping* is a great way to detox your tissues and often relieves tension to boot. Cupping is an ancient Eastern practice of applying suction cups to areas of the body to draw toxins out of the muscles and lymph and into circulation to be eliminated via one or more of your "exits."

Dry skin brushing is common in many European spas. It involves brushing the skin in the direction of the heart, which helps push lymphatic fluids and waste back toward the heart to be recirculated and excreted. Although the benefits are similar to cupping, dry skin brushing is easier to use on your limbs. Cupping, on the other hand, is more suited to wide areas, such as the torso. Dry skin brushing is often done in conjunction with *hydrotherapy*—plunging in alternating pools of hot and very cold water—which is helpful in stimulating circulation. You can do this at home using buckets of water for your lower legs or filling the bathtub with hot water and taking a cold shower.

You may have heard about *castor oil* from your parents or grandparents since it was once popular as a drink to help purge the bowels. Midwives also sometimes recommended it for getting labor going. In the context of do-it-yourself cleansing, it is used topically as a means to increase circulation and break down junk that has accumulated in the liver and gallbladder. The process involves applying castor oil to the right side of your abdomen (liver) and covering it with a thin cloth (cheesecloth or paper towel). Then apply a heat pack (water or electric is fine) over the area and relax for 30 to 45 minutes. Note that this same approach can be used to dissolve ovarian cysts by performing the routine on the lower pelvic region. You can buy a "castor oil kit" from health stores or online (organic preferred), or you can make them yourself with castor oil and a thin cloth (preferably cheesecloth).

Structuring Your Day

Before walking you through each week of the cleanse individually, I first want to impart some tips on making the diet work for you.

In order to get the most out of this program, you'll want to combine it with the tips from the preceding Big Four chapters, especially those you found most relevant to your unique fertility profile. For example, if you suspect that insulin is the main culprit behind your fertility struggle, apply all of the lifestyle tips in chapter 5 in addition to the diet plan presented here.

It's incredibly important to be strategic about *when* you eat, not just *what* you eat. Breakfast sets the foundation for your day. Don't skip it! Eating a breakfast rich in either protein or fat (or both) within an hour of waking helps you feel more satiated for longer. Incorporating nuts or avocados into your breakfast or making a protein smoothie is a great way to do this, hence why the cleansing protein smoothie option has become so popular.

The window for lunch should be three to four hours after breakfast and fall in the late morning or early afternoon, ideally between 11 a.m. and 2 p.m. Carving out 10 to 20 minutes on a busy day can provide space for you to relax, chew, and digest properly. Many of us start to associate eating with bloat because of scarfing in a hurry. It doesn't have to be this way! Sit down for a breather, absorb all the benefits of your food, and avoid the pain.

The evening is for rest of body and mind, digestion included. To best aid your body's natural rhythm, strive to finish a light dinner by 7 p.m. Eating more and/or later will leave excess sugars and carbs in your system that you can't burn off (unless maybe if you're going out dancing).

> Remember, your digestive energy is strongest in the early morning and weakest at night.

Hunger pangs between designated meals may tempt you to reach for the closest thing available regardless of whether it falls within the diet's parameters. The best way to avoid this is keeping a smart snack handy, such as almond flour crackers, an apple, a cleanse-friendly smoothie, leftovers, seaweed snacks, nuts, or pumpkin seeds (see appendix D for additional healthy snack ideas).

Helpful Hint

Look for restaurants that accommodate vegan and gluten-free options. These spots will list "GF" (gluten free) or "DF" (dairy free) on their menus. They're also generally less likely to give you a hard time about any inquiries.

Last but not least, prioritize quality sleep to keep sugar and caffeine cravings at bay! Take some lead time to wrap your mind around the program (a week should do) so that you are mentally prepared to dive in. Now let's jump into how exactly to apply the diet week by week.

Your Three Weeks of Bliss

Changing food habits can seem like a complex, confusing, and sometimes emotional process. The following week-by-week instructions are designed to simplify that process with sample menus, recipes, snack suggestions, and other useful tips.

The Quick Version

Feel like you are running out of time? If you are already in the midst of fertility treatments and don't want to slow down or postpone, then I suggest a modified version of this program. You can reap at least some of the benefits without feeling like you've been put on hold.
Here's how it works:

1. Spend four days following the week 1 instructions.
2. Spend three days following the week 2 instructions.
3. Spend three days following the week 3 instructions.

Let's start by breaking down what you can and cannot eat during the cleanse.

SHOPPING CHEAT SHEET

The Conception Cleanse is centered around the three clean eating principles outlined above. Throughout the 21-day elimination cleanse, choose your daily meals based on the Conception Cleanse shopping list (see also table 8.1). If you look at this list and say, "I don't know how to make meals out of this?," don't worry. It's not as daunting as it seems. To prove it, I've provided a list of cleanse-friendly recipes in appendix C in addition to the sample days provided in this chapter. I also have a full course, including cooking demos, called Eating for Optimal Nutrition, available on my website (https://naturnalife.com or christinaburns.com).

Read Labels Carefully

When you make a grocery trip to prepare for your first week of detox, check the labels on anything that comes in a can, box, or bag. Just because something is "allowed" on the diet doesn't necessarily mean a packaged version of it follows all of the guidelines. Often, chemicals and additional ingredients, such as flavor enhancers and preservatives, are added to packaged foods. As a general rule of thumb, if you don't know what the ingredient is, it's not a good sign. Put the package down and walk away.
Examples of what to look for are the following:

- Cornstarch in baking powder and any processed foods.
- Corn syrup in beverages and processed foods.
- Vinegar in mustard is usually from wheat or corn.
- Oats that aren't labeled "gluten free."
- Many canned tunas contain textured vegetable protein, which is from soy; look for low-salt versions, which tend to be pure tuna, with no fillers.
- Multigrain rice cakes are not just rice (they may contain wheat or other gluten-containing grains). Purchase plain rice cakes.
- Additives like MSG, dyes, and natural flavors.
- Added sugars like maltodextrin.
- Sugar alcohols like erythritol. Look for "-ol."

Table 8.1. Foods to Include and Exclude in the Conception Cleanse

Include	Exclude

Fruits
    Whole fruits (berries, cherries, pears, and apples preferred—those that are domestic to northern states); unsweetened, frozen, or water packed.
	Tropical Fruits
	    Oranges and orange juice, mango, pineapple, and banana (these are more acidic and higher in sugar).

Dairy Substitutes
    Rice and nut milks, such as almond milk, hemp, macadamia, and coconut milk (unsweetened).
	Dairy and Eggs
	    Milk, cheese, eggs, cottage cheese, cream, yogurt, butter, ice cream, frozen yogurt, and nondairy creamers.

Non-Gluten Grains and Starch
    Brown rice, gluten-free oats, millet, quinoa, amaranth, teff, buckwheat, yams, and butternut squash.
	Grains
	    Wheat, corn, barley, spelt, kamut, rye, triticale, semolina, and couscous.

Animal Protein
    Wild, fresh, or water-packed fish (preferably low in mercury [i.e., sole, flounder, and pollock] and high in monounsaturated fat [i.e., salmon, herring, and sardines]), duck, organic poultry, and game meats, such as lamb, bison, and venison.
    During the lead-in and lead-out of the program, you can consume fish, game meats, and poultry two or three times per week each. The 10-day intensive portion should contain fewer or no animal proteins.
	Animal Protein
	    Pork, beef/veal, sausage, cold cuts, canned meats, frankfurters, and shellfish.

Vegetable Protein
    Chickpeas, black beans, split peas, lentils, and legumes (dried beans) other than soybeans.
    Consume two or three times per week max and less if you have IBS.
	Soybean Products
	    Soy sauce and soybean oil in processed foods such as tempeh, tofu, soy milk, soy yogurt, and textured vegetable protein.

Include	Exclude
Nuts and Seeds Walnuts, sesame seeds, pumpkin seeds, sunflower seeds, hemp seed, hazelnuts, pecans, almonds, and nut butters, such as almond, sunflower, and tahini. *Make sure nut and seed butters don't contain extras like sunflower oil, palm oil, or sugar. Sprouted nut and seed butter are best.*	**Nuts** Peanuts and peanut butter, cashews, and pistachios.
Vegetables Any raw, steamed, sautéed, juiced, or roasted vegetables.	**Vegetables** Corn, creamed vegetables *Eat fewer nightshades such as eggplant, tomato, zucchini, and potato and eliminate them altogether if inflammation was your main Big Four culprit.*
Cold-Pressed Oils Olive, flax (do not heat), sesame, almond, walnut, pumpkin, coconut, pumpkin seed, and macadamia oils.	**Oils** Hydrogenated and processed oils (safflower, sunflower, peanut, grape seed, corn, and soybean), butter, margarine, shortening, salad dressings, mayonnaise, and spreads.
Drink Filtered or distilled water, non-/decaffeinated herbal teas. *Nettle, raspberry leaf, and red clover are good feminine teas. Can combine with berry, hibiscus, or citrusy teas to spruce them up.*	**Drinks** Alcohol, seltzer (high acidic), coffee, and other caffeinated beverages like soda.
Sweeteners None! You are retraining your palate to taste the natural sweetness in your foods. Better to use fruit purees/compotes or add sweetness from herbs such as cinnamon or vanilla.	**Sweeteners** Refined sugar, white/brown sugars, sucanat, honey, maple syrup, high-fructose corn syrup, evaporated cane juice, agave nectar, coconut sugar, brown rice syrup, tapioca syrup, and inulin/chicory syrup

(continued)

Table 8.1. *Continued*

Include	Exclude

Condiments and Seasoning
   Apple cider vinegar and all spices (excluding pepper), basil, cinnamon, cumin, dill, garlic, ginger, mustard, oregano, parsley, rosemary, tarragon, thyme, and turmeric.
   It is best to eliminate salt, BUT if you must use it, then sprinkle on food AFTER cooking only. You'll find if you eat good-quality produce, herbs, spices, and meats, you won't need to add salt.
	Condiments and Seasoning
	   Ketchup, relish, chutney, soy sauce, barbecue sauce, teriyaki, chocolate, and other condiments.

Soup
   Clear, vegetable-based broth, bone broth, homemade vegetarian soup with chicken or turkey, and miso soup (miso not made with gluten or soy; i.e., chickpea miso is okay)
	Soup
	   Canned or creamed soup; any with glutinous flours, grains, or corn. *Be wary of cubed soup stock, as it often contains MSG or gluten.*

The most effective way to prep for each week of the Conception Cleanse is to stock up on healthy groceries and batch some meals. Fill your freezer with proteins and frozen veggies so that you have those handy in case you run low. Root veggies and squashes have a relatively lengthy shelf life, so you can keep carrots, beets, parsnips, butternut, and sweet potato varieties on the counter or in the fridge for a while. Any greens will have to be bought once or twice per week, but that could be a really quick grocery pit stop if you already have the other items. Try to do a little extra cooking on your days off so that you have meals for a couple days. Consume leftovers within three days or freeze individual portions and thaw on demand. This is to avoid ingesting the bacteria that grows on food after it's been sitting—yes, even in the refrigerator.

Whenever possible, buy local. Go to your local farmers market on the weekend and stock up for the week. This ensures you're eating food that's fresh and in season. Theoretically, your local selection also contains the exact nutritional components you need to stay healthy in your environment.

Of course, shop organic or "no spray" whenever possible, too. If you're eating in restaurants, investigate whether their ingredients are local or organic, especially if their business is a convenient, quick option for you.

Flavoring Your Food on the Cleanse

Eating simple meals doesn't mean it has to be tasteless and plain. Want to add complexity without conventional sauces? Try these:

- Fresh squeezed lemon
- Coconut aminos
- Pressed olive oil
- Coconut oil

- Ginger
- Fresh and dried herbs
- Sesame oil
- Lemon or orange rind

WEEK 1

You're in it now. You're committed. Starting on day 1, completely cut out everything that isn't in the program. To help ease you into the adjustments, I am giving you a list of transitional foods that you can swap out for your favorite meals and snacks (see table 8.2).

In reality, not everyone will take to the kitchen. As a New Yorker, I find takeout is the rule for most rather than the exception. In the event you can't get around to cooking or you find the very idea repellent, you will have to dedicate time to exploring the restaurant and delivery options in your neighborhood. Ask them clarifying questions about preparation at each place you select. For example, "Does this contain butter? Is it gluten free? Is this deep fried?" For some, this may feel more troublesome than preparing food at home. Just know both options are there. No matter your preferred source of food, it's still helpful to pick out a few takeout options in advance of the cleanse so that you don't get yourself into a situation where you are starving and will eat the closest thing available.

In this chapter and in the appendices, I'll do my best to provide you with as many tips as I can and make this as easy and straightforward as possible. However, the truth of the matter is that it will take effort and ingenuity on your end. You are learning a new way of doing things, and sometimes the initial learning curve is steep. Start off by figuring out a few go-to recipes to integrate into your routine and then build from there. Knowing your options and having some recipe ideas certainly cuts back on confusion and being overwhelmed at the beginning. Not to worry, as that feeling of being overwhelmed will quickly transform into empowerment.

Table 8.2. Transitional Foods

If You Love	Try This
Crackers	Nuts and seeds, paleo crackers made from almond flour, and seaweed snacks.
Chips	Make your own in the oven with olive or coconut oil and sea salt. Try colorful potatoes instead of white ones and slice them thinly. Another option is homemade kale chips in the oven or dehydrator.
Pasta	Whole grains like buckwheat (kasha), quinoa, brown rice, and millet.
Yogurt	Coconut yogurt (try Anita's, Coconut Cult, or COCOYO). These are the cleanest brands I have found. There should be nothing in the yogurt besides coconut and probiotics.
Burgers	Bison, venison, lamb, turkey, fish, or veggie patties made from beans. You can make your own or buy organic frozen ones in health food stores or the farmers market.
Pizza	Try making a dairy-free cauliflower crust with sliced roasted tomatoes, basil, and olive oil. If you are absolutely craving something cheesy, then try cashew cheese or nutritional yeast.
Candy	Berries or a poached apple or pear. Your sweet cravings will dissolve after a few days on the program, so fret not.
Potatoes	Beets, sweet potatoes, yams, and parsnips.
Cold cuts, sandwiches	Nori-wrapped sandwiches with avocado and protein of choice. Dehydrated coconut wraps and flax wraps are also an option.
Eggs	Substitute the eggs in the recipe for 1 tbsp of ground flax or chia seeds, 2 tbsp arrowroot powder, or agar with a bit of water.

Your Detox Arsenal

- Detox protein smoothie powder
- Fiber powder
- Greens powder
- Detox herbs/vitamins (omega-3 fish oil and vitamin D3)

I've done this cleanse many times myself, and I've supported many women through it. One thing I've noticed is that if breakfast is taken care of, the rest of the day falls into place much easier. The quickest and most satisfying breakfast is what I call the "detox smoothie." The main components are water or some kind of vegan milk, one to two scoops of detox protein powder, one scoop of greens, and one tablespoon of flaxseeds or chia seeds. Make a substantial-sized shake for breakfast so that you have some left over for a morning or afternoon snack. The detox smoothie powders are packed with nutrients and are easy to digest. (You can find my preferred brands in appendix E.) They are sold by licensed integrative medical doctors, acupuncturists, and naturopathic doctors. If you aren't currently under the care of a practitioner, then you can purchase from christinaburns.com or https://naturnalife.com. When using a detox smoothie, I advise adding a fiber to the mix to latch onto toxins for easier elimination. Try a premade fiber powder, or you can opt for a tablespoon of chia or fresh ground flaxseeds. To spruce up the taste, try adding other diet-friendly foods to your blender, like blueberries, steamed pumpkin, cinnamon, almond butter, coconut, spinach, avocado, or hemp milk. A well-balanced smoothie will contain nutritious and colorful veggies, fruits, healthy fat, and a liquid such as water or unsweetened vegan milks (almond milk, coconut milk, and so on).

In addition to smoothies, incorporate plenty of cleansing herbal teas throughout all three weeks. Burdock, dandelion, and milk thistle are great for your liver, while nettle, raspberry leaf, and red clover are wonderful for your

Smoothies Not Your Jam?

Here are some other detox supplements that are incredibly effective at digging out and eliminating toxins while supporting your organ systems rather than taxing them:

1. *Unda drops.* This is a gentle homeopathic preparation to help the liver, digestive system, and kidneys drain out junk. Daily dosage is five to 10 drops three times per day.
2. *Gentian root.* This Chinese herb is a heavy-duty liver detoxifier. It also helps to kill off yeasts and bad bacteria. Daily dosage of this bitter tincture is 10 drops twice per day. Seek out a qualified practitioner to help you pair it with a Chinese herbal formula. Virtual and in-person consultations are available through naturnalife.com or christinaburns.com.
3. *Gemmotherapy.* This type of herbal medicine uses a combination of remedies to assist elimination at a cellular level in the liver and kidneys. Examples are *Juniperus communus*, *Rosmarinus*, and *Ribes nigrum* at a dosage of 50 drops three times per day. It's best to have a prescription from a trained professional.

reproductive health. These herbal beverages are cleansing and nutritious and can be consumed liberally during your three-week program. Drink two or more cups per day and feel free to try any number of combinations. You can also add dried hibiscus flowers, rose petals, mint, or lavender and cool the tea to room temperature if you want a souped-up version of iced tea.

In all honesty, you may feel awful this week. It could involve a foul mood. I'm talking *hangry*. Also, don't be surprised if you experience headaches, body aches, and fatigue, especially if you are typically a heavy caffeine drinker or a sugar hound. The icky feelings are a withdrawal response. To reduce their severity, drink extra water and try out an acupuncture session. You'll probably have urges to quit, and those around you may tell you

> Consult your health care practitioner if any of the initial symptoms become overwhelming or if you have any concerns.

to jump ship. Don't be fooled. These are all signs that your body is detoxifying. After the initial feeling of lethargy, most people report increased energy, better mood, clearer skin, and improved sleep quality. Many also drop a few pounds of unwanted weight.

Remember why you're doing this and keep your eye on the prize. Slap a sticky note on your laptop, set reminders in your phone, and tape a mantra to your mirror. Surround yourself with positive affirmations and reminders that you are on the right track. Do not

> Incorporate mindfulness into your daily routine via guided or quiet meditation. It will help you stay centered and focused.

let little bumps psyche you out. Feeling like crap means it's working.

Week 1 Pro Tips

Try out one or more of the following to help combat the potential for fatigue, cravings, or low mood you may encounter this week. These enhancements also encourage your body to process and eliminate those toxins faster:

- Acupuncture sessions one or more times per week.
- Thirty-minute sessions of any moderate, low-intensity exercise three times per week. Yoga preferred.
- Ear seeds. Ask for the National Acupuncture Detoxification Association protocol or purchase through an online vendor.

A Snapshot from Week 1

This week, try getting up 10 or 15 minutes early, giving you plenty of time to whip up a breakfast smoothie and throw snacks in your bag. If strapped for time or uninspired by your blender, you can just throw a couple scoops of smoothie powder into a jar or travel cup with some nut milk, greens, and fiber. Shake and voila! Your meal is ready.

Sample Day:

Breakfast: Smoothie or broccoli and feta omelet with toast (recipe in appendix C)
Snack: Pumpkin seeds, blueberries
Lunch: Quinoa salad (recipe in appendix C), dandelion tea
Exercise: Thirty minutes of a yoga or barre class
Snack: Leftover smoothie
Midday detox booster: One acupuncture session
Dinner: Baked salmon and veggies (recipe in appendix C) with steamed broccoli or bone broth
Vegetarian option—ultra-alkalizing vegetable soup (recipe in appendix C)
Evening booster: Castor oil pack, 30 to 45 minutes
Reminders: Drink two quarts of water and reduce animal protein portions to two to three ounces

WEEK 2

You've made it through week 1. Congratulations! This is the week things start turning around. You are adapting well, and your resolve is strengthened. When doubts creep in, envision the results you're working toward: an elated mood, plentiful energy, increased focus, and a baby bump!

> Should low energy and fatigue persist into this week, avoid strenuous physical activity.

Week 2 is your vegetarian week. We eliminate all animal products except for your cup of broth. Detox smoothies, nuts, and legumes are your sources of protein this week. Less animal foods help to reduce the burden on your digestion and allow for a deeper detox.

Portions are the next thing to cut. Reduce your typical breakfast and lunch by one-third and aim to have soup or broth for dinner. Try to make the soup or broth yourself to avoid the salt and additives you'll encounter in store-bought versions. It's also imperative to

> This week, increase your smoothie intake to twice daily. Drink the first as breakfast. The second can be either lunch or your afternoon snack (I recommend the latter, as most people have a blood sugar dip that requires nourishing in the mid- to late afternoon).

consume bone broth fresh or not at all. It's a high-histamine food that can become increasingly inflammatory if left to breed bacteria. Even homemade broths shouldn't sit in the fridge longer than three days. For convenience, freeze individual portions for a lengthier shelf life.

> If you're naturally on the skinny side and find it harder to gain weight than lose it, a restrictive diet can make you too trim. You want to focus on *maintaining* your weight, not shedding pounds. So pay extra attention and add more rich fats like seed butters, avocado, and coconut to your diet if you feel the cleanse may cause you to drop too much weight.

You will likely feel hungry this week, and snacks will seem very appealing. You'll want to minimize the noshing to allow your digestive system to cleanse and rest. This is where more liquids come in. Lots of lemon water, broth, herbal tea, and smoothies will keep you satisfied. Remember, your body often mistakes thirst for hunger. If you want a little something more, add almond or another vegan milk to herbal tea (herbal chai, rooibos, or chamomile) to satisfy the cravings. It doesn't sound like it will do the trick, but it really does. Your willpower just has to get you through making the cup of tea.

Keep up your acupuncture and exercise sessions from week 1. These practices not only make you feel great but will also dramatically reduce cravings. If time and budget allow, add a cupping,

> Ask your acupuncturist for ear seeds to curb your hunger pangs and control cravings.

infrared sauna, or lymphatic drainage session to assist the detox process.

Although challenging, this is the week you'll likely start feeling (and looking) much better. The sense of accomplishment is also very satisfying. Seeing the results will make the process more bearable.

A Snapshot from Week 2

This week, make sure you drink more fluids so you have fewer urges to snack. Make heartier smoothies and soups to further curb your hunger.

Sample Day:

Breakfast: Cleansing smoothie or coconut yogurt fruit parfait (recipe in appendix C)
Lunch: Alkalizing soup, steamed or roasted veggies (recipe in appendix C)
Midday detox booster: Acupuncture session or an infrared sauna
Snack: Cleansing smoothie (assorted recipes in appendix C)
Dinner: Broth, soup, cooked veggies, and herbal tea

WEEK 3

Now you're feeling great, and you know what you're doing. You've got this. Stay the course. You are already through most of the heavy lifting. Carry on with the one or two detox smoothies daily and continue to hydrate with water and tea. There are only a few minor adjustments for this week:

1. You can reintroduce animal foods three times total this week (two- to three-ounce portions), testing your reaction to them.
2. Add one deep-tissue or lymphatic drainage massage to your one or two acupuncture sessions and one or two sauna sessions.
3. As you move closer to the end of the week, you can start to increase your portions but ask yourself if you need to fully return to your old norms. We North Americans are famous for overeating, and the body often does better with less. There is a saying in India: "To overeat is to feed disease." The point is that if you know you were overdoing your portions, don't go back to that just because it is familiar. Be aware of your choices, beliefs, and habits. The Conception Cleanse is as much for your mind as it is for your body.

This week, you'll feel excellent, so take some time to relish it.

A Snapshot from Week 3

By now, you've got a handle on things. Stick to what makes you feel the most satisfied and pay close attention to how much food you need to feel full so you don't overdo it.

Sample Day:

Breakfast smoothie: Cleansing smoothie
Snack: Nuts, seeds, chia pudding, or coconut yogurt for emergency cravings
Lunch: Soup *or* baked chicken or fish with quinoa and sautéed greens
Midday detox booster: Deep-tissue massage or yoga session
Snack: Cleansing smoothie
Dinner: Roasted veggies and soup

Slow and Steady: Coming Off the Cleanse

Where to go from here? You recognize that you feel (and look) amazing on the cleanse, but continuing a full detox diet for the rest of your life may sound like some form of cruel torture. If you don't think it's sustainable in the long term, that's okay; this type of lifestyle isn't for everyone. You do, however, want to avoid overindulging, or you run the risk of quickly reversing some of the positive changes you've achieved. It's important to come off your detox slowly. Your body is no longer used to eating the way you did before, so if you reintroduce all your old favorites suddenly, you may experience uncomfortable stomach pains, diarrhea, and so on. Yo-yo diets or cleanses will give only momentary benefits and may cause more harm than good.

Instead of swinging the pendulum back to where you started, I recommend an 80/20 percent rule: 80 percent sticking with the program and 20 percent flexibility to play around. This will keep you empowered and on track. Clarity and emotional health are key in helping you to cope with the fertility journey.

To best maintain your newfound state of reproductive health, add in originally restricted vegetables and fruits the first few days. After a few more days, reintroduce a red meat. Several days later, you might try a refined grain product, such as bread or pasta. If you notice irritation, like bloating, abdominal pain, gastrointestinal issues, and so on, it means your body is giving you a loud and clear signal that these foods might trigger inflammatory responses in you. This phase is the perfect opportunity to explore hidden food sensitivities by gradually reintroducing one food (such as wheat, milk, cheese, or sugar) on one day and then waiting three to five days before trying another. You will learn a lot about your compatibility with various foods and drinks if you do opt for this gradual reintroduction method. By reintroducing one new thing every three to five days, it's easier to form a clear picture of which foods are hindering your health. Avoid adding in multiple foods from different categories all at once. For example, on your first girls' night out after finishing the diet, don't reintroduce pasta, wine, and gelato in the same meal.

Dairy, gluten, and sugar are items that I recommend keeping very minimal, if you must consume them at all. Refined sugar should be avoided completely. If consuming gluten, then lean into sprouted, sourdough, or spelt items, as they are generally less of an offense to your system. Adjusting your intake to small amounts of organic, grass-fed, raw dairy is acceptable. Kefir and unsweetened yogurt are also okay in moderation as long as you don't have a dairy allergy (mild or otherwise). They are easier on the stomach because the lactose and proteins have been broken down by beneficial bacteria and/or yeasts. Feta and sheep or goat cheeses are also less reactive in similar fashion.

If you suffer from autoimmune or inflammatory conditions like endometriosis or PCOS, you may want to consider staying on a modified version of this diet to best care for your health moving forward. These conditions are greatly influenced by what you consume. Eating clean will help your fertility as well as diminish unpleasant symptoms.

Easy does it. Relax, rearrange your diet slowly, and celebrate the fact that you've reset your entire system in just three weeks.

Delayed Gratification

The Conception Cleanse is a major step forward in clearing subtle barriers to conception. My hope is that in discovering a newfound state of health, some of the principles you've learned here will carry over into your everyday life.

Halfway through the cleanse, you will be feeling much improved. By the end of three weeks, you'll feel brand new. A great deal of healing has taken place, and you've likely broken some bad habits and formed new, healthy ones. Your body will begin functioning with more ease, creating a more ideal environment for conception.

The key to moving forward is sustainability. Since most of us don't foresee being on a cleanse forever as a viable option, I've dedicated the next chapter as a guide on how to eat in sync with your cycle to optimize your hormonal health and fertility.

CHAPTER 9

Woman Food

Food has the ability to hinder as well as to heal. I have witnessed this statement's truth on many levels, both personally and professionally. When I began incorporating more dietary counseling into my sessions, my clinical results improved dramatically. Similarly, my own body was healed largely through conscious diet changes.

There is an ancient Chinese proverb that eloquently states, "To neglect the diet is to waste the time of the physician." No medication out there will make your daily food habits obsolete. We rely far too much on conventional medicine to provide solutions via pharmaceuticals and invasive procedures while rarely pondering how our daily choices might be playing a role in our struggles.

Our bodies respond in amazing ways when we take in the proper nutrition. In this chapter, you'll find an informative melding of Eastern dietary principles and Western science-based nutrition to guide you. You'll get the scoop on fertility-boosting foods and how to eat to optimize the phases of your cycle.

Food has the power to do the following:

- Improve ovulatory function
- Improve egg quality and implantation rates (Nehra et al. 2012)
- Reduce incidence of miscarriage
- Improve IVF outcomes
- Improve mood, energy, sleep, and so on
- Lower inflammation
- Lower immune disturbances
- Balance blood sugar
- Reduce stress
- Improve sperm quality

Nutrition Basics

There are two key kinds of nutrients: *macronutrients* and *micronutrients*. The macro (aka "major") nutrients are fats, carbs, and proteins—the three most basic components of any diet.

Carbohydrates give you energy and can take many forms, such as sugars, starches, and fibers commonly found in grains, fruits, vegetables, and dairy products. Fiber-rich and low-glycemic carbs are preferred. Fibrous food flushes toxins and xenoestrogens, while low-glycemic (aka less likely to spike blood sugar) foods have been linked to improved fertility (Chavarro et al. 2007c).

> Healthy carb sources are fibrous greens like collards and brussels sprouts as well as low-glycemic foods like quinoa, sweet potatoes, and apples.

Proteins are the building blocks in foods such as meat, eggs, nuts, and beans. They are essential in building and maintaining healthy cell tissue. When choosing your proteins, aim for a blend of plant and animal. In fact, higher amounts of vegetable-based protein in place of animal-based protein is associated with a nearly 50 percent lower risk of infertility (Chavarro et al. 2008).

> Some of the best protein sources are lentils, almonds, and wild salmon.

Fats are the body's tools for building nerve tissue, like the brain, and hormones. The type of fats you consume matters a great deal. Trans fats like hydrogenated vegetable oils or charred animal fats are bad for fertility, reducing your chances of conception by more than 50 percent (Chavarro et al. 2007a). This is thanks to the inflammatory response they trigger. Instead, choose hormone-healthy food rich in omega-3s from seeds, nuts, and fish (Nehra et al. 2012).

> The best fats for fertility are omega-3s. You'll find them in foods like wild fish and flaxseed.
>
> Nehra et al. (2012)

It's from a balance of these three macronutrients that you derive energy for all your body's processes. A diet deficient in macros can lead to fatigue, low immunity, neurological disorders, and reproductive issues, such as ovulatory infertility, low-quality eggs, or poor embryo growth (Chavarro et al. 2007c).

When you hear the word "nutrient," you probably think of vitamins and minerals. Those are "micronutrients," such as iron, magnesium, vitamin C, and folic acid. You need far lesser quantities of micronutrients than macronutrients, but maintaining healthy ratios of vitamins and minerals is essential to overall

Minding Your BMI

Our weight can be a determining factor in how quickly and easily we get pregnant. As a general rule, it's best to stick within the following parameters:

- Low BMI (<20 kg/m²)
- High BMI (>25 kg/m²)

Veleva et al. (2008)

health and fertility. For example, magnesium regulates the DNA and RNA synthesis necessary to produce a chromosomally normal egg. It also regulates sleep cycles, inflammation, and production of the most potent antioxidant, glutathione. These factors translate to a healthier environment for eggs to develop and embryos to implant. Micronutrient deficiency can manifest as fatigue and weakness, heart palpitations, depression, tingling in the muscles and joints, poor concentration, and menstrual issues, such as anovulatory cycles or very heavy periods.

In the pages to follow, I outline a system to guide you on what specific foods and nutrients are most important to support the hormones present in each cycle phase.

An Eastern Perspective

In place of the macro- and micronutrient principles, Eastern medicine describes food energetically. Foods are categorized using the Five Natures, which denote the properties: nourishing, warming, cooling, moving, and contracting. These principles are incredibly helpful for treating women's health and fertility because the descriptions of the foods' "natures" easily match up with the needs of a woman's cycle. Each phase has its own energetic qualities. The menstrual phase is assisted "moving," "warming," or "cooling"; the follicular phase is building resources for "nourishing" the egg; ovulation is rooted in "moving" the egg; and the luteal phase focuses on "warming" the uterus for implantation.

Next, all foods are classified under the Five Flavors, or the "taste" of each food: pungent, sweet, sour, bitter, and salty. The Flavor defines the action the food takes in the body. For example, pungent flavors fight cold and flu and move circulation, while salty flavors soften masses and promote bowel movement. Everybody needs a different combination of these actions in order to best balance their body's unique energetic makeup.

Getting in Sync

Syncing these nutritional principles to promote hormonal balance is a powerful way to enhance fertility. It helps you connect with the phases of your cycle and become better attuned to your body's needs throughout the month.

Phase Recap

- **Menstruation (days 1 to 3):** Hormone production slows down to reboot.
- **Follicular (days 3 to 13):** Estrogen begins to steadily rise and take over.
- **Ovulation (days 13 to 15):** Estrogen reaches its peak, and LH surges to release that egg.
- **Luteal (days 15 to 28):** This is the progesterone-dominant phase wherein your body readies a cozy place for a fertilized egg to implant.

Reminder: Your cycle may look slightly different in terms of the exact days you enter each phase, but this is a guideline for the general progression of the phases. Varying hormonal profiles require their own unique nutritional profiles. Track your cycle to get the clearest picture of when you're experiencing each phase.

SUPPORT THE FLOW

Menstruation is the phase when your hormones flatline and reboot. The sudden nosedive in progesterone and estrogen levels causes you to shed your lining to start anew, resulting in the arrival of your period. The nutritional approach for this phase can be broken down into the following principles:

Macro focus: healthy fats and lean protein
Micro focus: iron, vitamin C, omega-3
Nature focus: moving and building

Most women are prone to iron and other mineral deficiencies during menstruation because we lose nutrients via our menstrual blood. Those dealing with heavy periods may become more deficient or even anemic. That said, if you have very light periods, it makes sense to address why your body didn't have the resources to build a healthy lining in the first place.

Eastern medicine focuses on "moving" and "building" blood during the menstrual phase. Therefore, your diet during menstruation should be packed with mineral-dense foods, vitamins, and nutrients to help replace the nutrition lost through menses. It's also helpful to assist the circulation in your uterus with "warming/moving" spices and castor oil with heat packs (see appendix C).

Inflammation has a tendency to rear its ugly head in the menstrual phase. The massive drop in hormones may bring with it heavy or painful periods, fatigue, headache, and/or body pain. For this reason, when adjusting your diet to suit the menstrual phase, it makes sense to select foods that assist in reducing inflammation. Foods rich in omega fatty acids are ideal, such as flaxseeds, sardines, and wild salmon (the skin of the salmon is actually where most of the good fats reside).

> Cinnamon and ginger can soothe your period pain. Boiling these yummy herbs can help with microcirculation and reduce pain for those with rough periods. For the best effect, combine it with a piece of rock sugar in your cup.

Consider also supplementing with the oil from flaxseeds if you tend to experience really bad periods. Avoid the inflammatory foods listed in chapter 4 both leading up to and during your period.

Nutrient Spotlight: Iron

Our body requires optimal levels of iron to perform many important functions—the production of red blood cells and the distribution of oxygen throughout the body, to name a few. Inadequate levels may cause fatigue, low mood, anxiety, sleep disturbances, and a tendency to bruise easily. For some, it may also be correlated with an inability to lose weight given its relationship with thyroid function. As it pertains to fertility, iron deficiency can cause irregularities in ovulation and cycle length, making your fertile window harder to peg. Low levels of this key nutrient also hamper our ability to receive and nurture a pregnancy. It may also be an underlying factor in poor egg quality

> Remember to eat alkaline! Eating high amounts of acidic foods might impact the growth of yeast and bacteria that deplete hormone levels and throw off hormonal balance.

and embryos that fail to thrive. The statistics of iron-deficiency anemia during pregnancy are staggering at 35 to 50 percent of women. Many women enter pregnancy already borderline anemic because their levels appear normal but are in the lower range. If you suspect a deficiency, ask to have your ferritin tested. Low ferritin is an early indicator that your iron stores are low. If levels come back within normal limits, then determine whether it's at the low end of normal. If so, I recommend giving it some attention *before* it falls out of normal limits. Lab tests aside, iron-rich foods are amazing for women's health.

The richest sources of heme iron (the more absorbable form) are found in lean meats and seafood. Organic chicken liver is one of the best sources, though it's understandable why this may be a turnoff for many. If organ meats are too adventurous, eat the dark meat of chicken, as it's higher in iron than the white meat (i.e., breast). Organic, grass-fed bison, venison, and lamb are great additional sources. The less absorbable form, nonheme iron, is still worth seeking out and can be found in nuts, beans, and vegetables. Soaking and sprouting nuts and beans in advance of consuming them can help make their nutrition more absorbable. If you are a vegetarian, then aim to incorporate beet powder into smoothies and eat lots of spinach and sprouted pumpkin seeds.

Table 9.1. Food Sources of Iron

Foods	Amount	Iron
Bison and lamb	3 oz.	3.2 mg
Nuts (cashew, pine, hazelnut, raw red-skinned peanut, almond)	1 oz.	1.7 mg
Dark leafy greens	1 cup	6 mg
Dark chocolate	1 square (29 g)	5 mg
Beans	1 cup cooked	6.6 mg
Pumpkin seeds	1 oz.	4.24 mg

Supporting Nutrients

Other important nutrients for the menstrual phase are those that assist the absorption of iron and support the rise in estrogen as we transition into the follicular phase. During our monthly flow, we are building resources that benefit the growth and development of our precious eggs.

Vitamin C

In addition to aiding proper red blood cell formation, vitamin C increases the absorption of iron, especially from plant sources (nonheme iron). It is also highly anti-inflammatory and reduces free radical damage to cells (i.e., egg quality!).

Antioxidants such as vitamins C, E, and A fend against oxidative stress associated with menstruation and painful periods. They also help create a happy environment in which your eggs can grow.

Table 9.2. Food Sources of Vitamin C

Foods	Amount	Vitamin C
Red peppers	½ cup chopped	95 mg
Kale	1 cup	80 mg
Brussels sprouts	½ cup cooked	48 mg
Broccoli	½ cup cooked	51 mg
Grapefruit	½ cup	43 mg

Omega-3

These fats have long been touted for their incredible health benefits. In more recent years, the research has expanded beyond cardiovascular health into the realm of fertility. Omega-3s pack potent anti-inflammatory and antioxidant effects and are excellent for soothing period pain. They provide building blocks for healthy hormone production and growth of eggs. Omega-3s are natural blood thinners that aid in implantation. These essential fats also enhance the development of baby's IQ in utero. With all these benefits, I suggest consuming omega-3–rich foods from the beginning of your cycle. Think fatty cold-water fish, nuts, and seeds to boost your reserves. Find more on the benefits of these magic fats in chapters 11 and 12.

Table 9.3. Food Sources of Omega-3

Foods	Amount	Omega-3
Sardines	3 oz.	2 g
Anchovies	3 oz.	1.4 g
Walnuts	1 oz.	2.5 g
Chia seeds	1 oz.	5 g
Flaxseeds	1 tbsp.	1.8 g

Menstruation Munchies—Wisdom from the East

Traditional Chinese medicine suggests the following iron- and mineral-rich foods to "build blood." The recommendations also include "moving foods" to increase circulation, reduce inflammation, and promote a full discharge of the uterine lining. These foods are intended to be added in small amounts to an overall recipe. Most of the foods listed would be prepared in soup, congee, or stew:

- **Veggies:** Squash, sweet potato, turnip, eggplant, beets, spinach
- **Fats:** Ghee, coconut milk, anchovy, chestnut, almonds, black sesame, coconut oil, pumpkin seed oil
- **Fruits:** Date, longan, papaya, peach, hawthorn berry, blackberries, cherries
- **Proteins:** Black beans, lentils, aduki bean, egg, trout, chicken, eel, prawns, sturgeon, sardine, tuna, salmon, pumpkin seeds, duck, venison
- **Grains:** Oats, rice
- **Flavors (small amounts):** Amasake, apple cider vinegar, nutmeg, ginger, chive, coriander, fennel, basil, black pepper, turmeric

FOODS TO AVOID DURING MENSTRUATION

Menstruation is the female body's monthly cleansing process. As such, what you eat in this phase should be easy to digest and assist the cleansing. The body's energy is naturally lower and less tolerant of misbehavior in this phase. This means ignoring those period cravings and laying off foods that are heavy, greasy, or rich in refined sugars and carbs.

Recap

1. Eliminate foods that irritate and inflame.
2. Reduce the burden.
3. Aid elimination.

Nutrient Blockers

To fully reap the benefits of your new diet, you want to assist your body's absorption of the iron-rich foods you're eating. We've talked about foods that aid absorption, but we must also touch on substances that block absorption so that you consume less of them. The major culprits are tannins, oxalic acid, phytates, gluten, and calcium. These compounds are found naturally in foods and drinks such as bitter teas (black, green, and rooibos), coffee, corn, grapes, whole grains (wheat and barley), legumes, alcohol, nuts, seeds (sprouted versions okay), chocolate, and dairy products. So what's left to eat, right?! My recommendation is simply not to gorge on the previously mentioned foods during your menses, but

Recipe No-Nos—Wisdom from the East

Eastern nutrition categorizes some foods as "cold" and some as "warm." When trying to conceive, especially when in the menstrual phase, you should generally aim for more "warming" types of foods since infertility in Chinese medicine is often classified as a "cold" uterus. Foods that are "warm" in nature can help to increase circulation and reduce period pain. "Cold" types of foods are thought to lead to more clots, cramping, and pain. Raw or icy items in any food group should be avoided. For the smoothest sailing through your menstrual phase, keep the following to a minimum:

- **Veggies:** Mushrooms, radishes, seaweed, cabbage, celery, bean sprouts
- **Fruits:** Bananas, strawberries, tomatoes, pineapples, melons, mandarins, lemons
- **Proteins:** Tofu, oysters, crab, clams
- **Fats:** Dairy products

a serving here and there is fine. Also, in many cases, these unwanted substances can be reduced by timing your consumption, such as not eating calcium-rich foods like cheese or yogurt in the same meal with iron-rich meats, seeds, and greens. Finally, seek variety rather than relying on one or two foods to give you your full iron and mineral intake.

NOURISH AND BUILD

In the *follicular* phase, your hormones power back up, and estrogen takes the lead. Your pituitary gland releases FSH to tickle those ovarian follicles (eggs) to grow. The technical term for this steady build is "anabolic" mode. In this phase, we want to impart the proper building blocks for your hormones and proper DNA and RNA synthesis for healthy eggs. Nutritional principles for health development of eggs include the following:

Macro focus: Fats and protein
Micro focus: Folate, vitamin B12, vitamin D
Nature focus: Cooling, sweet

Healthy proteins and fats are the macronutrient focus of the follicular phase. You can get away with eating more animal foods at this stage, so meat lovers can enjoy high-quality products such as grass-fed beef, lamb, bison, venison, ostrich, dark meat chicken, duck, and turkey. All are rich in iron and B vitamins. Fatty fish are great here, too. If you are a vegetarian or simply prefer to eat less meat, you can turn to plant sources such as sprouted legumes, nuts, and seeds. Both diet preferences come with pros and cons. In one large study, plant-based diets were associated with fewer anovulatory cycles. However, animal proteins pack high levels of vitamin B12, iron, and other supporting micronutrients. Eastern traditions almost always recommend consuming animal foods. The problem with our culture is that we eat highly inflammatory factory-farmed meat and too much of it. Animal proteins are nutrient dense, but they are hard to digest in large quantities and are far more acidic than plant foods.

> The type of protein matters! One study found that women who consumed most of their protein from dairy sources (cheese, eggs, yogurt, and so on) had lower AFC. Yes, that translates to lower egg counts!
>
> Souter et al. (2017)

Personally, I'm an advocate for more veggies and less meat, but it's important to note that as a vegan or vegetarian, you'll have to be very deliberate to get adequate protein, iron, and vitamin B12 in your diet. Unless you are vegetarian for religious or philosophical reasons, I recommend eating small amounts of animal protein a few times per week while maintaining a primarily plant-based diet.

Estrogen is on the rise in this phase, but not all estrogens are equal. To best support the follicular phase, we want to consume healthy phytoestrogens. They're plant compounds that can bind to estrogen receptors and foster healthy estrogen production while blocking the negative effects of bad estrogens (i.e., xenoestrogens). They help you steadily increase your levels to foster egg growth as you approach ovulation. The good

> Flaxseeds supply healthy phytoestrogens and fiber that facilitate the removal of estrogens and improve the ratios of the good to bad estrogens.

kinds are found in oats, flax, apples, alfalfa, carrots, pomegranate, and herbs such as red clover, licorice, and Dang Gui.

Your micronutrient focus for the follicular phase is on vitamins that encourage healthy egg development and estrogen synthesis. For this, we turn to B vitamins such as folate and B12 as well as the "sunny" vitamin D. Let's look deeper into how to get adequate amounts of these through whole foods.

> Near the end of the follicular phase, you'll want to lighten the load of proteins and fats so that your liver and digestive system can better metabolize the shift in hormones that ovulation brings. As you near your ovulation phase, switch to leaner proteins and less saturated fats. This is especially important if you are undergoing IVF or a medicated IUI, as you have more hormones in your body to process.

Yin and Blood Foods—Wisdom from the East

In the follicular phase, your red blood cell counts should be back on the rise, but it never hurts to give them a boost. In Eastern teaching, blood and all bodily fluids are yin substances, which translate to nourishing healthy estrogen levels. The following yin foods will help you achieve the optimal nutritional balance to support the activities and promote optimal hormonal balance in the follicular phase:

- **Veggies:** Zucchini, squash, sweet potatoes, string beans, beets, mushrooms, spinach, carrots
- **Fruits:** Pomegranate, apples, coconut, peaches, melons, grapes, cherries, plums, tomatoes
- **Protein:** Mackerel, egg, rabbit, sardine, octopus, tuna, duck, grass-fed, organic pork and chicken
- **Fats:** Black sesame seeds, almonds, flaxseeds, olive oil, flaxseed oil, almond oil, coconut oil and milk
- **Grains:** Millet
- **Flavors:** Parsley, molasses, nettle, marjoram, vegemite, kelp, spirulina, wheatgrass, miso

Nutrient Spotlight: Folate

Folic acid (aka vitamin B9) is essential in the creation of red blood cells. It's also a major player in the chromosomal development of eggs, and according to research, women taking high levels of folic acid are three times more likely to conceive. In one study, women who took it before IVF produced higher-quality eggs that led to a higher proportion of well-developed embryos, not to mention that 70 to 80 percent of neural tube defects could be avoided by supplementing folate (Boxmeer et al. 2009).

> Vitamin B9's best allies for absorption are vitamins B12 and B6.

You'll find this super vitamin in green foods.

Table 9.4.   Food Sources of Folate

Foods	Amount	Folate
Spinach (boiled)	½ cup	131 mcg
Asparagus	4 spears	89 mcg
Avocado	½ cup	59 mcg
Dried beans	½ cup	50 mcg

Seed Cycling

This nutritional approach to supporting the phases of your cycle uses the rotation of seeds to help you balance your hormones. It suggests using whole food nutrient sources to power the manufacturing and breakdown of hormones. Simply put, you eat flaxseeds and pumpkin seeds during menstruation and the follicular phase to support estrogen production and metabolism. During the ovulation and luteal phases, you eat sesame and sunflower seeds to support progesterone and improve estrogen/progesterone ratios.

In one study, the addition of 5 or 10 grams of ground flaxseed significantly increased urinary 2-OHEstrogen in postmenopausal women, suggesting that there are components of flaxseed capable of inducing estrogen. The lignans in flax also increased the length of the luteal phase in premenopausal women, increasing the chances of a successful implantation. In several other studies, substituting sunflower seeds in place of soybeans in the diets of beef cows both reduced body weight and increased chances of conception.

You can add the seeds to your morning smoothie or your salad, or try raw sprouted seed butters.

Instructions:

- Menstrual/follicular—one tablespoon ground flaxseeds and one tablespoon ground pumpkin seeds daily
- Ovulation/luteal—one tablespoon ground sunflower seeds and one tablespoon ground sesame seeds daily

Inoue et al. (2013)

Supporting Nutrients

Vitamin B12

Like folate, vitamin B12 is necessary for the production of red blood cells. Without it, you can't effectively carry iron and oxygen through your blood to nourish vital reproductive processes. Vitamin B12 deficiency is associated with miscarriage, irregular cycles, poor embryo quality, male infertility, and neural tube defects. Low levels most commonly manifest as fatigue and poor focus, though more severe neurological symptoms have also been noted.

Vitamin B12 is essential in the utilization of folic acid. This is why quality folic acid supplements are combined with vitamins B12 and B6 for best absorption. These three nutrients are needed to break down homocysteine, a naturally occurring amino acid, that in excess causes a great deal of inflammation and potentiates blood clot formation. High levels of homocysteine are implicated in implantation

Table 9.5.   Food Sources of Vitamin B12

Foods	Amount	Vitamin B12
Sardines	3 oz.	3.2 mcg
Grass-fed beef	3 oz.	1.7 mcg
Tuna	3 oz.	6 mcg
Lamb	3 oz.	5 mcg
Salmon	3 oz.	6.6 mcg
Eggs	1 large	0.44 mcg

failure, miscarriage, and pregnancy loss. Vitamin B12 is found mostly in animal sources such as organ meats, beef, lamb, salmon, tuna, and clams. Vegetarians may source it from eggs, nutritional yeast, and fortified foods and drinks. In some cases, supplementation might be helpful to achieve optimal levels.

Vitamin D

This vitamin packs a punch when it comes to fertility, immunity, and mental health. According to research, sufficient vitamin D levels are correlated with a quicker path to conception, while low levels are associated with low fertility. Studies show that women with PCOS benefit from additional vitamin D since lower levels in this population are correlated with delayed conception. Vitamin D deficiency in women with PCOS has been associated with a 67 percent reduced chance of follicle (i.e., egg) development (Lerchbaum and Rabe 2014). In IVF cycles, adequate vitamin D is associated with a thicker endometrial lining and better chance of implantation.

It is sometimes tricky in this day and age to get sufficient amounts of vitamin D through sun exposure. Indoor jobs, polluted skies, and dreary weather can keep us D deficient. Thankfully, it is also found abundantly in fatty fish such as mackerel and salmon as well as in cod liver, beef liver, egg yolk, and some nutrient-enhanced foods like cereals and nut milks. Although I still suggest getting outside as much as possible, it is advantageous to source from food as well as sunlight. I can't begin to tell you how many more women I see become pregnant or have better IVF results in the sunnier months of spring and summer or after a beach vacation!

FOODS TO AVOID DURING THE FOLLICULAR PHASE

The follicular phase is the time of your cycle where healthy fats and protein from fish, organ meats, dark meats, eggs, nuts, and seeds can be plentiful. It is in this

Recipe No-Nos—Wisdom from the East

From an Eastern perspective, eliminate foods that have a "hot" or "pungent" nature. That does not mean giving up heated foods. The hot nature rather correlates to spicy, acidic, or highly sugary foods. Pungent foods are those that can aggravate an already distressed gut or immune system. Here's a short list of hot and pungent foods to eat less of during the follicular phase:

- **Veggies:** Onion, radish, raw spinach
- **Fruits:** Lychee, mango, dates, oranges
- **Protein:** Beef, charred or fried meats, prawns
- **Flavors:** Ginger, garlic, chilies, pepper, cloves

phase that your body will be least reactive to what you eat, giving you the most freedom to play. As in the menstrual phase, avoid high-inflammation foods that will create oxidative stress for the growing eggs (alcohol, fried foods, charred meats, pesticide-treated fruits and veggies, and so on). As you move closer to your fertile window, you'll want to reduce the heavy proteins and raw veggies and lean into lighter, cooked, plant-based options.

HARMONIZE THE TRANSITION

Ovulation is a short phase characterized by a peak in estrogen and a surge in LH, the hormone that "triggers" ovulation. Given the significant transition of hormones at this juncture, place your dietary focus on light, alkaline foods to assist easy digestion. We are avoiding an excess of heavy proteins or fats from red meat or dairy and instead eating warm, cooked plant foods to enhance the free flow of circulation and support the release of the egg. Nutritional principles for ovulation include the following:

Macro focus: Fibrous carbs such as broccoli, brussels sprouts, cauliflower, artichoke
Micro focus: Zinc, vitamin B6
Nature focus: Warming, moving, aromatic

Healthy fiber-filled carbohydrates are your go-to macronutrient in the ovulatory phase. You want to eat foods that are easy to digest so that you can aid your liver and gut as they filter and process the dramatic shift in hormones. Estrogen that built up during the follicular phase will need to be processed by the liver and eliminated through the bowels, hence the focus on fiber-rich foods. If not properly processed, retained estrogen will lead to inflammation, water weight, and nasty PMS in the luteal phase. If you have gas, bloating, or breast tenderness during ovulation, then your liver and guts may benefit from the Conception Cleanse in the prior chapter. Choose light, cooked, and aromatic foods to enhance circulation and elimination. Cooked vegetable sources such as steamed broccoli, cauliflower, brussels sprouts, and kale

> For optimal digestion, you can build good gut flora through small doses of prebiotics and probiotics from artichoke, asparagus, apple cider vinegar, and dandelion.

cleanse the liver with the added benefit of providing fiber that sweeps out estrogen metabolites. Aromatic spices are those that typically assist digestion and improve bloat (refer to box below).

Improve Qi and Embrace Aromatics— Wisdom from the East

A steady flow of energy and circulation assists with a smooth release of the egg. In Eastern medicine, energy is "qi," and the concept of "qi flow" is intertwined with the function of your liver and bowel elimination. If qi is stagnated and the organs of elimination are backed up, your hormonal balance can pay the price. Getting bloated or gassy during your ovulation? These are signs of gut bacteria imbalance, pancreatic insufficiency, and/or liver congestion. We can use healthy, "qi-moving" food choices to prevent these backups and reduce bloat, assist digestion and elimination, and balance your estrogen-to-progesterone ratio in the upcoming luteal phase. Aromatic and lightly pungent foods are good additions because they have a warming and "moving" nature that helps move out congestion (mucus, bad bacteria, and yeast), reduce bloat, and improve circulation:

- **Veggies:** Broccoli, kale, brussels sprouts, cauliflower, mustard greens, cabbage, turnip, dandelion greens and root
- **Fruits:** Lemon, grapefruit, tangerine peel (dried and made into tea)
- **Spices:** Cardamom, basil, cilantro, arugula, coriander seed, fennel, turmeric, cayenne pepper, rosemary, spearmint, thyme, garlic, scallion, ginger, apple cider vinegar, saffron, hawthorn berry (Shan Zha), green tea, raw onions, tarragon, scallions, white and red radish, ginger, peppers, wasabi (dry mustard), horseradish, garlic

Your micronutrient focus in the ovulatory phase builds nicely on what was introduced in the follicular phase. Ovulatory issues have been associated with iron and vitamin B deficiencies, so the previous micronutrient recommendations still apply here. Additions include zinc and B6 for optimal hormone balance. Specifically, zinc aids in the production of LH to help your ovaries "eject" the egg(s), and B6 supports progesterone production for a healthy transition into the luteal phase.

> Selenium is a great boost for sperm quality. Have your partner incorporate chicken, Brazil nuts, and shrimp to improve his motility and morphology. Selenium is also a great nutrient to incorporate in cases of low thyroid function.
>
> Moslemi and Zargar (2011)

pH Balance and Fertility

An overly acidic uterine environment during ovulation can kill off sperm before they reach your egg and allows bad yeasts and bacteria to multiply rapidly. This can worsen endometritis, fibroids, polyps, and other infections that could result in implantation failure or miscarriage. Keeping the pH levels of your uterus alkaline (over 7) through ovulation and into the luteal phase is essential for breeding better egg quality, fertilization, and implantation.

There are tons of great alkaline options in all food categories, but the general rules are as follows.

Consume more:

• Fresh and cooked vegetables
• Cold-pressed oils
• Raw sprouted nuts and seeds
• Water

Consume less:

• Red meat and shellfish
• Oil-roasted nuts and seeds
• Beer, wine, coffee, tea

Nutrient Spotlight: Zinc

Zinc is an incredible mineral for the reproductive health of both women and men. Healthy zinc levels combat male factor infertility by improving sperm parameters. On the female side, zinc plays a significant role in egg maturation and

Table 9.6.   Food Sources of Zinc

Foods	Amount	Zinc
Oysters	1 medium	8.6 mg
Grass-fed beef	1 oz.	3.0 mg
White beans	1 cup cooked	2.9 mg
Lamb	3.5 oz.	4.7 mg
Shiitake mushrooms	1 cup cooked	2.0 mg
Lentils	1 cup cooked	3.0 mg
Pumpkin seeds	1 oz.	2.11 mg

fertilization because of its influence on synthesizing FSH and LH. Zinc *deficiency* in women is implicated in bad PMS, low progesterone, and pregnancy complications such as miscarriage, toxemia, and birth defects (Favier 1992).

Supporting Nutrients

Vitamin B6

This crucial B vitamin is essential for a smooth transition from ovulation into the luteal phase. Vitamin B6 reduces inflammation and hormone chaos that can occur premenstrually by helping to process and eliminate estrogen and to develop the corpus luteum, which is responsible for producing progesterone in your luteal phase. Its diuretic properties assist in managing the fluid retention that may occur around ovulation and the luteal phase. Additionally, it's a necessary cofactor in the production of happy neurotransmitters such as GABA and serotonin. Low levels of these will leave you sleeping poorly and feeling anxious or low. B6 is found in seeds, nuts, poultry, and beans.

Table 9.7.   Food Sources of Vitamin B6

Foods	Amount	Vitamin B6
Turkey breast	3 oz.	0.7 mg
Pistachios	¼ cup	0.5 mg
Pinto beans	1 cup cooked	0.4 mg
Avocado	1 raw	0.4 mg
Sunflower seeds	¼ cup	0.25 mg
Sesame seeds	¼ cup	0.25 mg

FOODS TO AVOID DURING OVULATION

During ovulation, it's important to scale back on heavy fats, heavy proteins, and raw veggies. Raw foods will cause more bloat and gas, creating discomfort and dysbiosis. Oily, fried, and dense fatty foods are too weighty for the liver and gut as they try to work through the significant hormonal transition. These heavy foods require more resources to digest, hindering the "free flow" of energy and circulation required for the smooth release of an egg. If you have estrogen-dominant conditions such as PCOS, cysts, fibroids, or endometriosis, then it's especially important to eat light, fibrous foods and up your hydration for easier elimination in this phase. Without healthy elimination, you may experience miserable side effects such as bloat, weight gain, breast tenderness, painful periods, and mood issues. Sweet, sugary foods and refined carbohydrates also wreak havoc by increasing bad bacteria in the gut and spiking insulin. Besides making you bloated, moody, and pimply, refined foods and sugars can delay ovulation, lead to cyst formation, and diminish uterine receptivity.

What you drink matters as much as what's on your plate. Water is your ally in aiding elimination and cleansing your system. Aim to consume two to three liters daily of purified water.

Limit This Mineral

Not all minerals are wonderful nourishment for the reproductive organs. In excess amounts, some, like sodium, can harm fertility. A diet rich in sodium is associated with increased risk of ovulatory issues. To control sodium intake, you can break the habit of adding salt to your foods, eat at home more, and avoid high-sodium sauces and packaged foods. Restaurants often add a lot of salt to make the food "tastier," so it's tough to avoid when eating out.

Recipe No-Nos—Wisdom from the East

Sweet, cloying, and damp foods, in an Eastern sense, can typically be identified by their sticky texture. Unsurprisingly, many sugary treats fall into this category. Foods of a sweet or cloying nature block the free flow of circulation by creating an excess of inflammation, yeast, and mucus, all of which make you feel bloated and yucky (not to mention that sticky foods are associated with accumulation of masses such as cysts and fibroids):

- **Fruits:** Dried fruit, banana, or excess consumption of any fruits
- **Carbs:** Bread (wheat or white), sticky rice, mochi, cookies, cakes
- **Fats:** Cheese, trans fats

NURTURE THE NEST

The *luteal* phase is marked by the increase in progesterone levels and higher body temperature. This is your "incubation" phase. Progesterone and estrogen are peaking, and your body is primed for implantation. It's a magical time, but it often comes with unwanted symptoms. The luteal phase is when imbalances in the ratio of estrogen and progesterone rear their ugly head (aka estrogen dominance). If you deal with extreme PMS or you're prone to bloating and puffiness during this phase, your gut and liver are asking for some assistance. The symptoms of insulin resistance, thyroid issues, and inflammatory conditions such as endometriosis, fibroids, and PCOS tend to become pronounced in the luteal phase if you are off your mark with nutrition and lifestyle. To keep yourself in balance, eat mostly plants in this phase, with a strong emphasis on cooked leafy greens and healthy starch sources such as butternut squash, sweet potato, and lentils. You'll also find a great improvement in PMS by avoiding inflammatory triggers, eating a moderate amount of healthy fats, and eliminating caffeine and booze altogether. As mentioned in the prior section, you'll benefit if your elimination is on point. Nutritional principles to support a healthy luteal phase include the following:

Macro focus: Fibrous carbs, healthy fats
Micro focus: Magnesium and vitamins E, B6, and C
Nature focus: Dry, warming

Carb Cravings

Many of the women I see report serious carb and fat cravings during the luteal phase. Theoretically, this could be a result of insulin resistance and/or low serotonin. I previously mentioned the research conducted on diabetic women that revealed that they required more insulin during the luteal phase to control their diabetes (Pulido and Salazar 1999). Another study on menstruating women found that those experiencing PMS had trouble controlling their intake of refined foods and sugars. PMS is characterized partially by low mood and anxiety. One of our happy hormones, serotonin, is more deficient in the luteal phase for some women. Those women may crave fast carbs because they provide a temporary boost of serotonin and a consequent feeling of elation (Gil et al. 2009). The problem is that the high comes crashing down and transforms into a low (in both mood and energy). In a similar fashion, fats create a feeling of comfort and satiety, and you are inclined to reach for them when feeling low or stressed. The trouble is that in excess, those heavy fats can be hard to process, leaving you sluggish in body and mind.

For a healthy carb fix, try incorporating complex (slow-burning), high-fiber carbs with lots of water to aid elimination, such as starchy veggies like artichoke, butternut squash, or pumpkin. Get in those healthy fats with cold-pressed olive oil, small amounts of ghee, coconut oil, or sprouted seed and nut butters.

The macro focus in this phase is on high-fiber carbs and healthy fats. Carbs rich in fiber are slow burning and help you produce serotonin, keeping you feeling happy and at ease. The fiber (and water) flush excess estrogens that inflame and aggravate, meaning less discomfort and a better progesterone-to-estrogen ratio. Healthy fats reduce inflammation, thin the blood for enhanced circulation, and satiate you when you are most hungry. Aim to consume lots of dark leafy greens for cleansing, sprouted seeds for hormone balance, and fish for a light, mineral-rich protein. Small amounts of dark meat poultry or game meat are also okay.

Wisdom from the East—A Note on Warmth

The luteal phase is your nesting phase, when any fertilized egg(s) will seek out a place to latch on and nestle in for nourishment. It's essentially incubation, and our food emphasis should support warmth and healthy circulation. We also want to combat "dampness," meaning the formation of excess yeast and bacteria that can occur with luteal hormonal changes. The following foods assist in supporting circulation, warmth, and optimal bacterial balance:

- **Veggies:** Celery, lettuce, scallion, turnip, squash, sweet potatoes, yam, pumpkin
- **Fruits:** Raspberries, dates, figs, longan, cherry
- **Proteins:** Aduki beans, lamb, pistachios, shrimp, anchovy, beef, venison, chicken
- **Fats:** Walnut, chestnut, pistachio, pine nut
- **Grains:** Oats, amaranth, quinoa
- **Flavors:** Licorice, basil, chive seed, dill seed, garlic, sage, star anise, cinnamon bark, fennel seed, ginger (dried), thyme, clove, nutmeg, rosemary, fenugreek seed, peppermint

Your micronutrient focus revolves around optimizing uterine receptivity for the best chances of implantation. In your luteal phase, seek out sources of vitamins E and C to support progesterone production and improve circulation to your uterine lining. For your preferred mineral, turn to magnesium,

> Remember that vitamin B6 helps break down excess estrogen, regulate mood, and diminish fluid retention.

which helps improve bowel movements, increase circulation, and calm the nerves that tend to arise over the two-week wait.

Nutrient Spotlight: Magnesium

Magnesium plays an essential role in creating energy, protein, and DNA. It's an especially helpful nutrient in the luteal phase because of its role in tissue growth.

Table 9.8. Food Sources of Magnesium

Foods	Amount	Magnesium
Avocado	1 medium	58 mg
Cashew	1 oz. dry roasted	82 mg
Black bean	1 cup cooked	120 mg
Tofu	3.5 oz.	53 mg
Spinach	1 cup cooked	157 mg
Banana	1 large	37 mg
Salmon	1 fillet	106 mg
Chia seeds	1 oz.	95 mg

Magnesium is therefore vital in the formation of a healthy uterine lining. Given its more than 300 functions in our body, including a role as a nervous system "conductor," healthy levels are crucial for hormonal balance, sleep, digestion, stress relief, and more. In the luteal phase, it will help you stave off that carb-fueled insulin resistance by acting as an insulin sensitizer. It has also been shown to positively influence IVF suc-

> Sunflower and sesame seeds help you metabolize sex hormones during the luteal phase to keep progesterone and estrogen in balance.

cess rates and assist thyroid function (Stuefer, Moncayo, and Moncayo 2015). Magnesium is found in nuts, seeds, legumes, avocados, and dark leafy vegetables.

Supporting Nutrients

Vitamin E

Vitamin E is an antioxidant that dilates blood vessels to increase circulation and thicken your uterine lining. It also helps form the placenta after implantation. Maintaining healthy levels will aid immune system function while lowering inflammation and oxidative stress. Deficiency of this nutrient, on the other hand, can lead to poor estrogen detoxification. Women with low vitamin E levels often have elevated estrogen levels, which increases the risk of growths such as cysts, fibroids, and endometriosis,

> Antioxidants may prevent or delay cell damage.

not to mention breast cancer! The blood-thinning effect of this fatty nutrient is helpful to build uterine lining and foster implantation. Up your vitamin E intake by adding nuts, seeds, and vegetables like pumpkin and squash to your meals.

Table 9.9. Food Sources of Vitamin E

Foods	Amount	Vitamin E
Spinach	½ cup cooked	1.9 mg
Tomato	1 medium	0.7 mg
Almonds	1 oz. dry roasted	6.8 mg
Hazelnuts	1 oz. dry roasted	4.3 mg
Kiwi	1 medium	1.1 mg

Remember, vitamin C is a potent protector against free radical damage. In the luteal phase, it offers the added benefits of supporting progesterone production, boosting immunity, and reducing inflammation.

Henmi et al. (2003)

Tips for Treating Estrogen Dominance

By the midway point of the luteal phase, if your body isn't effectively metabolizing estrogen and/or you are under-producing progesterone, you are likely to face the unpleasantness of estrogen dominance: painful periods, mood issues, and fluid retention. The following estrogen detoxifiers work great in conjunction with a high-fiber, alkaline diet:

- *Magnesium.* This mineral supports two major estrogen detox pathways, but women are often deficient in magnesium due to dietary and hormonal issues. Adding 250 to 300 milligrams before bed helps you break down estrogen and reduce PMS symptoms.
- *I3C.* This natural compound protects estrogen-sensitive tissues as well as helping you metabolize estrogen.
- *Vitamin B6.* Not only does this vitamin get rid of estrogens, it can also decrease the sensitivity of your estrogen receptor, decreasing your body's inflammatory response to estrogens and the consequent side effects.

Trister (2013)

Veggies and Goitrogens

Cruciferous foods like broccoli, kale, and brussels sprouts are healthy foods great for alkalinity, fiber intake, and cleansing nutrients. However, the raw forms commonly contain goitrogens, which can hinder your thyroid's ability to use iodine, a key building block for hormones such as T3 and T4. Excess consumption of goitrogenic food can result in hypothyroidism and even grow a goiter! (That's a lump in the front of the neck commonly seen in malnourished populations.) Cooking them reduces the goitrogens while allowing your body to more easily access their nutrition.

FOODS TO AVOID DURING THE LUTEAL PHASE

During the luteal phase, constipation, mood issues, and bloat are very common. Maintaining healthy elimination, lowering inflammation, and keeping insulin balanced is the crux of improving hormonal wellness in this phase. Steer away from acid-forming foods and drinks like chocolate, coffee, seltzer, wine, beer, or anything deep fried to keep inflammation under wraps. Make sure to also keep insulin-spiking and yeast-forming foods like ice cream, bread, cookies, cakes, or excess tropical or dried fruits to a minimum.

Itchy Lady Parts before Your Period?

If you find yourself scratching more in the luteal phase, the culprit could be yeast overgrowth (aka candida). In Eastern medicine, this is referred to as "dampness." The proliferation of yeasts and bacteria is caused by overconsuming "sweet" foods, refined carbohydrates, alcohols, and some fermented foods. Overeating raw or cold foods can also contribute to yeast infections by stagnating digestion and nutrient absorption. The following foods cause candida overgrowth:

- **Veggies:** Sweet potato, yam, taro
- **Fruits:** Lychee
- **Carbs:** Beer, wheat
- **Fats:** Peanuts, cheese
- **Other:** Ice cream, wine, kombucha, vinegar, yeast, mushrooms

Feeling Fat? Reduce the Salt!

High salt intake is associated with high FSH in the follicular phase (leading to poor egg development) and low progesterone in the luteal phase (implantation issues, fluid retention, and estrogen dominance) (Kim et al. 2018). Packaged foods like frozen dinners and chips contain alarming amounts of sodium. If you need a salty kick, sprinkle a bit of sea salt onto your food only *after* cooking. Even better, kelp, dulse, and celery salt add a salty taste without adding sodium.

Hunger tends to be an issue for many in this phase. This is generally due to issues with insulin sensitivity brought about by the hormonal shift. If you've already eaten yet find yourself trolling the cupboards, try first reaching for an herbal tea, glass of water, broth, or soup. If the craving feels insatiable, then I find a date dipped in almond butter can do the trick.

Green tea is a good option to curb appetite, control weight, and give you a mini caffeine boost. I prefer the clean, extended energy that it gives over the high from coffee. In addition to its amazing antioxidant capacity, green tea is anti-inflammatory, controls insulin resistance, and contains probiotics that help you poop.

Sync Up

Your body is designed to create and nurture life. Sustaining a diet that supports the natural rhythm of womanhood is one of the best ways not only to speed the path to conception but also to support your hormonal health for the long haul. Although the nutritional advice is broken down into phases, I want to emphasize the importance of eating a varied diet and getting all these nutrients throughout the cycle. For example, zinc is listed in the ovulation phase, but having adequate amounts of zinc in advance of ovulation is necessary for the healthy growth of eggs, not to mention it helps fight PMS in the luteal phase. Similarly, magnesium is listed in the luteal phase, but it is beneficial for egg maturation in the follicular phase. Eat a variety of healthy foods throughout your cycle, and don't get stuck in the weeds trying to sync things perfectly. By incorporating some of the information you've gleaned in this chapter, you can start making food work for you and your fertility. In the next chapter, we'll explore how to adopt a lifestyle conducive to conception via exercise and mindfulness.

CHAPTER 10

The Yin and Yang of Your Daily Routine

Eastern medicine maintains that disease begins when there is disharmony in one's daily habits and lifestyle. The *Huang Di Nei Jing*, the earliest and most respected text on traditional Chinese medicine, describes how your environment, your spiritual health, and your lifestyle work together to dictate the quality of your entire existence. The theory holds that, for the most part, we have the power to manage our health with mindful decision making. In essence, taking charge of your fertility means taking responsibility for your daily choices.

But in true modern fashion, we all want results fast. Dr. Google says there's a quick fix for everything. Bandage solutions are only one search or click away. Fad diets, cure-all vitamins, gimmicks, and gadgets abound, all claiming to solve your problems in a snap. These speedy schemes exist in every niche, and fertility is no exception. But no singular app, diet, workout, supplement, prescription, or procedure is going to solve everything. After uncovering the hidden effects of the Big Four, you're now aware that your habitual lifestyle has a huge impact on your reproductive health.

Receive, Conceive

The symbol of yin–yang has become a recognizable emblem in the West but few actually understand its meaning and philosophy. I'll give you the short version. In Taoism, yang is activity, and yin is quiet reflection. Sounds a lot like the two nervous system modes we talked about in chapter 6, right? Go Mode correlates to yang, while Chill Mode embodies yin. The latter is our more fertile state, in which we stop "doing" so

> Yin is defined as female energy, so it's no wonder that nurturing quiet contemplation in your life is favorable for fertility.

169

that we are able to "receive." It's in Chill Mode that we send circulation and resources to our reproductive organs. While there is no contesting that activity fosters health, you must have both modes in equal parts to keep your body and mind balanced and harmonious.

Although it seems logical that neither yin nor yang is more important than the other, that's not how we behave in the modern day. I can tell you that New Yorkers are functioning at 99 percent Go Mode, be it mental or physical exertion. Many of us base our opinion of self on how much we're able to accomplish. We worry about putting in enough hours, meeting the deadline, getting fit, and keeping up with endless meetings and appointments. When someone asks us how things are going, we list off recently completed tasks and social events. Rarely do we mention catching up on rest, meditation, mindfulness practices, or general relaxation.

The Attributes of Yin and Yang

The spheres of yin and yang coexist to create balance in the universe. Here are just a few qualities attributed to each:

Yin	Yang
Dark	Light
Passive	Active
Woman	Man
Night	Day
Quiet	Loud
Inward	Outward
Rest and digest	Fight or flight
Solitude	Productivity

Have you ever noticed that rest makes us perform better physically and mentally? It keeps us balanced emotionally, too. Without incorporating purposeful "pauses," we don't process all the day's sensory information, not to mention you can feel enslaved by your routine. The reality is that you will be more creative and efficient if you pause, assimilate, and regroup. It's the same principle as stretching before you participate in your favorite physical activity— golf, dance, volleyball, you name it.

The philosophy for wellness that I'm proposing in this book is that we exist as a whole, interconnected system. Therefore, enhancing fertility starts with balancing the yin and yang of your routine, thereby creating the balance you need to conceive. You may also discover a newfound joy in areas where you had become less inspired.

You picked up this book because you may be encountering frustrating, unexplained obstacles that are preventing you from conceiving. In this chapter, we explore how to bring activity and rest into alignment for optimal fertility.

The Right Kind of Activity: Exercise Guidelines

Exercise is an essential health practice and immensely important to hormonal wellness. The type and frequency of exercise, however, can either enhance or hamper our efforts to conceive. Many of us use intense exercise as an outlet for burning away stress as well as calories. The euphoria that follows a hard workout or a long run may alleviate nervous energy temporarily, but in excess, this short-term solution can be detrimental to fertility.

So what's a healthy level of physical activity? If you're already seeing a fertility doc, he or she may have told you not to exercise at all, which often leads to confusion over how to relieve stress and care for yourself, not to mention how to address the bloat and weight gain that are common side effects of fertility treatment. Fear not. In the pages to follow, you'll gain useful direction on how to proceed with your fitness programming. But first, let's give some context with Sarah's story.

Sarah was a workout junky, frequenting intense New York City exercise classes such as Barry's Boot Camp and SoulCycle. Her physique was important to her, but like many of my type A ladies, Sarah also used the exercise as stress relief. It was a major focus of her life outside of work. I knew I had to be careful and fact focused when addressing the topic of exercise with her. Those sorts of workouts provide the body with an endorphin high that can be quite addictive. I worried that suggesting she cut it out entirely might result in a panic attack, followed by grief and despair. Sarah was in her third IUI cycle (the two previous had failed). She was taking Clomid in hopes that an extra follicle or two might increase chances of pregnancy. As is common for many women, Clomid made her feel nuts and disrupted her sleep. She felt more than ever that the workouts were a necessity for her emotional health. While I understood where she was coming from, I explained that the type of exercise she was doing had high potential for deleterious effects. For example, Clomid can actually thin your uterine lining, and Sarah already had trouble building her lining before going on the medication, as indicated by her light periods. My hunch was that the intense workouts were flooding her system with so much cortisol that it was causing an underproduction of the lady hormones necessary to build a healthy lining. As we touched on in chapter 6, adrenaline and endorphins will actually downregulate the production of reproductive hormones. The longer and more frequent your endorphin highs are, the sleepier your ovaries can become. And since Sarah was undergoing fertility treatment aimed at producing an additional egg or two, ovarian torsion was another concern that made her brand of exercise a potential hazard.

I recommended Sarah scale back on the intense exercise and explore other ways to maintain her sanity. Her response: "But what if I gain weight?! And besides, it's the one thing that helps my anxiety. Not to mention that I already have a child, and I worked out back then, too." I counseled her on how our bodies can change, so that what worked in the past isn't necessarily right for the present. We talked

> Beware of ovarian torsion! If you are undergoing IVF, you are likely taking medications to stimulate egg production, which enlarges the ovaries. Exercise can sometimes cause them to twist (aka ovarian torsion), causing extreme pain and potentially sending you to the hospital for emergency surgery! During an IVF cycle, stick to walking and add an incline or a few stairs to get your heart rate up if needed.

through mindfulness techniques and the possibility of exchanging the high-impact, adrenaline-fueled workouts for low-intensity options three times per week. Although she wasn't happy about it at first, I ensured her that these methods would provide the much-needed outlet for stress *and* keep her fit. There was also the distinct possibility that *not* attending those boot camp classes might provide stress relief by reducing the amount she was rushing around town to make a time slot. Instead, she could take some chill time or run errands that she'd normally have to cram in later. Finally, I prescribed Sarah some Chinese herbs and raspberry leaf tincture to build her lining and some magnesium to help calm her nervous system. Within two months, she was pregnant (and still looked great).

Every woman's body is different, and depending on your body type, constitution, and current workout habits, you may need a slightly different routine than Sarah. Let's jump into some tips on how to evaluate what sort of exercise is right for you while actively trying to conceive.

EASY DOES IT

It's a common misconception that you need to be in the best physical shape of your life before you get pregnant. In reality, anything that's going to make you look like you're the cover girl for a fitness magazine is probably not ideal for your fertility. In one study of 40 female participants attending a training course at the Korea Third Military Academy, an intense workout regime decreased the women's waist sizes but also decreased thyroid hormones and caused 70 percent of them to develop irregular periods (Cho et al. 2017). All had regular menstrual periods before the training began. The researchers conducting the study also noted an increase in cortisol levels and a decrease of corticotropin-releasing hormone (CRH) at the end of the study, most likely from fatigue. CRH release is increased during physical or mental stress, and this secretion has been directly related to elevated resting cortisol levels, meaning cortisol lingers in your system long after the exercise is over. Furthermore, increased CRH has been shown to decrease the release of GnRH (which releases your follicle-stimulating hormone) in the hypothalamus and reduce LH (our ovulation hormone) levels. In essence, the intense exercise dulled the brain's activation signals to the ovaries. Without the brain's cues to grow and release an egg, the ovaries become sleepy. You may end up with irregular cycles or no cycle at all! I've observed patients clinically whose short or irregular cycles were likely induced by intense exercise. In some of these cases, the women ovulated early and thus had a short follicular phase. In other cases, their luteal phases were shortened, and their implantation and "incubation" were affected. Most, however, had very delayed ovulation, making their attempts to conceive few and far between.

The Pregnenolone Steal

High-intensity exercise triggers your fight-or-flight response, turning on Go Mode. Spending an extended time in this state taxes the adrenals and affects our sex hormones, throwing estrogen, progesterone, and testosterone out of balance. If we had primarily low-stress, relaxed lives, an occasional intense workout wouldn't matter much. But since the vast majority of us are already under daily stress of some sort, a high-intensity workout could be the straw that breaks your fertility.

High-intensity training and long bouts of cardio are thought to cause the endocrine system to commit an action called the "pregnenolone steal." Pregnenolone is a major building block for an array of sex hormones, including estrogen and progesterone. The demands of intense exercise will cause your body to convert pregnenolone into cortisol rather than progesterone. A deficiency of this hormone can cause implantation failure and early miscarriage, not to mention fatigue, bad PMS, bloat, and poor muscle development. Kind of defeats the point!

Having some body fat is far more favorable for hormone production than being too lean, and in the fertility game, your hormonal fitness is far more important than a super toned bod, right? Exercises and sports that emphasize leanness, such as ballet, long-distance running, gymnastics, and figure skating (or any type of exercise where there is a calorie deficit involved), can lead to low estrogen levels. Essentially, these regimens suppress the hypothalamus, meaning less GnRH, which then limits the secretion of LH and, to a certain extent, FSH. This causes a prolonged follicular phase or the absence of an LH surge mid-cycle, which can lead to delayed menstruation, period irregularity, delayed ovulation, and long cycles (Warren and Perlroth 2001). On the flip side, strength training, wherein you focus on gaining muscle mass rather than reducing fat, can cause an excess of male hormones. Generally, if testosterone goes up, your lady hormones (estrogen and progesterone) may go down.

Low to mid-intensity workouts strike that ideal balance, getting your blood flowing without causing strain on your system. These lower-impact workouts are meant to warm your muscles and joints, increase circulation, and aid in detoxification without causing an energy (or hormone) deficit.

Dos and Don'ts: Rules of Thumb

1. Feel like there are not enough minutes in a day? Well, then, this recommendation is going to relieve some stress. *Keep your exercise to around 30 minutes per session.* This is a tricky one for those of you who love long-distance runs. Running can be made more fertility friendly by practicing a run–walk method where you run for 10 minutes and walk for three or run for five and walk for one. Even in these shorter intervals, you'll get the calorie burn, detoxification, circulatory, and stress relief benefits. The difference is you'll also avoid flooding your system with the cortisol and adrenaline that can limit ovarian function.
2. *Temper the intensity.* Keep your heart rate below 140 beats per minute and ditch all high-intensity programs such as high-intensity interval training, CrossFit, Barry's Bootcamp, and SoulCycle. If you're into weight training, the aim would be to do more repetitions with smaller weights. Think barre classes, not massive dumbbells. Intense weight training can result in a significant inflammatory response because you are essentially tearing muscles fibers so that they grow back stronger. If you overdo it, you may zap your body's resources.
3. *Walking is always a therapeutic go-to* for calorie burn, mental health, and overall wellness. In times when your body and mind are under siege with stress, fertility treatments, and the like, walking in lieu of a workout can help you conserve your baby-making resources. Aim for 30-minute walks per day at a minimum, preferably outside.

A FINE LINE

Weight control is a balancing act for many, and there are some considerations to keep in mind for optimal fertility. For example, a very lean body may not manufacture enough hormones to grow eggs and ovulate. On the other hand, too much weight is implicated in insulin resistance, inflammation, and toxin accumulation.

Healthy weight is really an individual matter. Many a thin or soft woman have perfectly healthy fertility parameters. As a general rule, you want to maintain a healthy BMI between 20 and 25. It's also good to maintain a body fat

Exercise and Ovulation in Women with PCOS

PCOS and insulin resistance are known to pack on the weight as well as block or delay ovulation. Activity is essential for women with PCOS to help cleanse, shed pounds, and improve fertility. A study conducted on eight overweight/obese women (aged 18 to 30) with PCOS evaluated the success of individualized aerobic exercise training at lowering their symptoms (Redman, Elkind-Hirsch, and Ravussin 2011). After 16 weeks, there was a significant increase in their insulin sensitivity (meaning a reduction of insulin resistance) and a significant decrease in cysts. Additionally, the women lost weight and improved their cycle regularity. In obese patients with PCOS, it has been shown that a reduction in body weight of at least 5 percent leads to significant improvements in menstrual cyclicity, ovulation, and biochemical hyperandrogenism as well as improved glucose tolerance and reduced risk of cardiovascular disease. At the end of the 16-week study, aerobic exercise led to a 40 percent higher rate of ovulation (25 versus 65 percent) compared to dietary constriction.

In another study, 31 women with PCOS were randomly assigned to high-intensity interval training (HIIT), strength training, or a control group (Almenning et al. 2015). The exercise groups exercised three times weekly for 10 weeks. During this time, the researchers assessed whether their insulin resistance reached or progressed toward a state of homeostasis. For both exercise regimes, fat percentages decreased significantly, without changes in body weight. However, insulin resistance homeostasis improved significantly in the HIIT group (by 17 percent) rather than the strength training groups. The study also found that there was significantly reduced insulin resistance and improved endothelial function after 10 weeks in the HIIT group. While this is valuable information to note about PCOS, high-intensity workouts and long bouts of cardio are not recommended forms of exercise while actively trying to get pregnant. Instead, use these methods as part of a preconception plan (starting six months before trying to get pregnant) to get the initial weight off. After that, transition to mild or moderate forms of exercise on a maintenance plan. For example, if you're on an elliptical, don't crank the resistance or the incline up to 10. Keep it low (at 2 or 3) and then apply interval training tactics by increasing the incline or your pace for a minute or two. If you don't have the luxury of time and you are already in the thick of your fertility endeavors, stick with this gentler version of interval training.

composition of 18 to 25 percent. You can calculate these yourself with free tools online or ask your general practitioner/internist.

Maybe you know you are a few pounds above where you'd like to be. If you are overweight, meaning a BMI of 25 or above, your fertility might well improve by trimming down a tad. Unless you are obese, it's unlikely that you've been told by your doctor that you'll get pregnant if you *lose* weight. However, an interesting observation I've made over the years is that many women describe their body "going crazy" if they get even a pound over their homeostatic weight. For example, they would feel okay anywhere up to 165 pounds, but if they hit 166 or above, they would start swelling, feel stressed all the time, get pimples, experience accelerated weight gain, have menstrual irregularities, and so on. Everyone has their own tipping point. Only you will know where exactly that falls. If the number on the scale rises, so should your activity level. I recommend daily walks plus light interval training three to four times per week. That interval training can be a simple circuit of short bouts of cardio and strength training that uses your own body weight (stairs, planks, lunges, squats, and so on). This method helps to quickly sensitize insulin and shed BMI points. Other options are dance, hatha yoga, bicycling outdoors, or barre classes.

Are you on the other end of the spectrum where keeping weight *on* is more the issue? If you tend to lose weight too easily, then use caution when implementing changes to your diet and exercise regime. Irregular or absent periods can signal that you need to put on a few healthy pounds (likely not much, say, two or three). Being skinny isn't the problem. Rather, it's being "too thin" to manufacture hormones that poses an issue. Many willowy women have made babies. Try not to select exercises that will make you leaner, such as long-distance running or cycling. Stick to yoga, tai chi, dance, walking, NIA, and other balancing forms of exercise.

The Yin to Your Yang: Balance Improves Everything

Fourteen years ago, I went on a quest of sorts to find medicine master, kung fu monks in the holy mountains of China. I was convinced I'd find them existing just as they were in the old kung fu movies that I so adored or perhaps à la Uma Thurman in *Kill Bill*. The core objective of my stay in remote Chinese monasteries was actually to study Taoism and discover the true essence of old Chinese traditions. In this way, I would capture the magic of Chinese medicine beyond its modes of practice in Chinese hospitals. I believed these monks, with their centuries of passed-down knowledge, could impart the deep wisdom behind the methods. I was not disappointed. I stayed at several monasteries along my journey and witnessed the practices of several different "lineages" of Buddhist and

Taoist martial arts masters and healers. Many of the monasteries housed groups of children, either orphaned or sent by their parents to study martial arts. Not only could they practice some amazing kung fu, but they were also trained in tai chi, qigong, and quiet meditation. Their master taught them that in order to excel at external yang practices, like the tumbling, splits, and swordplay they were all so eager to try, they were to engage in the more meditative, slow-flowing movements characteristic of tai chi and qigong. It did, in fact, improve their quicker movements! In the West, we've placed the value almost entirely on constantly being active, missing out on the enhancing effects of slowing things down. Consider, for a moment, that this balance can awaken something amazing in you and create the physiology needed to conceive a healthy pregnancy.

YOGA

It's probably fairly clear at this point that I believe yoga is a fantastic option for your baby-making exercise plan. Yoga is both a spiritual practice and a form of exercise. You'll have the benefit of toning, detoxing, enhancing blood flow, and relaxing all at once. Its advantages go far beyond weight management. Yoga is good for any body shape, constitution, or personality type.

Tried it and didn't like it? I suggest you try again. There are many different forms of yoga, and the teacher also makes a huge difference. Try a few different teachers until one "lands" with you. With some experimentation, you can find a philosophy or approach that suits you.

Already into yoga? Awesome! Just keep in mind that twisting poses are out after ovulation. They are highly detoxifying, which is great for wringing out your organs, but if you're in the implantation phase, it's not ideal. Twisting poses are down bearing and can place a lot of pressure on the uterus, acting somewhat like an eject button. Last but not least, the risk of ovarian torsion is high during an IVF or medicated IUI cycle. Slow-flow and restorative classes are best for these circumstances. More vigorous vinyasa can be practiced in unmedicated cycles.

No matter the phase, I do *not* recommend hot yoga. The heat brings with it an intensity that may stress the body. While hot yoga does detoxify, it does so too quickly, releasing a flood of toxins the body will struggle to process, not to mention the potential for dehydration. Fertility-friendly yoga is akin to the type traditionally practiced at cooler times of day, with a focus on balancing the body's energy.

Here are a few fertility-enhancing poses:

1. *Paschimottanasana (seated forward bend).* Sit on your mat with your legs extended and together. Start with hands on your thighs, then as you inhale,

raise your arms over your head. On your exhale, bend forward and reach for your toes, bringing your chest toward your thighs and your head toward your knees. Hold your breath here for five seconds and then inhale to resume the starting position. This pose wonderfully compresses your pelvic region, massaging your reproductive organs and enhancing toxin removal. Forward bends like this one have the added benefit of calming the mind. Avoid during the implantation phase.

2. *Baddha Konasana (butterfly pose).* For this amazing hip opener, start seated with your legs straight, then bend them inward so that the soles of your feet touch each other. Keep them close by holding your toes. Make sure you're sitting straight and practicing your normal yoga breath, then gently bend forward or use your elbows to apply downward pressure on your thighs. This pose enhances circulation in your pelvic region, flushing toxins and loosening blockages that might impede blood flow.

3. *Setu Bandha Sarvangasana (bridge pose).* Lie flat on your back with knees bent and feet pressed to the mat, stacking knees over ankles. With arms flat at your sides and palms pressed to the mat, inhale and raise your pelvis. Lift your chest toward your chin, keeping your chin pointed to the sky (don't do a crunch with your neck). You will support yourself with your shoulders, arms, and feet. While you breathe comfortably and slowly, flex your buttocks to keep your thighs parallel to the floor. Stay here as long as you can without discomfort, then descend slowly on an exhale. This is a wonderful pose to open circulation in your hip flexors and pelvic region. It can also benefit your thyroid, helping you regulate hormone production.

4. *Viparita Karani (legs up the wall pose).* Lying flat and straight, gradually raise your legs 90 degrees in line with a wall while maintaining your yoga breathing. Repeat five to eight times, remaining in the position as long as you can without discomfort. With the assist from gravity, this pose cleanses the lymphatic and circulatory systems in the legs and reproductive system by sending blood back to the core, where it is then filtered and recirculated. It also relieves tension in your hips and hamstrings, stretching the lower back and thighs. Avoid during your period, as we want the gravity at this time to assist blood flow outward.

5. *Bhujangasana (cobra pose).* Lying on your stomach with legs together and extended, place your hands in line with your rib cage. As you inhale, press up, lifting your torso off the mat. Stretch as far back as you can without force or discomfort, curving the spine and tilting the chin toward the ceiling. Hold for 30 seconds, retaining your steady yoga breathing, and slowly descend on an exhale. Cobra pose elongates the colon for better elimination and gently increases blood flow in the pelvic region.

TAI CHI

This ancient "internal" martial art is slow, steady, and fluid. The movements are designed to relax, focus, and balance the body's energy. Tai chi sequences massage the internal organs and help improve their function. Consistent practice will also assist with stress reduction and enhance overall well-being. Tai chi ticks all the boxes because it has some aerobic benefits and aids circulation, but it's low impact and low intensity. Believe it or not, it's actually an extremely effective martial art. Speed up some of those movements in a street fight, and your opponent better watch out!

QIGONG

Qigong's guiding principle is the cultivation of energy. You're channeling qi from within yourself and from nature. The movement sequences of qigong are designed to connect with your body's natural energy pathways. Breathing and strong mental focus are integral to the practice. Qigong is incredible for circulation, organ function, stress management, and too many disorders to list! It's also used as a form of energy healing similar to Reiki.

DANCE

While tai chi and qigong focus the mind's energy with meditation-like practices, dance sets the spirit free. There is more than one way to find your bliss. Dance forms like salsa, modern contemporary, hip-hop, or even Zumba offer fun cardio and can generally be done at your own pace to keep it fertility friendly. Dance allows you to let loose, giving us an opportunity to shake off the stress of infertility. Just make sure you don't get too carried away!

Wisdom from the East—Your Exercise "Type"

When structuring your ideal workout routine, Eastern philosophy can provide deeper insight than BMI charts. While your BMI and percentage of body fat act as great guidelines, a generalized chart or number range is not always 100 percent accurate. In Eastern philosophy, everyone has a unique "type," or "constitution." It includes appearance, personality, tendencies, and health characteristics. In traditional Indian medicine (Ayurveda), your constitution is referred to as one of three "doshas" that create your identity or tendencies: Vata, Pitta, and Kapha. These types help determine how you can best find internal balance. Vatas are naturally slender types who can sometimes lose weight too quickly; Pittas are strong, athletic types with a medium physique; and Kaphas are softer body types with naturally larger womanly curves. The doshas help determine which exercises are best for you. The thinking is that catering recommendations to fit your dosha will create better results than a one-size-fits-all approach. For example, if you are a Kapha dosha and you tend to gain weight easily, then you won't do well with recommendations that work for the naturally thin Vata women. Vatas should stick to the lightest, slow-flowing or "yin-centric" routines, while Kaphas should take on slightly more intense interval training options, with Pitta falling in the middle. You may feel you're a mix of doshas, which is exactly right. Every woman is a unique combination of the three, and your dosha balance can fluctuate depending on your habits, stress levels, and environment. However, we all generally have one dominant dosha, which helps guide the recommendations for our lifestyle choices.

Kapha is the dosha that finds it harder to keep the extra pudge at bay. If you currently need to shed a few pounds, take the first step from the starter routine below and add some stair climbing, cycling, and elliptical in short bursts with rest periods in between. Get your heartbeat up for three to four minutes and let it rest for one to two minutes. This low-impact form of "interval training" is incredibly effective for sensitizing insulin and sizzling fatty deposits. No-contact martial arts, dance, and swimming are also great options.

Pitta types are your quintessential alpha-wired personalities. They have a competitive streak and a tendency to get frustrated and stressed. If exercise is overdone, it can flare the stress response more. For Pitta types, vinyasa flow yoga, barre classes, and Pilates are great options. Barre classes involve longer repetitions with lower weight and breaks between reps. You'll work your muscles enough to tone, but you'll calm down your nervous system (and the cortisol) with the breathing and stretching breaks in between. More assertive forms of tai chi, such as Chen style or trying out a kung fu, aikido, or karate class, could be fun. And any kind of dance besides break dancing or swing is also good unless it's at a competitive level. Opt for shorter, 30-minute classes and make sure you focus on optimizing the breaks as much as the work.

Vata types are naturally slim, so if you fall within this dosha, your exercise routine should focus on maintaining your current weight. Lean into yin-type exercises like hatha yoga, walking, NIA, tai chi, and Pilates. Tai chi and qigong may seem like they're for old people, but they are highly sophisticated techniques that cleanse organs, increase circulation, and balance the mind. Since Vatas tend to struggle more with anxiety and lack of focus, these meditative practices help to balance both body and mind. They are mindfulness and exercise rolled into one, perfect for promoting the optimal sleeping patterns Vatas require.

Need a "catchall" starter routine to keep things simple? Here you go!

1. Work out for no more than 30 to 45 minutes three or four times per week (unless doing restorative yoga or tai chi). Stick to gentle and somewhat "feminine" options such as barre, Pilates, and dance.
2. Either daily or on "off" days, integrate a quick yoga routine of 10 rounds of sun salutations followed by three resting poses for two to three minutes each. You can opt to go to a class, follow an app, or self-motivate if you've memorized the sequence. Choose from child's pose, butterfly pose, savasana, paschimottanasana, lotus, or modified lotus (cross-legged meditation pose) after your initial 10 minutes of vinyasa flow.
3. Walk daily for 30 to 60 minutes, preferably outside, to benefit from fresh air and vitamin D. Aim closer to 60 minutes if you are not engaging in the exercise options in step 1. Walking is also the exercise of choice during an IVF cycle.

Exercising for Your Cycle

Just as your nutritional needs change with the phases of your cycle, your exercise should shift as well. Aligning your workout routine with your body's natural rhythms helps you glide through your hormonal transitions and enhance your fertility along the way.

PHASE 1

During the beginning days of your period, lean into gentle forms of movement, such as walking, qigong, or restorative yoga. Focus on passive stretches, long holds in comfortable positions, and basic breathing techniques. It's best to stick to these less strenuous options during your monthly flow. You are losing minerals and nutrients through your blood, and your body is working overtime at half capacity to manage the massive shift in hormones. Avoid taxing yourself in this phase so that you can gather resources to support the growth of your eggs as you enter the follicular phase.

By the fourth or fifth day of your period, if you're bleeding very little, you can start some more active forms of exercise. Stick with mild to moderate options like the previously mentioned vinyasas, NIA, tai chi, and walking and limit your sessions to 30 to 45 minutes.

PHASE 2

By day 6 or 7 of your cycle, your period has (hopefully) come to an end, your energy levels are restored, and your estrogen levels are on the rise. Now you can switch to those moderate, 30- to 45-minute exercises like barre or Pilates classes and interval training, swimming, or dance.

PHASE 3

When you reach ovulation, increasing circulation is key. Cardio in the form of dance or a vinyasa flow can assist in the smooth release of your egg by promoting the free flow of blood circulation to the reproductive organs. Active forms of exercise will also lend a helping hand to the liver and digestive system, assisting healthy elimination, reducing bloat, and facilitating a smooth transition into the luteal phase.

PHASE 4

Once you've entered the luteal phase, the plan changes. Exercise is still required for circulation, removal of waste, and stress relief, but we have to make sure not to overdo it. It's a catch-22 because exercise is helpful to combat many of the issues we face premenstrually. The liver becomes more congested in this phase, bowel movements may slow down, and bloat is likely to increase. You may be wondering at this point how much is too much. My advice is to behave as if you are already pregnant. You can safely do mild to moderate interval training (two minutes raising your heart rate and one to two minutes bringing it down) or short bouts of cardio (10 to 20 minutes) on the elliptical, bike, or treadmill. Hatha yoga, light weights, barre classes, tai chi, or dance are also fine as long as you don't find yourself heaving for air. Keep your sessions to 30 minutes and always do a thorough cooldown by stretching or walking until both sweat and heart rate decrease. Stay out of the heat, avoid contact sports, and remove twists from your yoga. Finding a "yin–yang" balance within your physical activity is best practice when it comes to fertility. Note that if you have just done a "retrieval" of eggs via IVF, walking, slow elliptical, and light weights are the way to go.

Table 10.1. Quick-Look Workout Chart

Menses (yin)	30 minutes or less	Restorative yoga, qigong, meditation, and mindful walking
Follicular (yin)	30 minutes or less + 10-minute cooldown	Barre, Pilates, interval circuits or cardio, Vinyasa yoga, dance, and martial arts
Ovulation (yang)	30 to 45 minutes + 15-minute cooldown	Free-flow movement like dancing, Vinyasa yoga, and tai chi
Luteal (yang)	30 minutes + 15-minute cooldown	Interval pace cardio (3 minutes increased heart rate and 1 to 2 minutes to restore resting heart rate; outdoor cycling, elliptical, hatha yoga, dance, and one or two sessions of barre and Pilates weekly)

Deep Yin: Practicing Mindfulness

When you're struggling to get pregnant, you want concrete answers. You're looking for actionable information on what to eat, how to exercise, and which supplements to take. Less obvious but equally as important is taking time for yourself to pause and process your thoughts and emotions. Just like our exercise routine, we need to be deliberate about our "inner work" in order to find a place of calm. The quieter side of our nervous system is more often where magic happens for conception.

You may be avoiding quiet time for fear of the unpleasant thoughts that dance around in your mind. There may be some "unpacking" to do concerning the thoughts and fears that stem from this process. Infertility hurts. It's frustrating, exhausting, and often crushing. That said, you will be surprised by how much the time dedicated to quiet reflection will actually help you cope with the emotional ups and downs. By tapping

> Harmony is found between "doing" and "pausing."

into a deeper place within ourselves, we may start accessing a different frame of mind, one characterized by a deeper knowing and trust that things will work out, perhaps also letting go of the desire to control every aspect of the journey and instead tuning in to what you truly need here and now.

Mindfulness and Menstruation

One of the most important times to engage in a quiet, positive dialogue with yourself is during the menstrual phase. For a woman hoping to conceive, the arrival of your period brings with it the devastating reality that you are not there yet. Take the time to grieve the loss and check in with yourself. What was successful this past month? Where could you have improved? Try to avoid numbing with booze, shopping, talking, or other methods of distraction. Once you feel you've rested, set an intention for this next cycle. Integrate a healing habit, be it fertility-friendly food, movement, mindfulness, or otherwise.

If the idea of accessing your internal dialogue through meditation makes you recoil, you are not alone. That said, becoming an observer of your own mind is incredibly empowering. You'll come to find that *your mind will lie to you*. Mental chatter is *not* your inner truth. Your thoughts are a product of your experiences, deepest fears, and/or insecurities. Lack of sleep, excess caffeine, sugar, stress, and the like influence the nature of your thoughts. I know mine turn quite ugly under these circumstances, and it's

> Meditation helps you to pause and assess *before* reacting.

nice to know that the negativity is likely a reflection of the imbalance and not objective truth. Even better is that we can transform our mind-set with the right lifestyle habits. Exercise is an effective outlet for many women, but you may find that, if given a chance, mindfulness practice is a powerful and very efficient way to access inner calm. Even five minutes of meditation can completely change the inner dialogue. And since meditation is the queen of all mindfulness practices, let's delve into how you can make this ancient tradition work for you.

MASTERING YOUR MIND

The definition of meditation varies by tradition. Some focus on a recited mantra, while others use a "body scan" technique. What they all promise is a deeper exploration of "self" and a connection to the "divine." Proponents of meditation, myself included, believe that it is the most effective means of connecting with your deeper truth and taking control of your mind. You'll often hear of the concept of "oneness" applied to the practice. In meditation, you connect to a higher level of consciousness, where your emotions are less likely to get the best of you and you can access ongoing clarity and calm.

When practicing meditation, you allow the world to go on around you without you having to interact in it for a time. This gives you a chance to focus inward and takes strain off of your mind, allowing you to switch off and go into

Chill Mode. In this state, you access deeper healing, creating a more harmonious environment for conception.

The research teams at the Benson-Henry Institute for Mind Body Medicine at Massachusetts General Hospital and the Beth Israel Medical Center studied relaxation practices like meditation, yoga, and breathing techniques. They found that these techniques not only reduced anxiety but surprisingly also improved the expression of genes in the immune system, the metabolism, and insulin secretion sites.

Easier said than done? Maybe, but it is my firm belief that anyone can get the hang of meditation if you just give it a try. Many first-timers say meditation makes them feel crazy. Their thoughts bounce around, and they can't focus. I was one such person. Daily practice, however, transformed my view. It's now a blissful experience for me. That said, I still have to remind myself to do it daily! In true alpha fashion, it's more appealing when I remind myself that stopping for a moment makes me better able to tackle my to-do list.

Immersion Therapy

Some women do well developing their meditation practice by incorporating a 10-minute pause into the day. I, however, had a lot of trouble with meditation until I did a 10-day, fully immersive, silent meditation retreat. During these 10 days, you don't speak (yes, silence all the time). You eat two small vegetarian meals per day and are woken at 4:30 a.m. each morning to start meditation practice. Walking is the only form of exercise allowed and only for five minutes between one-hour meditation sessions. I had lived with monks for a year in the mountains of China and India, I had been a yogi for years, and I had attended weekly gatherings to practice meditation throughout. But for my monkey mind, only the total immersion of the retreat would do it. If time allows, consider trying it for yourself. Ten days is a big commitment, but there are also weekend retreats available all over the United States and all over the world.

If you don't want to call it "meditation" because you don't fully identify with it philosophically, try something like "quiet sitting." Let the world pass you by for that short time, then jump right back into what you need to do. Remember, we are trying to offset the effects of the stress that thwarts your fertility efforts.

Meditation and mindfulness work only if you give them a real shot. So many of us suffer from "busy brains" that prevent us from focusing on one thing at a time thanks to the constant rush of modernity. To set yourself up for success, find a quiet place to find comfort and turn off all your nearby devices.

There are many different types of meditation and mindfulness techniques. Trust that there is one out there that works for you. It may be formal training through a Transcendental Meditation center or a vipassana retreat or a casual practice integrated into your day, such as a guided meditation from iTunes or an app. Last but not least, there are free meditation "challenges," like the 21-day session offered at chopracenter.com. The following list offers widely available options to assist you in finding your preferred technique.

TYPES OF MEDITATION

Transcendental Meditation (TM)

Brought to the West by Maharishi Mahesh Yogi and popularized by celebrities and business moguls alike, this simple and effective form of meditation is easy to learn and gets you results fast. It is a form of meditation that utilizes a mantra, a word or phrase, to focus the mind and sink deep into meditation. TM foundations in your area will offer paid one-on-one sessions to help you choose mantras and grow comfortable with the practice.

Mantra Magic

Mantras owe their origins to Buddhist and Hindu faith, so most who have been "assigned" a mantra by their teacher are given a Sanskrit phrase. A mantra can be a sound (like the classic "om mani padmi om"), a word (such as "fertility," "healing," or "peace"), a phrase (such as "My body is strong" or "My womb is fruitful"), or a prayer (such as "Grant me peace and healing so that I may thrive"). The word or phrase is essentially repeated internally throughout the meditation.

The objective, as with pretty much all meditation techniques, is to simply refocus the mind if it strays. Over time, it will get easier to withdraw from the mental chatter and access a quiet place within.

Vipassana Meditation

Vipassana is a Buddhist form of meditation that involves the use of a "body scan." In the initial stages of learning this technique, you are told to focus on the small area between your nose and your upper lip and observe the in breath and out breath. The study then progresses to a full-body scan, whereby you consciously drift your attention over one body part at a time until you've traced your entire form several times.

Vipassana retreats are a tad more rigorous than some other teaching methods. It involves sitting day after day in total silence and stillness, shutting out everything. While living abroad, I attended a 10-day silent vipassana retreat. Interestingly enough, at that time, I hadn't had my period for almost a year, and it finally returned a few days into the retreat. Coincidence? Perhaps. But I've seen countless examples of the reproductive system waking up when we reach a deeper state of calm. It happens with acupuncture all the time!

Unlike TM, these retreats are by donation (any amount that fits your budget) and are held all over the world. If you have the time to spare and want to break through a mental barrier or your own, I highly recommend them. But I understand this isn't going to be everyone's cup of tea. As an aside, the first time I heard of this kind of retreat was almost a decade before I actually had the courage to do one. It did, however, turn out to be one of my life's most transformative experiences to date.

Twice Daily to Blissful Consciousness

Seemingly every tradition of meditation recommends meditation twice daily for 15 to 20 minutes (more is also completely fine). Usually, the first session should be practiced when you rise in the morning, prior to drinking caffeine or eating. This will set the tone for your day. Another session in the afternoon will give you a chance to assimilate, unpack, and process all the information that your senses experienced (i.e., everything you saw, heard, and felt that day). It also provides a chance to consciously interrupt unconscious thought patterns and gain control over your mental chatter. Last but not least, it's an amazing recharge. For more information on the physiological benefits of meditation, I highly recommend Emily Fletcher's *Stress Less, Accomplish More*, Eckhart Tolle's *The Power of Now*, or Joe Dispenza's *Becoming Supernatural*. If 15 to 20 minutes seems like an eternity, then start with five to 10 minutes. An interesting side effect of the meditative calm is that it makes you feel as if you've *gained* time in your day. This is the effect of reversing the rushing sensations that build up in your body and mind over the course of the day.

Body Scanning

This mindfulness technique is used in many forms of meditation, vipassana being one of them. Similar to the use of a mantra, you have a "task" to focus on. A body scan goes something like this: Simply sit on the floor or lie on your back and begin breathing deeply. Make sure you're filling your lungs to capacity. Your belly should puff up with air. Then let it out as slowly as you can. Once you've settled into a breathing rhythm, you continue that practice as you focus your mind on one body part at a time. With your eyes closed, drift your awareness over the contours of your body. Start with your left toes and move slowly up the front of your leg until you reach the pelvis. Then return to your right toes and move to the pelvis again. Imagine warmth and light around your uterus and ovaries. Carry on up the torso, scan your arms, and then move up the neck to the top of your head. Once you've reached your apex, you can follow the same course all the way back down. Imagine your breath moving in a wave from head to toe and back again. This scanning practice will calm your mind and bring a great deal of awareness to sensations and blockages in your body.

Progressive Muscle Relaxation

This is similar to body scanning but with an addition. This technique requires the more involved "task" of consciously tensing and relaxing your muscles, making it best suited for alpha-wired women who have trouble focusing in other techniques. It's ideal for stressed-out women because it teaches you to recognize the difference in the sensation of a tensed muscle and a relaxed muscle at a conscious and subconscious level. If you repeat this practice often enough, you will learn to recognize when you're tensing during the day and then consciously relax that tension.

To get started, lie on your back and begin your deep breathing, just like in body scanning. Now focus on both feet at a time and tense the muscles of each foot together, holding for a few seconds and then releasing. Then you move upward to all the major muscle groups on each side, tensing and relaxing them together: calves, thighs, buttocks, abs, fists, forearms, biceps, shoulder, neck, jaw, and so on. After you've finished with all the muscles of your face, tense your whole body in unison, squeezing as tightly as you can, and then release as a unit.

Yoga to the Rescue

If you try traditional meditation a few times and find it tough, try using yoga to prepare your body and mind. Yoga is actually meant to prepare you for meditation by limbering up your body and calming your mind. The syncing of movement to breath mimics the essence of meditation. Try the 10 rounds of sun salutations suggested earlier, followed by three resting poses of your choice. The stretching will allow you to sit more comfortably, and your mind will be less likely to jump around. Try moving from your preferred yoga routine straight into meditation and see if you shift into quiet reflection easier.

Mudras

Mudras are hand and finger "poses" that have various effects on the nervous system. They are often seen as an add-on to your meditation and yoga but can be used on their own. The word *mudra* means "seal" in Sanskrit, and these positions are meant to seal in the intention or desire you're focusing on while meditating. Below is a short list of mudras that are meant to bring peace, calm, and clarity. You can choose one to help you

> **Fun Fact**
>
> Using the same mudra each time you meditate will help you sink into meditation more quickly. The mudra will signal Chill Mode via muscle memory once your brain associates the pose with your meditative state.

drift into quiet meditation with ease and maintain focus throughout the session.

Anjali Mudra is said to foster deep self-reflection and bring clarity to a troubled mind. Put your hands together at your heart and then turn your fingers away from your body, pressing the wrists and heels of your palms against your sternum between your breasts.

Prithivi Mudra is a stabilizing position that makes you feel grounded, secure, and at peace. This makes it a great option on days when you're doubting yourself or feeling scattered or fearful. Gently press the tips of your ring fingers to your thumbs on each hand, keeping all the other fingers raised. Rest your hands on your knees or lap.

Pushan Mudra specifically targets the nervous system to calm and relax you. It's great for days when your stress levels are through the roof. On your right hand, press together your thumb, index finger, and middle finger, with the remaining fingers raised high. On your left hand, press together your thumb, middle finger, and ring finger.

The Pushan Mudra was especially helpful for my patient Kristin. As an interior designer who traveled a lot for her job, she was one stressed-out lady. At 34, she'd been experiencing irregular periods after quitting birth control pills. Her fertility doctor diagnosed her with PCOS and suggested she start with a round of Clomid and IUI. Kristin wanted to see what other options were available before going this route. Her doctor kindly referred her to me to start with a more natural approach. She noted that her follicular phase was super long at around 25 days, meaning that she wasn't ovulating until around day 26. Her luteal phase, on the other hand, seemed to be only around eight days long, which was on the shorter side and might not be sufficient to hold a pregnancy. I suspected that her estrogen stayed low well into her follicular phase and that her progesterone levels were too low to keep the lining intact. Recall from chapter 6 that stress may lower hormone levels. Kristin admitted that her anxiety was hard to manage. Her outlet of choice was going to 5 a.m. SoulCycle classes six days a week. I cautiously suggested that she needed a new routine for the time being, explaining that the intense cardio might be at least partially to blame for her hormone troubles.

Kristin wasn't too keen to change things up. Meditation was intimidating, and she said she'd never really liked yoga. She agreed to start with 10 rounds of sun salutations (i.e., vinyasa flow) followed by sitting quietly for five minutes. She soon came to enjoy the yoga and even asked for more pose recommendations. I gave her the Pushan Mudra and three yoga poses to do in the morning and at night to calm her mind and wind down. For supplements, I prescribed an herbal blend with chasteberry (supports progesterone), ashwaganda (controls stress), and rehmannia (supports estrogen). I also gave her vitamin B6, magnesium glycinate, NAC, and myoinositol to lower anxiety and treat her irregular cycles. Within two months, she was ovulating by day 18, and her luteal phase was 12 days long. By the third month, she was pregnant. Not only was she ecstatic to have conceived, but she had transformed her notion of a stress "outlet" into something that would provide easy access to calm at any stage of the reproductive process.

Need Guidance?

If meditating and other mindfulness techniques seem too overwhelming to tackle on your own, an expert guide could be the key to success. There are many programs and institutions that can help. Here are a few options to explore:

1. *Local yoga studios.* You can receive guidance on poses, connect with others, and explore meditation classes.
2. *Center for Mind-Body Medicine groups.* Their programs provide a variety of relaxation techniques, like hypnosis, mindfulness, meditation, yoga, breathing exercises, imagery creation, body scanning, journaling, etc.
3. *Buddhist or Taoist monasteries.* They offer meditation training and classes that are often free.
4. *TM centers.* Their programs help you learn Transcendental Meditation within a guided structure.
5. *Vipassana centers.* If you're interested in taking an immersion retreat, this is where to turn.
6. *Ashrams.* These monasteries or spiritual retreats, with available living quarters, are another great place to learn about yoga and meditation with 100 percent immersion.
7. *Guided meditations on iTunes or other sites.* Stay at home with my top recommendations, which include Belleruth Naparstek's Health Journeys audio library (for a wide variety) and the Circle + Bloom website (for fertility-specific guidance).
8. *Apps like Headspace.* This is an easy-to-use resource that you can use as an introduction to mindfulness.

Your Version of Balance

It's true that slowing down may sound highly unappealing to many of the driven, tenacious women holding this book. I'm not suggesting you abandon your career to go on a yearlong retreat in the mountains. Exercise, crush those deadlines, and be the boss you are. I'm simply recommending that you remember to balance your output with adequate downtime.

In the past, I too have been known to push the boundaries by always being on the go. It took my getting to the point of hormonal and stress burnout before I learned the importance of finding balance. I'm grateful for the hormonal and fertility challenges I faced because it gave me an opportunity to understand this about myself. That knowledge now helps me dial it down before things get out of hand. Similarly, I understand when activity is needed to get out of a funk. Learn your own limits and design your life accordingly.

Keep in mind that the guidelines offered throughout this chapter are simply suggestions. The essence of sustainability is that it needs to work for you. Forcing yourself into a routine that doesn't match your personality will never be tenable. The guidelines are a calling for you to reevaluate your current routine and tinker with your habits to achieve a greater state of balance for your fertility. The path to healing starts with tuning in. And for that, sometimes we need to slow down. Only by observing will you understand what your body needs. With mindful execution of your daily routine, you'll find an equilibrium that heals you at a deep level and creates space for your baby.

CHAPTER 11

Your Guide to Natural Fertility Solutions

The first steps into the world of natural medicine can feel like wandering into a noisy crowd. With so many options, where does one begin?! Then the pressing question arises: Does it really work? Despite the controversy of opinions in mainstream thinking, there are great advantages to exploring these lesser-known areas of medical practice. Many swear by the answers they found while venturing this path and enthusiastically share their success stories. With a bit of an open mind, there is so much that natural medicine can offer you. Imagine a world of solutions that you didn't know were even an option.

Natural medicine gives each of us the opportunity to elevate our health and wellness—achieving a greater state of physical, emotional, and spiritual well-being. Attuned to the connections between mind and body, a holistic approach takes into account all things that could be affecting your fertility. That "big-picture" starting point is then whittled down to a treatment plan based on your individual struggles, circumstances, and goals. Therein lies the greatest strength of this approach: it is highly customized for *you* to achieve best results.

All said, without guidance, it's hard to know where to start in such a vast array of options. Fret not; this chapter will be your trusted guide in your quest for a baby. The wide and wondrous world of natural medicine awaits you, and I am quite sure you will be pleased—if not dazzled—by the incredible power it holds.

Trusting Your Innate Ability to Heal

Maybe you've heard success stories from friends. "I swear by acupuncture. I got pregnant two months after starting!" And now you're excited. Maybe you're disillusioned with the conventional methods that have tried and failed and you are looking for an extra something to up the odds. Or perhaps, like many, you are at the end of your rope and ready to try anything from snake oil to walking on hot coals to get the job done. Whatever your reason for considering this route, you won't be disappointed. Most everyone will reap rewards, and some people will experience heightened benefits. Many fertility challenges, such as PCOS and endometriosis, respond incredibly well to lifestyle changes and alternative medicine. In fact, many gynecologists and fertility specialists refer their patients to my clinic to receive counseling in nutrition and complementary methods as a means to improve their fertility. If you already know what is going on, a qualified practitioner can help you proactively address that issue from all possible angles. If you are at a loss, practitioners of natural medicine will seek to identify the issue at its source. While I'm all for the benefits of modern fertility treatment, I believe the power of natural methods is greatly understated. When it comes to your fertility, it could be just the thing to get you over the hump. But don't just take my word for it. Let's explore Jen's story.

Jen came to see me after she had consulted every fertility doctor in Manhattan and was, as of yet, unable to conceive her second child. Jen was hysterical. She couldn't understand why conceiving the first child was so easy but the second was proving impossible. Every fertility doctor she consulted told her to go the donor egg route. Jen was 39 and had very high FSH (64 or higher). To put it into perspective, most doctors will tell you your ovaries are kaput when the FSH is over 20. But Jen was determined to have her second child from her own eggs, and she refused to take no for an answer. She knew there must be at least one good one left in there.

During her intake, I learned that she was a vegetarian, had Hashimoto's disease, didn't really sleep, loved carbs, was not on any vitamins, didn't exercise, and overall wasn't on any kind of health regimen. She ate gluten and soy (terrible for Hashimoto's) daily and a lot of processed foods. She had regular menstruation but an irregular ovulation, even showing signs of ovulation during her menstrual period. I suggested she get monitored to confirm when exactly her egg was dropping. One very open doctor agreed to work with her just to monitor her cycles. I prescribed Chinese herbs, a cleansing diet, acupuncture, and supplements.

Jen had the hardest time with the nutritional portion of the program. She literally cried in my office each week about the difficulty. Emotional ties to food can be very triggering, but I encouraged her to stick with the program. Sure enough, she persisted in replacing packaged foods with more whole, organic foods. She was also apprehensive about the acupuncture, but she trusted the process and kept coming for her appointments. Four months later, she was pregnant. Hysterical again (Jen was a crier), she was so grateful that she stayed the course. Nine months later, she delivered her second healthy child without complications.

Jen's story is not a fluke. There are many others who have experienced miracles at the hands of natural medicine.

Open Your Mind

Yes, there is still healthy skepticism surrounding natural medicine. That is to be expected. In the Western world and beyond, we have come to view modern scientific approaches to medicine as the only trustworthy solution. Few of us have been taught to respect nutrition, natural medicine and simple lifestyle tweaks as viable options. We even run to the doctor for things like a common cold, which is more effectively treated with rest and home remedies than with antibiotics. No longer is wisdom being passed down from elders, at least not in our culture. In this chapter, I aim to provide a compelling case that alternative medicine is worth exploring. Conventional medicine has made amazing advances from which we have seen great benefit. IVF, for example, provides a solution for many women and couples seeking to conceive that wouldn't be able to otherwise. But for those who have experienced several failed attempts, natural medicine has the potential not only to improve outcomes but also to attend to your overall health and well-being in the process.

WHERE IS THE EVIDENCE?

Natural medicine is rooted in deep traditions spanning thousands of years. It's a wonder why so many long-standing, clinically proven techniques haven't yet been accepted by the mainstream. But things are changing. Many people who aren't finding the answers they need in conventional medicine, are seeking help elsewhere.

"Wellness," which encompasses a variety of natural approaches, is now a billion-dollar industry, and that's unlikely to happen without solid results to substantiate their use. Research studies show that women using holistic care for fertility are reporting positive outcomes with increasing frequency and are even requesting that medical facilities in their area offer alternative methods (Hinks and Coulson 2010). For example, between 2002 and 2012, the number of acupuncture users in the United States ballooned by 50 percent (Cui et al. 2017).

The system is set up for us to see a conventional doctor from the moment we enter the world, and consequently we are never led to explore natural medicine. Most of our beloved doctors are not educated on the topic, so unless we happen on it ourselves, we must rely on only one perspective. And while modern medicine has provided many amazing solutions, it does not effectively attend to all of our needs.

Our modern world requires science to validate the use of any medical approach. But many fields of natural medicine predate scientific thought by hundreds, if not thousands of years, not to mention that they are highly customized to the individual, making it hard to standardize protocols with which to conduct studies. It's part of what makes natural medicine so effective, but it's also what gets in the way of proving its worth. Also noteworthy is that money is a natural driver of many industries, and pharmaceuticals are much more profitable than herbs and acupuncture. Resources will go to funding the research that generates income. There is no issue with that other than when it clouds the ability to see other viable options.

Although there is still a long way to go in conducting research, the studies that *have* been done show promise, which is one reason why alternative medicine is growing exponentially. I suspect it has more to do with word of mouth than research, but I'm delighted to have both working toward the greater good.

No one form of medicine can provide all the answers. Natural medicine has advantages over conventional approaches and vice versa. The best paradigm for health care is for us to team up and work together.

Wholeness

Inherent in the philosophy of natural medicine is the belief that optimizing your body and mind will smooth your path to conception. Our belief is that you can establish a fertile internal environment using methods that work *with* your body rather than wrestling it into submission. Applying holistic strategies like proper nutrition, acupuncture, herbal medicine, or a personalized supplement program has been shown to shorten the duration of time dedicated to "trying." There's also ample evidence to suggest that these strategies complement and optimize IVF, but we'll get to that later.

Practitioners of natural medicine are focused not on life-or-death situations per se but rather on one's quality of life. The philosophy is, first and foremost, to *prevent* disease through proper lifestyle practices. However, in many cases, natural medicine also has the power to slow down the progress of disease and/ or reverse it.

Holism views body and mind as one. To achieve wellness is to treat the person rather than an ailment. We look for more subtle drains on fertility and overall health and address the imbalance through natural means. In this chapter, I'll walk you through the modalities that I've found most clinically effective in the treatment of infertility.

Eastern Medicine

When it comes to wellness, perhaps no one does it better than the East. Traditional Chinese medicine (TCM) is a field of natural medicine that dates back thousands of years and is revered by many. This highly effective system has the power to address myriad health conditions. Although the wisdom has been passed down over millennia, practitioners of Eastern medicine continue building on the foundations established by their ancestors, adapting ancient methods into the modern world to great success. In fact, many of the ancient Chinese herbal formulas and acupuncture approaches used thousands of years ago are still proving incredibly effective today. Only in more recent years has research been conducted to support the use of Eastern medicine, but the clinical efficacy is traceable for thousands of years. It is tried, tested, and true.

The philosophy fueling TCM is that overall wellness can be achieved via three basic steps. First is the implementation of prevention strategies to ward off illness. Second is the timely diagnosis of illness to prevent the disease's progression. Third is the creation of a long-term, sustainable treatment to prevent relapse. TCM tunes into subtleties of imbalances in the body's energy and organ systems. It takes into account the interplay of physical, mental, and emotional factors and how they affect our health. As it was developing, the doctors didn't have access to the tests we have now, so they became highly skilled in observation of the patient to understand body functions and make a diagnosis. Practitioners of Eastern medicine see disease before it fully manifests so that we can effect change before the illness takes hold.

Under the TCM umbrella, which covers a wide array of natural treatments, the most mainstream is the incredible art of acupuncture.

ACUPUNCTURE

Acupuncture is among the oldest of all Eastern healing practices, first originating in ancient China more than 2,500 years ago. Today, the practice of acupuncture has spread throughout the world, widely accepted as an effective and trusted method for a variety of conditions.

Many of my patients ask me how inserting needles into our body could possibly have any positive effect. For starters, research has been conducted to show that the body's natural painkillers, such as endorphins and peptide opioids, are released during acupuncture treatment, resulting in pain relief and a feeling of elation. One study conducted on 607 mothers in labor showed that the group who utilized acupuncture for pain relief and relaxation requested significantly fewer pharmaceuticals and invasive pain relievers during delivery (Borup et al. 2009).

When you lie down on an acupuncture table, a skilled specialist gently inserts very thin needles into specific points around your body to stimulate a healing response. Those special pressure points are called acupoints. Electroacupuncture is a variation that attaches a small device to the needles, passing a mild electrical current through them for improved stimulation. Both forms are generally painless unless you are seeing a practitioner whose style is to manipulate the needle to intensify the "sensation." From my observation, most of the people who've experienced acupuncture report feeling a sense of peace and tranquility wash over them during and after the session.

In the ancient TCM school of thought, acupuncture heals, soothes, and relaxes the body by tapping into unique pathways called meridians to smooth the flow of qi (pronounced "chee"). Qi is our vital energy, and a balanced flow is essential for health and wellness. It drives all body processes from circulatory function to digestion to immune processes. In Chinese medicine, the causation of disease is based primarily on the obstruction of energy flow, or disrupted qi. By stimulating acupuncture points, you regulate the flow of energy.

Acupuncture is thought to regulate the nervous system. Nerve impulses carry sensory messages to and from the brain to initiate commands and create a desired effect. Acupuncture can regulate body systems by normalizing communication between the brain and the various systems in the body.

Acupuncture is amazing at increasing circulation in your reproductive system. A study on 10 infertile women showed that electroacupuncture (two times a week for four weeks) significantly increased blood flow to the uterine arteries after just eight sessions (Stener-Victorin et al. 1996). Acupuncture harmonizes the circulation in your reproductive organs, clears obstructions, and improves blood supply to your ovaries and uterus. This abundant blood flow provides oxygen and nutrients for your developing eggs and helps build a thick, highly receptive endometrial lining (Maughan and Xiao-Ping 2012). That said, blood flow is only the tip of the iceberg when it comes to acupuncture's health benefits.

Alternative Solutions for Heavy/Painful Periods

Many women consider painful periods a normal fact of life, but period pain is actually a sign of underlying issues such as inflammation, toxicity, endometriosis, and hormone imbalance. Severe pain and erratic bleeding is your body warning you that something is not quite right.

The conventional medical solution is birth control pills or, if you're trying to conceive, painkillers. In some severe cases, a doctor may suggest laparoscopy to investigate the possibility of endometriosis, which may result in surgery to remove scar tissue. This may be a necessary procedure for some to conceive, but a caveat is that the tissue will likely grow back. Whether you undergo a surgical procedure or not, it will be beneficial to apply diet modification, acupuncture, and herbal medicine. Not only will your periods improve, but you'll also reduce the inflammation that might be blocking your fertility.

Acupuncture is shockingly effective and quick acting for a variety of health challenges. I suggest pairing it with a fertility-supportive diet and lifestyle for best effect. However, even without a lifestyle overhaul, it packs amazing healing potential.

> **Pro Tip**
>
> For painful periods, apply castor oil packs on your lower belly (see chapter 8 for a refresher).

Here are just a few things that acupuncture can tackle:

- It *battles inflammation* by widening blood vessels, which activates neuropathic connections that tell your brain to send healing cells to inflamed areas (Zijlstra et al. 2003).
- Low-frequency electroacupuncture helps *reverse insulin resistance* by stimulating fibers in the spine and aiding the transport of glucose without the need for insulin. Another way it fights insulin resistance is by helping your insulin receptors react appropriately to the secretion of insulin (Liang and Koya 2010).
- It *knocks out stress* through the release of serotonin and other mood-balancing neurotransmitters (Cabioglu 2012).
- It *reduces toxicity* by assisting the function of eliminatory organs for clearer detoxification pathways.

It Takes Two: Acupuncture for Your Partner

Feel like your hubby could be doing something? Indeed, he could. Your partner can also use acupuncture to improve your chances of conception. Why not work on both sides of the equation to best optimize fertility? If he is resistant, try firing some convincing evidence at him, such as the study by Siterman et al. (2000) that found that acupuncture can improve the sperm density of men suffering from low sperm counts, especially if the cause of the low numbers is genital tract inflammation (very common). Acupuncture can also improve sperm motility by improving the effectiveness of the sperm's tail, which allows it to swim faster and with better endurance (Kwon et al. 2014). Last but not least, acupuncture reduces the amount of abnormally shaped sperm, making it easier for those little guys to penetrate and fertilize the egg.

Pei et al. (2005)

REIKI

Reiki is a Japanese form of energy healing. The Japanese principle of life energy is called "ki" rather than qi, but it's essentially the same principle. Unlike acupuncture's use of needles, a reiki practitioner restores health by guiding your body's energy with the palms of their hands. It's a relaxation and healing technique that's gaining popularity. Some hospitals in New York City and other big cities now offer it as a way to provide comfort for inpatients. I've personally found it very powerful, and I relax deeply (snoring a little) during my sessions.

MOXIBUSTION

If you're deathly afraid of needles and can't get past the idea of traditional acupuncture, there is still more that Eastern medicine has to offer. The word "moxibustion" is derived from the Japanese word *mogusa*, which means "burning herb." In a moxibustion session, an herb called mugwort or moxa is burned over carefully selected acupoints. The burning moxa warms the meridians (energy pathways), stimulating circulation and a smoother flow of energy. From a physics perspective, the herb burns at a high temperature that deeply penetrates the tissues to enhance circulation and reduce inflammation. The resulting increase in blood flow helps to enhance function of hormone-producing glands such as the adrenals, thyroid, and ovaries. If you are already doing acupuncture, moxibustion boosts its effectiveness, making the two an ideal fertility treatment combo. In fact, the Chinese character for acupuncture ("zhen") is tied to the character for moxibustion ("jiu"), implying that traditionally they are best used together. With or without acupuncture, moxibustion is an effective option that you can learn to do on yourself at home.

Moxibustion for Your Man

Male reproduction can benefit from moxa smoke as well. Utilizing moxibustion in conjunction with acupuncture twice a week was found to help produce normal-formed semen in males, suggesting that certain acupoints associated with testicular function can be targeted to improve sperm concentration, sperm mobility, and progressive motility (Gurfinkel et al. 2003). That means his sperm could potentially be more numerous, move faster, and move in the optimal trajectory, essentially becoming more likely to fertilize your precious egg.

HERBAL MEDICINE

Over millennia, doctors of Eastern medicine have compiled *Materia Medica* describing the uses of thousands of herbs and herb combinations called "formulas." A skilled herbalist takes into account your symptoms, observes your tongue and pulse, and then selects a blend from more than 6,000 medicinal herbal substances for your prescription. These highly customized concoctions can be specially designed to address your fertility challenges. Since it can be tricky to find a qualified Chinese herbalist, we offer this service through our sister website https://junkjuicemagic.com. There you'll see the "bespoke" option, whereby you fill out a questionnaire to have a blend designed just for you. You can also contact https://naturnalife.com for an herbal consultation to see if this route is right for you.

Heard that a particular formula worked for a friend? Odds are that it won't work the same for you. These herbal combinations are carefully selected to heal *your* fertility woes. There are thousands of formulas, and your pattern of infertility (i.e., which of the Big Four are affecting you, to what degree, and in what way) is unique to you.

As with acupuncture, herbal medicine gives you the opportunity to get a fully customized prescription. *Do not self-prescribe.* Leave the mixing to your certified herbalist so as to not put yourself at risk. There is a reason why my fellow specialists and I went to school for years to learn this skill. Certain herbs can interact with medications such as blood thinners or antidepressants. Medications aside, if the formula doesn't match your Big Four pattern, you may experience side effects such as mood changes, gastric distress, or sleep trouble. Worse yet, you'll miss out on the effectiveness of this modality.

Herbal medicine is backed by thousands of years of practice and teaching, and it works. A meta-analysis in 2015 reviewed 40 randomized control trials, including more than 4,000 women (Ried 2015). Chinese herbal medicine (CHM) was shown to improve pregnancy rates with double the success of Western medical fertility drug therapy over a three- to six-month period. CHM achieved pregnancies 60 percent of the time, whereas Western medical approaches achieved pregnancies only 33 percent of the time. A separate meta-analysis of 15 studies involving 1,659 patients showed that CHM increased the pregnancy rate, reduced the miscarriage rate, increased the ovulation rate, and improved the cervical mucus score significantly more than the drug clomiphene, a commonly prescribed fertility medication (Tan et al. 2012). And China isn't the only country with herbal mixtures that produce results. Korean herbal medicine has improved pregnancy success rates in women over 35 (Heo et al. 2016). In fact, a retrospective analysis showed that older women actually had higher success rates with Korean herbal medicine than their younger counterparts. The research makes for a compelling argument to give it a shot.

Stick with Eastern Medicine Practitioners for Eastern Practices

Chinese medicine doctors have training in acupuncture and Chinese herbs far beyond that of those in other disciplines. Chiropractors, naturopaths, medical doctors, physical therapists, and the like can practice the ancient arts, but most courses available to them are short (i.e., a weekend workshop or a single semester) and pretty "bare-bones." When someone tells me acupuncture didn't work for them, it was often at the hands of someone who did not undergo the stringent training involved in a full program. You will, however, find "hybrids" such as myself who have done long-term training and apprenticeships in more than one arena. Ask questions!

Herbal treatments are created based on the Five Flavors discussed in chapter 9. However, herbs are also classified by the Four Natures, which denote the properties of cold, hot, cool, or warm. While these are similar to the Five Natures applied to food, they are not exactly the same. Each condition or ailment is associated with an excess or a lack of one of these Four Natures. Excess "heat," for example, can be caused by stress, hormonal imbalance, inflammation, toxins, illness, or an acidic diet. If this is part of your health picture, your herbalist may add "cooling" herbs to your remedy. Makes sense, right? We cool down the heat.

The Five Flavors in Action

Here's a quick recap of what the Five Flavors do for the body.

1. *Pungent* flavors disperse cold and flu and move circulation.
2. *Sweet* flavors have a nourishing and moistening effect.
3. *Sour* flavors aid the liver and have astringent effects.
4. *Bitter* flavors are dry and cool and treat infections and promote calm.
5. *Salty* flavors soften masses and promote bowel movement.

You can request your herbal remedy as a liquid tincture, pills, tea granules, or a bundle of herbs in their whole form to cook into a nutritious, soupy tea. At the Naturna Institute and https://junkjuicemagic.com, we take the guesswork out by cooking the herbs into a concentrated tea format and sending them to you individually packaged for daily consumption.

Your herbal formula can be modified as you go along to address the changes in your hormones and reproductive needs. A qualified herbalist will create adjustments to address anything from poor egg quality to a thin endometrial lin-

Dr. Christina's Favorite Fertility Formulas

My goal in providing you this list is simply to empower you with the names of my favorite formulas, to guide your research, and to give you direction for your herbal medicine consultation. This way, you can ask more informed questions and discuss these powerful formulas with your specialist. Once you're matched with your perfect formula, miracles can happen. Although each of the following formulas treats a variety of conditions, I've listed the conditions that I've found they assist in healing best.

1. Wen Jing Tang, "Warm the Valley decoction"—PCOS, amenorrhea, thin uterine lining
2. Ba Zhen Tang, "Eight Treasures decoction"—unexplained infertility, post miscarriage, chemical pregnancy/blighted ovum, failed implantation
3. You Gui Wan, "Restore the Right decoction"—hypothyroidism, LPD/low progesterone, embryos not progressing to blastocyst
4. Gui Pi Tang, "Restore the Spleen decoction"—premature ovarian insufficiency, unexplained infertility, high stress and anxiety affecting fertility
5. Gui Zhi Fu Ling Wan, "Cinnamon Twig and Poria decoction"—fibroids, adenomyosis
6. Xue Fu Zhu Yu Tang, "Drive Out Stasis in the Mansion decoction"—endometriosis, immunological infertility
7. Liu Wei Di Huang Wan, "Six Ingredient Formula"—male factor infertility, ovarian insufficiency
8. Zhi Bai Di Huang Wan—POF, high FSH

ing. We can even throw in herbs to regulate stress and improve sleep. Regular check-ins with an herbalist also ensures that what was working for you doesn't start working against you.

In addition to the formulas in the box "Dr. Christina's Favorite Fertility Formulas," there are countless other herbs and supplements that help fertility. For the sake of not making this chapter an encyclopedia, I've limited the list below to some favorites.

Licorice Root

Licorice contains plant-derived phytoestrogens that I've found effective in boosting egg growth and fortifying the adrenal glands. It is classically used in combination with other herbs to neutralize toxins and enhance the effectiveness of the formulas in which it is found. I typically prescribe it in IVF cycles when eggs aren't growing as they should with the medications prescribed, but it's also beneficial in natural cycles. As an adrenal tonic, it is perfect for anyone whose most troublesome fertility foe is chronic stress. Do not take in cases of hypertension.

Rehmannia

This one is rarely prescribed as a single herb but is found in many fertility-driven blends. It's highly nutritive for women (think iron) and makes a frequent appearance in formulas addressing anything from high FSH to recurrent miscarriage to unexplained infertility. I use it in cases where there is no good reason why a pregnancy just isn't "sticking" or when ovulation is occurring late or not at all. It is also effective in combination with other herbs for egg and sperm quality issues.

Ginger

Well known for its effective treatment of nausea, ginger has also been shown to significantly reduce sperm DNA fragmentation (SDF) in males thanks to its antioxidant properties (Hosseini et al. 2016). This may translate into improved embryo quality and a reduced chance of miscarriage. Ginger is great in cases where digestive function is weak and can assist in the digestion and assimilation of other herbs. If you have excessive hunger or a lot of anxiety, then I'd avoid big doses of this one, as it may aggravate those issues. Like licorice and rehmannia, ginger makes an appearance frequently in Chinese herbal formulas that enhance fertility.

Green Tea

This one's a favorite for PCOS. From an Eastern medicine standpoint, it "cools" the system when overheated, which translates somewhat loosely into "cooling" inflammation. It is a potent antioxidant and is very effective for insulin resistance, weight issues, and excess hunger. Green tea contains prebiotics that promote regularity of bowel movements. In Asia, it is used as a daily ritual to boost metabolism and prevent weight gain. Trade in your cup of joe for a lightly steeped (30 to 45 seconds) cup of loose-leaf green tea.

Alternative Solutions for Light Periods

Light periods sound delightful, right? Yes and no. The amount you bleed during your period can be directly related to the thickness of your uterine lining. A very light period may mean your lining isn't growing to the healthy, fluffy state that makes implantation more probable. Common causes of light periods are chronic stress, hypothyroidism, and sex hormone imbalances such as underproduction of estrogen and progesterone or overproduction of androgens and insulin.

Alternative methods address these hormone imbalances and Big Four issues most effectively. Try acupuncture to stimulate blood flow, blood-building foods outlined in chapter 9 to supply building blocks for hormones, and herbal medicine to tone the uterus and stimulate the hormone production. For structural conditions such as scarring in the uterine cavity, however, you'll likely need to integrate Western methods such as a hysteroscopy.

AYURVEDA

The ancient medical system of Ayurveda, or "the science of life," originated in India around 5,000 years ago. The practice's guiding belief is centered around prevention of disease and maintenance of health with the appropriate lifestyle choices—diet, exercise, meditation, and herbal and other therapies. Knowledge of Ayurveda teaches you how to live healthfully according to your "constitutional" profile, that is, the doshas discussed in the previous chapter (Vata, Pitta, and Kapha).

Much like TCM, Ayurveda is an ancient system that now has modern research to support its use. In 2010, a six-month study conducted on women with PCOS showed that Ayurvedic treatment regulated formerly spotty menstrual cycles, increased follicle maturity, improved immune health, and ultimately led to 75 percent of the patients conceiving. A whopping 85 percent showed complete reversals of all their PCOS symptoms (Siriwardene et al. 2010).

As with TCM, Ayurveda's *Materia Medica* encompasses thousands of herbs. Below are a few of my fertility favorites.

Panchakarma for Health

There are amazing holistic cleansing retreats around the world that offer comprehensive programs in Panchakarma. These Ayurvedic detox and rejuvenation programs help to bring balance to body and mind. Panchakarma treatments are designed specifically for your dosha (see chapter 10) and may consist of any combination of herbs, oils, massage therapy, yoga, nutrition plans, and cleansing techniques such as enemas.

Kaur, Danylak-Arhanic, and Dean (2005)

Ayur-Triphala

Triphala is a famous Ayurvedic remedy that is rich in vitamin C and possesses powerful antioxidant and anti-inflammatory qualities. It is a great formula to consider if PCOS or insulin resistance is playing a role in your infertility. A study on the effects of an Ayurvedic treatment regimen that used triphala as the first treatment phase revealed that it can reduce cysts, improve follicle growth, and regulate hormones like LH and FSH in women with PCOS (Siriwardene et al. 2010). Triphala also cleanses the entire digestive tract and improves elimination.

Shatavari

The literal translation of shatavari is "who possesses a hundred husbands" or "acceptable by many," which alludes to its power to enhance fertility. It is even said to promote love and devotion (Alok et al. 2013). Who doesn't need a little of that during a tumultuous fertility journey? It acts as an aphrodisiac and immunoregulator, reduces inflammation, treats nervous disorders, and remedies a variety of female reproductive conditions. It is overall considered a "tonic," or "strengthener," of the reproductive system and can help with follicular development.

ASHWAGANDHA

This herb is considered a medicinal tonic and has proven especially useful as a "nervine tonic" (think nervous system and stress regulation). It helps to rejuvenate overly taxed adrenal glands and is therefore an effective treatment for anxiety, insomnia, and the like (Singh et al. 2011). Ashwagandha also enhances mitochondrial activity, which may have a positive effect on egg quality. It can provide an amazing boost for women who lack enjoyment in sex due to dryness, inability to reach orgasm, or pain during intercourse (Dongre, Langade, and Bhattacharyya 2015). Although used frequently for female conditions, it's a powerhouse for improving sperm quality, so adding it to your partner's daily supplement intake can go a long way (Ambiye et al. 2013).

Eastern medicinal traditions offer remedies for just about every fertility-related condition. While some are eager to dive in, many more are hesitant to stray from science for their treatment. If you fall into the latter category, you may more easily buy into a system of natural medicine that maintains a basis in scientific thought.

The Naturopathic Way

If you prefer an approach rooted in science, naturopathic medicine can act as a smooth transition into the world of natural medicine. Not only is it a nice blending of several modalities, but naturopathic doctors explain natural remedies from a modern scientific paradigm, making it easier for the Western mind to grasp.

Naturopathy is somewhat of a hodgepodge of many of the other alternative practices included in this chapter, and it encompasses a holistic ideal as much as a method. Naturopathy is a discipline that emphasizes prevention, treatment, and optimal health through therapeutic methods such as herbal medicine, homeopathy, and nutrition. It was first developed in Europe, but when it came to North America in the 1800s, it was influenced by Native American herbal medicine, shaping it into the practice recognized today. Naturopaths help to guide their patients to wellness by teaching self-care practices combined with appropriate natural remedies. In some states, naturopathic physicians are qualified to be primary care practitioners, meaning they can tend to the yearly physicals and blood work that an internist would usually oversee. Naturopathy has seven guiding principles that are a good basis from which to understand the philosophy of various branches of alternative medicine.

The Naturopathic Principles

All certified naturopaths follow a set of principles that provide further insight into the practice and its multilayered approach to natural medicine:

Nature heals. Naturopaths believe that the body has an innate ability to heal itself. The naturopathic physician removes obstacles to healing while gently facilitating the body's own healing mechanisms via natural substances and health-conscious lifestyle changes.

Seek the roots. A naturopath is trained to seek the underlying cause of disease rather than only treating the symptoms to provide deeper healing and long-term solutions.

First, do no harm. Naturopaths use therapies that are gentle yet effective forms of healing and avoid more aggressive and invasive measures that may have negative side effects.

Treat the whole person. Naturopathy views the individual as a whole—a complex interaction of the physical, mental, social, and emotional spheres. Treatment aims to balance all aspects of the body and mind to "reset" the symptoms.

Physician as teacher. "Teach a (wo)man to fish." Rather than hand over a supplement and call it a day, a naturopath provides her patients with the necessary education and tools to facilitate their own healing.

Prevention is the best cure. Naturopaths specialize in disease prevention through education on nutrition and other lifestyle habits. When issues are caught in the early stages, they are more easily resolved.

Continual wellness. The naturopathic approach aspires to first establish overall wellness with lifestyle counseling and natural remedies, addressing disease as a secondary result.

As a highly individualized approach, the power of naturopathy is often best demonstrated through individual case studies. One such study placed a 37-year-old female with hypothyroidism and associated hyperprolactinemia on a naturopathic regimen for 18 months. By monitoring her TSH levels, researchers discovered that she had reversed *all* the hormonal imbalances associated with her condition. In the beginning, her TSH and prolactin levels were abnormally high, and her AMH was unusually low. Thanks to naturopathic interventions, including hydrotherapy, acupuncture, and yoga, she leveled out her TSH and prolactin and increased her AMH numbers to normal range (Nair 2016).

Naturopaths will often incorporate herbs in their treatment programs, which are selected on the basis of their patient's individual needs. They commonly use Western herbs in their prescriptions, though they are not averse to adding a few Eastern gems as well. Below are some of the naturopath-approved, Western botanical boosters I often prescribe. As with Eastern herbal medicine, proceed with caution. This section is meant more as an educational tool rather than a how-to guide.

Raspberry Leaf

This is a highly nutritive female herbal tonic. It contains all the important minerals needed to tone the uterus and regulate hormones. Most of the current research on this herb is based on its use during pregnancy to help induce labor. Raspberry leaf acts as a "tonic" on the uterine wall, making it a go-to for building uterine lining in preparation for implantation.

Nettle

I prescribe nettle, another highly nutritive tonic, to provide a gentle but profound boost to minerals such as magnesium and iron. Herbal lore categorizes nettle as a female tonic, but research supports its use as a remedy for male prostate issues as well. This is largely due to its anti-inflammatory and diuretic effect. It's an enjoyable sipping tea and also pairs well with rooibos.

Red Clover

Traditionally, red clover is considered a blood cleanser, meaning that it removes toxins and impurities from the blood. It's also a phytoestrogen powerhouse that's been studied as a replacement for estrogen therapy (Beck, Rohr, and Jungbauer 2005).

Chasteberry

This one is an herbalist's favorite for increasing progesterone and regulating PMS. You may remember from previous chapters that progesterone can be depleted by stress, estrogen dominance, perimenopause, PCOS, and myriad other issues (Westphal, Polan, and Trent 2006). Chasteberry is effective at improving the estrogen-to-progesterone ratio (Westphal, Polan, and Trent 2006; Grant and Ramasamy 2012). Use with caution in cases of PCOS or POF where LH hormone is consistently high.

Maca

For centuries, herbalists in the Andes of Peru have prescribed maca to boost fertility in women *and* men. It's popular among naturopaths as a remedy for ladies and gents with low libido, vaginal dryness, fatigue, irregular cycles, and unexplained infertility. There are many varieties of maca, and they all vary in benefits. Some are better for men, while others are good for irregular cycles or age-related infertility in women. Maca may boost egg quality according to research that demonstrated its ability to improve the quality of embryos in mice (Gonzales 2011). Based on the stellar results I've seen clinically, I'm confident those successful human studies aren't far off.

Á La Carte Naturopathy— Biotherapeutic Drainage

This approach focuses on healing through the flushing of toxins and consequent rejuvenation of organ function. Homeopathic remedies or gemmotherapy (young buds of various plants) are combined to assist the drainage of toxins through various emunctories (organs of elimination). The theory here is that disease is caused by toxic buildup and that healing is facilitated by eliminating toxins through excretory organs like the liver, large intestine, kidneys, lungs, and skin.

Homeopathy

Developed in Europe by German physician Dr. Samuel Hahnemann, homeopathy is based in the principle of "like cures like." It may sound crazy but remedies involve a dilution of the same substance that would have caused the symptom in the first place. For example, a bee sting would be treated with a dilution of bee venom. Belladonna is an herb that can cause headache, and thus the homeopathic cure for migraines is a dilution of belladonna. This is a tad oversimplified, but you get the point. Through years of testing natural substances on himself and healthy volunteers, Dr. Hahnemann logged reactions to 2,000 of these items. Using those *Materia Medica*, homeopathic specialists match the remedy to the symptoms. It sounds like these remedies would cause a reaction, right? Wrong. Homeopathic remedies contain the tiniest dose of the original herb or substance, diluted so many times that there is only a subtle energetic presence of the original remaining. Each remedy has a personality profile and funny quirks attached, meaning you'd have a remedy prescribed to you based on your habits and tendencies. It doesn't get more customized than that!

That Extra Something:
A Guide to Supplements

Supplements are a major buzz word in the infertility landscape. Traditionally, naturopathic doctors were the primary champions of supplementation, but now just about everyone is hopping onto the bandwagon. Evidence is mounting to corroborate the benefits of nutrient supplementation for fertility. Research suggests that micronutrient supplementation has a notable positive impact on improving success rates of women struggling to conceive (Schaefer and Nock 2019).

Supplement regimes are effective, but they don't replace healthy nutrition. Ideally, you'll be implementing dietary and lifestyle recommendations rather than simply throwing a vitamin pill at the problem.

Many people ask me why they can't just get their nutrients from food. I'd love to tell you that thoughtful attention to your daily habits is all you need. Sadly, modern farming practices and the globalization of food make that nearly impossible even if you're doing everything right. Mass production and shipping food all the way from Timbuktu depletes our food of nutrition. Even if you pluck it right from your garden, you'd have to eat a heck of a lot of certain foods to get the therapeutic dosages of nutrients that have shown promise for conditions like poor egg quality or PCOS. While I do believe that a healthy lifestyle would get you pregnant, it can take time. Catered doses of nutrients can in some cases act as a catalyst and quicken the path to conception.

Where *Not* to Buy Your Supplements

Be wary of buying supplements from Amazon or other online dealers. There is no way to know how they have been stored (i.e., near heat that could damage the product) or even whether it's the true product and not a knockoff that someone slapped a label onto. Scary, I know. Buy through a licensed practitioner or visit our online dispensary (https://wellevate.me/naturnainstitute or https://us.fullscript.com/welcome/naturnalife). You can also check appendix E for a list of brands that come highly recommended and order directly from their website.

I have done my best to pair dosage recommendations with the supplements to follow, but there are variables to consider, such as your body makeup (weight, genetics, current challenges, and so on) and the brand of supplement. For safety and the best optimal results, it would be best to have a custom-designed protocol by a qualified practitioner. Contact us at info@naturnalife.com if you can't find a qualified practitioner in your area.

CATCHALL FERTILITY ENHANCERS

Taking the right supplements from quality brands can be a great assist to your fertility journey. Below are just a few that are proven to shorten the time to pregnancy and prevent birth defects, with little to no side effects.

Multivitamins (aka Your Prenatal)

Beginning in 1991, one study followed 116,671 female registered nurses ages 24 to 42 over the course of about eight years. Those taking a multivitamin at least three times per week were much less likely to suffer from ovulatory infertility (irregular or absent ovulation) (Chavarro et al. 2008). The link has been noted in other studies that demonstrated higher pregnancy rates in women taking multivitamins (Westphal et al. 2004). I suggest taking a prenatal with high doses of B12, B6, methylfolate, and a variety of minerals and vitamins also mentioned in this section from brands like Thorne Research or Klaire Labs. They can be purchased through a reputable online dispensary from the link on our home page (https://naturnalife.com).

B Vitamins

The B vitamin family provides an impressive variety of important fertility benefits, but the following Bs are the most well researched in the areas of egg growth and development. *Folate* is responsible for making new copies of DNA and the building blocks of proteins. Most doctors recommend supplementing this nutrient since a deficiency may result in birth defects such as spina bifida. Adequate folate levels are important for egg quality and the chromosomal development of your embryo(s). Research conducted in England in 1991 determined that 70 to 80 percent of neural tube defects could be prevented with folate supplementation before pregnancy (Wald and Sneddon 1991). Similarly, women with twice the average amounts of folic acid were found to have a lesser risk of having a baby with Down syndrome (Hollis et al. 2013). An ideal dosage is one milligram per day. You'll want to seek out methylfolate since many women have trouble processing folic acid. Look for the bioavailable form called L-methylfolate and keep eating those folate-rich foods listed in chapter 9. Consuming the natural form of folate is especially essential for women with the MTHFR gene mutation, for whom folic acid may actually be toxic. Dose: 800 to 1,800 mcg daily.

Vitamin B6 assists in the absorption of folate as well as progesterone production and the elimination of excess estrogens. In a study conducted by Dr. Alayne Ronnenberg at Harvard Medical School, women with low levels of B6 were less likely to get pregnant and more likely to miscarry (Ronnenberg et al. 2007). Dose: 50 to 100 milligrams daily.

Vitamin B5 helps to support your adrenal glands and heal you from chronic stress, whether emotional, physical, or otherwise (Kelly 1999). Dose: 4 to 10 grams daily.

Vitamin B12 helps to absorb folate and iron. It is important in the prevention of anemia and allows the body to better utilize oxygen in the blood. According to a study from the Netherlands, B12 is associated with better embryo quality because it decreases homocysteine (Boxmeer et al. 2009), an amino acid in your blood that is tied to heart disease and blood clotting. Dose: 1,000 micrograms daily in the morning.

Pro Tip for MTHFR

Supplements that combine high levels of folate, vitamin B12, and vitamin B6 are the best combo for managing the deleterious effects of MTHFR.

Alternative Solutions for Fatigue

Constant weariness may be an indicator that you're nutrient deficient. More specifically, you may not be absorbing iron and B vitamins well or just not consuming enough of them. Fatigue can also be a result of a low-grade immune response to a toxin, latent bacteria, a virus, chronic stress, insulin resistance, or an imbalanced gut. Conditions caused by one or more of the Big Four may also tie into fatigue. If the body's energy is low, it may not be carrying oxygen, energy, or circulation well—all important factors in supplying an embryo the resources it needs to implant and thrive. It's also worth mentioning that withstanding a fertility journey when you're tired is incredibly difficult. The quest for baby can kick your ass emotionally. Try acupuncture to cleanse and de-stress, nutrition and supplements to restore nutrient levels, and herbal medicine if a boost is still required thereafter.

Minerals

Minerals like selenium, iodine, zinc, magnesium, and iron are essential micronutrients for everything from hormone production to egg development to fetal growth. Selenium and zinc are potent antioxidants, while magnesium and iron are necessary for more than 300 processes to occur in the body.

- Selenium has been shown to increase pregnancy rates in women with PCOS by 18.8 percent (Razavi et al. 2015). Dose: 50 to 200 milligrams.

- Iodine is a hormone naturally produced by your thyroid and is essential for its proper function. Dose: 100 micrograms.
- Zinc (along with calcium and magnesium) can help ward off preeclampsia (Jain et al. 2009). Low zinc in pregnant women has also been linked to low fetal heart rates, so supplementing can potentially help avoid miscarriage (Spann et al 2015). Dose: 30 milligrams.
- Iron helps prevent anemia and it is essential for distributing oxygen throughout the body. When supplementing iron, natural sources such as liver pills or botanical sources are preferable. They are more absorbable and have less likelihood of the side effects like constipation and inflammation commonly caused by synthetic iron. Dose: 10 to 25 milligrams.
- Magnesium helps tackle insulin resistance, stress, poor sleep, egg quality, and hormonal imbalance. Dose: 200 to 300 milligrams.

Many of these minerals are found in prenatal vitamins, but some should consider additional supplementation depending on your unique fertility challenges.

Vitamin D

Vitamin D has long been used for cardiovascular health and bone density, but in recent years, studies were conducted on its function in addressing female fertility. Research suggests that vitamin D can thicken your lining and strengthen the endometrium as a whole, especially in women with PCOS (Lerchbaum and Rabe 2014). There's also evidence that it potentially reduces the risk of neonatal diseases and complications if taken during pregnancy (Peña-Rosas et al. 2012). In the Harvard nurses study mentioned in the multivitamin discussion above, it was discovered that low vitamin D levels were associated with lowered fertility and that high vitamin D was associated with an increased rate of live births (Chavarro et. al 2008). In a similar university study, high levels of vitamin D increased pregnancy rates by 27 percent (Ozkan et al. 2010). Women with PCOS are more likely to have a vitamin D deficiency (44 percent compared to 11 percent) (Li et al. 2011). Since vitamin D deficiency is associated with significant metabolic imbalances, such as insulin resistance, it is important for women with this profile to consider supplementation. A dose of 2,000 to 5,000 international units (IU) daily is recommended.

Omega-3 Fatty Acids

These beneficial fats are found in fish, nuts, seeds, and algae. The preferred forms of omega-3s are eicosapentaenoic acid (EPA) and docosahexaenoic acid

(DHA). They reduce inflammation throughout the body, thereby improving the environment for an egg to grow and implant. Similar to vitamin E, omega-3 fatty acids act as blood thinners to improve circulation, ease swelling, and stimulate quicker healing (Kiecolt-Glaser et al. 2012). They also protect the nervous system of mom and baby in utero. Daily consumption throughout your pregnancy promotes a higher IQ in baby (Coletta and Bell 2010). For your preconception plan, aim for a combined dosage of around 1,200 milligrams daily to be taken with food.

Probiotics

Certain strains of probiotics are shown to reduce inflammation, improve insulin resistance, and improve the elimination of toxins and toxic hormones by improving gut health. I recommend choosing a probiotic from a company that specializes in probiotics, such as Genestra or Klaire Labs. Make sure to use the strains specific to you and to proceed with caution if you have inflammatory bowel disease, such as Crohn's.

Support Elimination with Prebiotics and Probiotics

Constipation is common in women with insulin resistance or hypothyroidism. Even loose stools can be considered a sign of constipation, poor nutrient absorption, and an irritated gut. Your body is telling you that something is awry, and it could be as simple as your food choices jamming you up. Some common dietary culprits are gluten, dairy, rice, bananas, chocolate, and eggs. Other factors, like stress, anxiety, and constant rushing, can also lock up your gut. Regardless of the cause, you're retaining waste in your intestines, which then reabsorbs toxins into your bloodstream and causes a cascade of inflammatory reactions. Yuck. Seek nutritional counseling, try acupuncture, and start a curated supplement program that includes prebiotics and probiotics.

FOR CONCERNS OF AGING AND EGG QUALITY

A poor egg quality diagnosis is painful and discouraging given that there is typically no concrete treatment known to "fix" the issue. Clinicians and researchers are, however, working to find solutions. Here are a few promising supplements that have some evidence to back them up.

The Damage of Oxidative Stress

Oxidants cause cellular damage in your eggs by reducing the mitochondria's ability to produce energy and keep the cell healthy. Each cell has oxidant defenses, including antioxidant enzymes to eradicate free radicals. However, as we age, our antioxidant levels decline, and oxidation damages our eggs. Interestingly, reactive oxygen molecules are found to be higher in women with unexplained infertility. One study showed that 70 percent of women with unexplained premature ovarian failure had elevated oxidation levels. Women with PCOS also have higher oxidative stress due to imbalanced insulin and the associated inflammation. Similarly, women with endometriosis have an increased oxidative stress due to immune disturbances and inflammation. To learn more about the sources of oxidative stress, jump back to chapters 4 to 6.

Ağaçayak et al. (2016)

Antioxidants

These free radical scavengers may have the power to slow or reverse the aging of your body's cells by protecting you against the damage caused by toxins, inflammation, stress, bad diet, and so on. Premature aging and damaged egg quality are often related to these (somewhat controllable) lifestyle factors. By boosting antioxidant levels, you can strengthen your cells and, as a result, your eggs. Conventional Western medicine currently offers very little in the way of reducing oxidative stress. Natural therapies like supplements, acupuncture, and herbs, on the other hand, are measures that you can take to boost your antioxidant levels. Let's take a look at the most potent antioxidants in supplemental form.

CoQ10

This fat-soluble supplement may assist in reversing the decline in egg quality that comes along with age or other factors. It works by improving the function of the mitochondria of egg cells. By jump-starting the powerhouse of the cell, studies show it may rejuvenate the eggs of older women or those with premature ovarian aging (Ben-Meir et al. 2015). There are some differences in opinion about the dosage required as well as which form is most absorbable: ubiquinol or ubiquinone. Ubiquinol was shown in one study to be slightly easier to assimilate and was recommended at a dosage of 600 milligrams daily. Both forms should fare similarly, though ubiquinol was shown to have higher absorption potential in an older study. More recently, companies have played around with technology to improve absorption to lower the dosage required. I recommend taking a minimum of 300 mg daily, up to 800 milligrams daily with an average of 600 milligrams spread across three doses over the course of a day. CoQ10 can also aid male fertility. A study published in the *Journal of Andrology* found that supplementation of 200 to 300 milligrams daily

> Take oily vitamins with food for best absorption.

improved sperm count and motility (Ko and Sabanegh 2011). It absorbs better when taken with food.

Vitamin C

Large amounts of vitamin C are naturally found in ovarian follicles, suggesting that it's an important nutrient for egg quality and development. For women of a healthy weight under the age of 35, studies have demonstrated that higher consumption of vitamin C results in a shorter time to pregnancy (Ruder et al. 2014). If you have allergies, you get bonus benefits because it's also a natural antihistamine and immune booster. Due to its potent antioxidant and anti-inflammatory qualities and its positive influence on the immune system, I prescribe it regularly for endometriosis and chronic stress. Typically, I recommend up to 2,000 milligrams daily. If you experience loose stools thanks to its laxative properties or if your frame is petite, then I suggest closer to 1,000 milligrams daily.

Vitamin E

This vitamin may be of assistance if you have past history of miscarriage or failed implantation, have an unexplained infertility diagnosis, or are over the age of 35. By reducing free radical damage in ovarian follicles, vitamin E supports the growth of healthy eggs. It also acts as a blood thinner or anticlotting agent to enhance blood flow to your uterus, which can assist in healthy placental development. In a study conducted on women over age 35, vitamin E supplementation led to a shorter time to pregnancy (Ruder et al. 2014). I recommend 400 IU daily.

Resveratrol

Similar to our own anti-inflammatory cytokines, resveratrol is an antioxidant produced by grapes and berries when they are under stress or attack, whether that be a fungal infection, bruising, or overexposure to light (Hasan and Bae 2017). So it's not surprising that this potent antioxidant can soothe hostile reproductive environments in cases of endometriosis where endometriomas (endometrial scar tissue) forms cysts in the ovaries (Taguchi et al. 2013). If you're an endometriosis sufferer, resveratrol may help with egg quality by reducing

Alpha-Lipoic Acid: Do or Don't?

This supplement is popular in some circles for its potential to improve egg maturation and embryo viability. However, there is conflicting evidence. In one study, a dosage of 800 milligrams of alpha-lipoic acid twice a day for 16 weeks showed improved insulin sensitivity and helped women with PCOS ovulate normally (Masharani et al. 2010). The downside is that it may have a minor negative influence on thyroid hormone levels. If on thyroid medication, avoid this supplement.

the oxidative stress the condition places on your developing eggs. Dose: 100 to 300 milligrams daily.

NAC

The supplemental amino acid cysteine may enhance egg quality and benefit fertility by boosting the activity of a critical antioxidant inside your cells called glutathione. Glutathione is produced in your liver and plays a major role in detoxification. It may also restore ovulation by regulating liver function and insulin response. NAC is one of my all-time favorite supplements for both fertility and treatment of anxiety. The ideal dosage is 600 to 1,200 milligrams per day. Lean into the higher range if you suffer from anxiety or have PCOS and/or high cholesterol.

Other Nutrients for Eggs and Beyond

Myoinositol

You can think of myoinositol sort of like a vitamin version of the diabetic drug metformin. If you suffer from insulin resistance and/or PCOS, this B vitamin is your new best friend. It's been shown to restore ovulation in women with PCOS over a six-month period as well as lowering insulin and improving blood sugar and pregnancy rates overall (Papaleo et al. 2007; Ciotta et al. 2011; Noventa et al. 2015). That means a lower risk of gestational diabetes and insulin resistance–related miscarriages. As with most supplements, it works better if started earlier in preconception planning, and I recommend a dose of two grams per day.

DHEA

The current theory is that DHEA improves low ovarian reserve, increasing the number of eggs resting in your ovaries. It does this by providing vital precursors to ovarian hormones needed for egg development (Kachhawa et al. 2015). However, some controversy surrounds it because it can also aggravate situations where women have higher androgen levels, such as in certain cases of PCOS. It can also make some women pimply, angry, or anxious. The lack of a large double-blind placebo controlled trial to test this possibility, which is the gold standard in traditional medicine, adds to the controversy. The recommended dosage according to an older study is 25 milligrams three times daily, but I often prescribe only 25 milligrams once daily in the morning for the previously mentioned reasons. If you have elevated testosterone levels or PCOS, avoid this one.

Supplements for Him

While you're grabbing your supplements, put these in the cart for your partner, too:

- Vitamin E, 400 IU daily, increases sperm potency by two and a half times and improves the pregnancy rates of previously infertile men (Moslemi and Zargar 2011).
- CoQ10, 200 to 300 milligrams daily, increases sperm parameters all around—higher sperm counts, improved morphology, and faster motility (Lafuente et al. 2013).
- L-carnitine taken in doses of two grams per day for two months has improved sperm count and motility (Mills and Yao 2016).
- Vitamin C combats the buildup of pollution and agricultural chemicals that lower sperm counts. It can reduce DNA damage by 91 percent (Fraga et al. 1991), reduce sperm abnormalities, and increase sperm count (Akmal et al. 2006). Try 2,000 milligrams daily.
- Zinc deficiency can lead to low semen volume and testosterone, so it's important for your man to retain normal levels. When combined with folate, zinc has actually been shown to increase sperm concentration (Mills and Yao 2016). Take 20 milligrams daily.
- Selenium is an antioxidant that can increase sperm motility and concentration. A daily dosage of just 0.1 milligrams over three months showed a motility increase of 29 percent in one study. When the dose was doubled over 26 weeks, increased concentration was noted (Mills and Yao 2016).
- Omega-3 is a fatty acid that's been shown to improve your man's overall sperm profile. It's been linked most prominently to better sperm count and concentration. I recommend 1,200 milligrams daily of EPA and DHA (Falsig, Gleerup, and Knudsen 2019; Safarinejad 2010; Jannatifar et al. 2019).
- NAC is an antioxidant that's improved semen parameters. One randomized study on infertile men conducted over three months showed significant improvement in sperm motility and concentration and significant decreases in DNA fragmentation. Their testosterone levels increased, and their FSH and LH levels were lowered to proper numbers (Jannatifar et al. 2019). Shoot for 1,200 milligrams daily.
- Korean red ginseng is an herb that's been shown to improve all three major sperm factors in infertile men: motility, morphology, and concentration (Mills and Yao 2016).
- Cumin is a plant rich in antioxidants that can help improve your man's semen volume as well as sperm count, motility, and morphology (Mills and Yao 2016).

Sample Supplement Plans

Based on the factors at play in your body, you'll want to prioritize certain supplements in your preconception plan. Here's a quick-pick guide for supplement combinations based on specific diagnoses or circumstances (note that these are in addition to a prenatal with high folate, B6, and B12):

- *PCOS.* Myoinositol, NAC, probiotics, omega-3, magnesium glycinate, alpha-lipoic acid, vitamin D
- *Endometriosis.* Vitamin C, probiotics, omega-3, pycnogenol, melatonin, vitamin D, resveratrol
- *35 years+.* Acai, ubiquinol, probiotics, vitamin D, omega-3, NAC
- *Low AMH.* DHEA, ubiquinol, omega-3, probiotics, vitamin D
- *Amenorrhea with high AMH.* Myoinositol, alpha-lipoic acid, NAC, omega-3, probiotics, vitamin D
- *High FSH.* Ubiquinol, omega-3, vitamin C, acai, NAC, L-arginine, vitamin D
- *Severe PMS and unexplained infertility.* Chasteberry, DIM, calcium D-glucarate, calcium and magnesium, NAC, omega-3, vitamin D
- *Late ovulation (day 18 or after).* Myoinositol, rehmannia, omega-3, probiotics, vitamin D

Explore All the Options

If you're new to this realm, a naturopathic doctor or practitioner of Eastern medicine will make a valuable first companion. This is especially the case if you're not certain where to begin or you aren't entirely convinced yet that natural medicine will offer anything of great value. Either approach would provide a great starting point because they are the most regulated of all alternative medicine fields in the United States. Becoming a certified specialist in these areas requires a minimum of 3,000 hours of study and a state-sanctioned license. There is ample evidence to support their use in fertility efforts, and both are covered by many insurance plans to boot. As always, choose what suits your needs and level of comfort.

Contrary to what some think, delving into the world of natural medicine doesn't mean you must choose it *over* conventional treatment. In fact, research is mounting that integrative medicine, wherein you combine natural and conventional treatments, has a lot to offer in the field of fertility. Evidence is mounting that therapies such as acupuncture, supplements, and nutrition can improve the outcomes of IVF and get you pregnant faster. They're also exceptional at lowering the adverse side effects of conventional fertility treatment. Getting started a few months in advance is best, but if you are already in the thick of fertility treatments, you'll still benefit by taking immediate action.

In the next chapter, we dive into all the details of integrative techniques for those of you going through or planning to go through ART or IVF treatments.

CHAPTER 12

Integrating East and West

Never in history have we had access to as much technology to navigate the world of infertility. I often think of what it would have been like for the women who were pronounced "sterile" in a time with little to no diagnostics and few viable solutions. Modern ART is giving babies to families who may not have been able to conceive otherwise. There is, however, a common misconception that technology is the answer to *all* fertility woes. I've seen so many women who delayed conception because, in their words, "I can just do IVF." Unfortunately, as advanced as these fertility treatments are, they're not foolproof, and your doctor can't always provide answers as to why. Even women who appear to be ideal candidates—with good egg count and under 35 years old with ideal hormonal profiles—still fail consistently. Making a baby involves a lot of mystery, and the path is at times unclear. This chapter is dedicated to teaching you how to make the most of the technology available. ART has incredible potential and natural medicine offers ways to improve the outcomes.

A Harsh Reality—ART Success Rates

- **IVF success rate for women 35 or younger:** 45 to 55 percent (National Summary Report 2022)
- **IVF success rate for women 35 to 37:** 40 percent (National Summary Report 2022)
- **IVF success rate for women 38 to 40:** 26 percent (National Summary Report 2022)
- **IUI success rates for women 40 years and up:** 0 to 5 percent (National Summary Report 2022)
- **IVF success rate (a cycle resulting in the live birth of a child) for women 40 to 42:** 12 percent (Bold and Bedford 2016)
- **IVF success rate for women 43 or older:** 4 percent

Modern medicine follows a mechanistic model of treatment whereby you break down the body into "parts" or "systems," and the treatment is aimed at addressing that singular part. In contrast, natural medicine is focused more on the body and mind as a whole of interconnected systems and parts. An imbalance in one, therefore, can easily affect another. Neither is wrong per se, and both are effective in their own ways. However, there are great advantages to using the strengths of both sides together.

In fact, integration of methods may be the key to a better patient experience and improved outcomes. Integrative medicine puts the patient at the center of the treatment and addresses a full range of physical, emotional, environmental, and spiritual factors that affect overall wellness and fertility. While conventional methods offer ways to circumvent many fertility challenges, natural medicine provides therapeutic methods that enhance the effectiveness of those treatments. Natural medicine also helps alleviate the emotional stress and unpleasant physical side effects of undergoing ART, such as bloat, pain, and sleep disturbances. Using complementary methods to reduce stress, inflammation, toxins, and so on, may in fact make it more likely that conventional methods such as IVF or IUI will lead to pregnancy and live birth.

East Meets West

In one study on 57 women, half of whom were given acupuncture during IVF treatment and half of whom weren't, the patients utilizing acupuncture had higher pregnancy rates across the board and reported lower stress levels throughout the process (Balk et al. 2010). In another study, 110 women suffering from harsh side effects of the drug clomiphene taken for PCOS were split into two groups. One served as the control, and the other was placed on a customized Chinese herbal protocol. The group using the herbs doubled their conception rates compared to the control, and they were found to have significantly thicker endometrial linings after treatment.

Jian-jun (2007)

Empowerment through Knowledge

Demand for an integrative approach is on the rise. The most popular fertility doctors/centers today are often the ones who offer progressive approaches and/or collaborate with practitioners like yours truly. Type A females want to know what they can do to up their odds of success. But we're not the only ones. Western doctors are referring their patients to natural fertility specialists like me with increasing frequency. These referrals reduce the physician's workload, freeing them up to do what they do best. When the doctor can integrate care alongside a nutritionist, acupuncturist, or therapist specializing in fertility, the patients get the extra support the doctor doesn't necessarily have the time or training to give. Doctors want to help in all areas, but in reality, they are usually spread so thin that they don't have time to devote to methods outside their specialty. They may not always have time to field all of a patient's questions, leaving the women in their care feeling rushed and anxious. As much as we want them to be, they can't be everything to everyone. When other practitioners are brought in, however, it ensures that you, as the patient, feel supported, informed, and empowered.

Over my years of practice, I've witnessed miracles when the two sides were integrated. One of the most memorable stories is that of my patient Jess. Like so many women who come into my office, Jess was tormented by the idea of childlessness. Every Mother's Day was agonizing, and each Christmas with her nieces and nephews was another sad reminder of the longing she felt. The prospect of childlessness consumed her to the point of paralysis. Jess had already been to several fertility doctors without success, and at 39 years old, she was 10 years into trying to get pregnant. The first doctor suggested IVF right away, but the cycle was canceled due to poor egg development. The next doctor suggested doing IUIs, only to find out, on further inspection, that Jess had blocked fallopian tubes. That meant that pursuing IVF was her only viable option. Jess panicked given her previous experience with IVF. Her doctor sent her my way in an effort to help prep her physically and emotionally for the next phase of treatment.

Jess was overweight and had some less-than-ideal lifestyle habits. She was a highly dedicated school counselor for children with special needs. She worked 7 a.m. to 6 p.m. and never stopped to eat or drink and barely to breathe! When she finally came home, she'd nosh on snacks while she cooked a hefty, late dinner. She skipped breakfast and lunch and calorie loaded in the evening. She had no time for exercise during the week and was too exhausted on the weekends to think about it. Jess was so fearful of not having children that it immobilized her decision-making ability. The prospect of another cycle failure made her shy away from even trying. Together, we made a game plan. I then worked alongside her very compassionate fertility doctor, who I knew had her best interest in mind. "Dr. Nice" (as we will call him) found clear evidence (laparoscopy) that Jess had fairly severe endometriosis, and the inflammation was flaring due to the excess estrogens and insulin characteristic of her weight problem. Dr. Nice agreed that we had to work on sensitizing insulin and reducing inflammation. I put Jess on a diet low in inflammatory foods (cutting out gluten, red meat, fried foods, chocolate, candy, pop, and dairy products). Jess wasn't boozy, nor was she a coffee drinker, so we didn't have to worry about those. Jess's biggest issue was she never slowed down long enough to develop good habits. I counseled her in quick breakfasts and protein powder smoothies that she could have for lunch on the fly if she really couldn't stop. It was an effort, but Jess was able to integrate both breakfast and lunch on a regular basis. She also began taking walks after school, and on weekends, she would jog.

While she continued with weekly acupuncture sessions, Dr. Nice and I settled on a supplement regime rich in antioxidants to combat the inflammation caused by the endometriosis. Jess's next IVF cycle was a success! She grew only five eggs, but one of her embryos made it to a day 5 blastocyst and tested normal with PGT-A (no chromosomal issues). Jess finally had a real possibility of becoming a mom. Sadly, this worsened her paralysis! She had tried so long and experienced so many disappointments that if this didn't work, she feared she might crack. Quite a bit of coaching went into mentally preparing her for implantation. In the days leading up to the insertion (aka transfer) of the fertilized embryo, Jess maintained the same dietary plan with the addition of some bromelain, probiotics, omega-3, and vitamin E to increase circulation to her uterus, reduce inflammation, and prepare her uterine lining. We also upped the acupuncture to three times per week for two weeks to beat down stress hormones and inflammation. Dr. Nice transferred the single embryo, and she carried it to term. Congrats, Jess! It was a long time coming.

The "When" and the "How"

Many of you are likely already pursuing IVF, IUI, or some other form of medical intervention to treat infertility. Or perhaps you've been trying for a while to no avail, and this is your next planned step. If you have the luxury of time leading up to your next treatment cycle, then I suggest introducing natural methods such as nutrition, acupuncture, and a supplement regime to get you prepped. It can take time for these methods to bear fruit, so the extra weeks or months of lead-up can be helpful. For example, the herbs and supplements that improve egg or sperm quality often require three to six months to work their magic. Acknowledging that many of you are already in the thick of treatment, start as soon as possible. It's still beneficial to integrate the Cycle Syncing Diet, acupuncture, and a supplement regime even if you are already actively entrenched in your fertility efforts.

A Play-by-Play: What to Expect at the Fertility Clinic

Embarking on your quest for baby is daunting, particularly because most don't really imagine they'll find themselves encountering challenges. Exploring treatment options can feel even more overwhelming given that you don't know exactly what you need or what to expect physically or financially. This next section is dedicated to getting your bearings in the land of ART (i.e., IVF, IUI, and so on). I've found that much of the anxiety melts away if you have a clear picture of what visiting a fertility clinic might entail. And since this chapter is your guide to integrating East and West, I've woven natural fertility-enhancing recommendations throughout to help you formulate a plan to improve both your experience and your outcomes.

Know Who to Ask

We want our doctors to be able to answer all of our questions. We are entrusting them with the most important quest of our lives. It is, however, important to note that most doctors have little to no knowledge of nutrition, supplements, and natural medicine, so their assistance in this area may be lackluster and at times counterproductive. Only 25 percent of physicians undergo even basic training in nutrition during the course of their medical schooling. Lessons on integrative or natural approaches to medicine might take the form of a guest lecture if at all. All this is to say that unless your doctor has taken an active interest in nutrition, supplementation, acupuncture, and so on, he or she is unlikely to be able to guide you on these topics. Many will disregard complementary therapies as fluff. This is mostly because they haven't explored the history of clinical efficacy or the new research in support of these methods. They've understandably been focused on their own craft, busy keeping up to date with the research and advances in their area of practice. Try not to be disheartened if your doctor pooh-poohs your natural medicine efforts; just know who to ask. You can find qualified practitioners via ABORM.org, the American Association of Naturopathic Physicians, or the World Naturopathic Federation. If your doctor is open minded, he or she may be able to refer you to someone in an alternative medicine field who is specialized in reproductive medicine.

ON YOUR MARK . . .

You've been worried something is off. Things aren't quite "taking" with your efforts at home. Perhaps you've researched your local fertility centers or have a recommendation from a friend. On your first visit, you'll have a consultation with a reproductive endocrinologist (REI) to discuss your history and help you determine your best course of action. Diagnostics are one of the places where Western medicine really shines. Your hormone levels will be evaluated with blood tests, and there are multiple imaging tools to check for obstructions, growths, and scarring that might be blocking your ability to conceive.

Tests to Expect

Here are a few of the preliminary, data-gathering tests your doctor may conduct during your consultation period:

- *"Day 2" test.* Conducted on or near the second day of your period. Your FSH and E2 will be tested via blood, and an ultrasound will be done to check the number of follicles. This "baseline" testing helps determine the amount of eggs one might produce during an IUI or IVF cycle.
- *Ultrasound.* Conducted to count your AFC (antral follicle count), which are the eggs that can be stimulated to grow. This number varies month to month.
- *AMH.* To assess your "ovarian reserve." It pairs well with the AFC to get a snapshot of how many follicles/eggs you have to stimulate.
- *HSG dye test.* Conducted to evaluate your fallopian tubes.
- *Saline sonogram.* Conducted to check the contour of your uterus for growths or scarring.
- *Thyroid (TSH).* A number falling between 1 and 2 is preferred to rule out the possibility of thyroid insufficiency or excess interfering with fertility.
- *Clotting and/or immune factors.* A screening sometimes done to assess your risk of failed implantation or miscarriage from genetic or autoimmune conditions.

When all the data are in, your doctor will suggest the best course of action based on your individual circumstances. The mildest option is monitoring (though this is rarely recommended as a stand-alone intervention). It involves going in several times throughout your cycle to draw blood and monitor your eggs with an ultrasound as they grow. This can help you home in on your fertile window and is especially helpful if you have an irregular cycle or OPKs aren't showing positive signs of ovulation. Monitoring is not generally recommended because the assumption is that you've probably already hit your fertile window. However, I've had patients who ovulate during their period! Without monitoring, they'd have no way of knowing that. Keep

> If your doctor is amenable, ask for your levels of vitamin D, ferritin, magnesium, and vitamin B12 to be assessed. Getting some intel on nutrient levels may give you a leg up in preparation.

in mind that you may have to suggest this to your doctor if you'd like to try it before proceeding with other interventions. Sometimes a "trigger shot" (i.e., Ovadril or something like it) is an add-on to a monitoring cycle. This injection is administered in your tush or thigh when your egg has matured to a point where it's ready to be released. The trigger shot forces the egg out and gives a more precise window for when to try naturally. Depending on your circumstances, it might make sense to skip this and jump to the bigger guns. However, I've seen women fail IUI, IVF, and every treatment under the sun only to then get pregnant with a combination of simple monitoring, nutrition, and acupuncture.

If option A doesn't cut it, next up are medications like Clomid or letrozole. You'll take them for five days of your follicular phase. This is often the first option your doctor will recommend in combination with either IUI or monitoring. The idea is to multiply the eggs available for sperm to fertilize in hopes that it will increase your odds of pregnancy. These ovary-coaxing drugs trick your body into thinking that your estrogen is low, thereby causing your pituitary gland to produce more FSH than it normally would. Note that this can result in pregnancies of "multiples" (i.e., twins or triplets), which are generally considered high-risk pregnancies. If you have a high egg count, then low dosages and lots of monitoring will be recommended to make sure you don't become the next "octomom." Both these medications help most women ovulate additional eggs, but only a fraction of them achieve pregnancy, prompting them to undergo the next stage of treatment.

The Caveat to Ovulation-Boosting Medications

These oral medications are frequently used as the first line of treatment to boost the amount of eggs ovulated. Although originally used with timed intercourse or IUI, they are now commonly prescribed in IVF protocols for women with low ovarian reserve. While so-called super-ovulation medications like Clomid and letrozole can be effective, they aren't guaranteed to lead to ovulation. Some women with PCOS or amenorrhea may not produce a viable egg with these meds alone. Another thing to note is that for some women, Clomid actually thins their uterine lining. In both cases, I recommend augmenting their effects with electroacupuncture and an herbal formula such as Wen Jing Tang (Warm the Valley Formula) or Ba Zhen Tang (Eight Treasure Formula). If you have PCOS, Letrozole is the preferred option as it is less likely to thin the endometrial lining. Also, beware of side effects, such as headaches, anxiety, insomnia, irritability, reduced ability to cope with stress, and so on.

That next phase is likely an IUI, although, in truth, this could also come prior to the medications mentioned in the box "The Caveat to Ovulation-Boosting Medications," especially if you're adverse to taking medications. Most commonly, IUI would come in conjunction with the previously mentioned ovary boosters. The process involves your partner providing his payload

Did You Know?

An IUI is usually prescribed for younger women with a diagnosis of "idiopathic" or "unknown cause" infertility. It is also routinely recommended to help patients meet the requirements of their insurance so that they can get coverage for IVF thereafter. Depending on your age, insurance requirements, and your diagnosis, you might continue IUI for three to six cycles.

a few hours in advance of the procedure. The clinic washes it, concentrates it, and shoots it into your uterus to bypass a potentially hostile cervical environment so that as many swimmers as possible are vying for the egg. Typically, an IUI is timed by monitoring the growth of your follicles/eggs. Once these are mature enough, you'll take the trigger shot (to release the egg or eggs), and 36 hours later, you come in for the procedure.

The fourth and most "advanced" intervention is IVF. It's a six-phase process that involves injectable and/or oral medications, manual insemination of the egg outside the uterus, and then the transfer of the fertilized egg back into the uterus.

Sample Plans for IUI

Natural IUI:

- Acupuncture one or two times per week.
- Sync up your nutrition with your cycle phases—refer to chapter 9.
- Nettle, rooibos, and raspberry leaf tea daily. Add herbal chai after IUI.
- Mindfulness practice daily two times per day.
- Low-intensity exercise (walking, light elliptical, or gentle yoga). Walk only when within 48 hours of IUI (day of and after).

Medicated IUI (less: Clomid, letrozole; more: Gonal-f, Menopur):

- Acupuncture two or three times per week leading up to and following the IUI (very helpful if you feel the medications affect your mental health and sleep).
- Sync up your nutrition with your cycle phases—refer back to the dietary guide in chapter 9.
- Eat an abundance of cooked leafy greens, herbal teas, and water around the time of trigger shot.
- Nettle and raspberry leaf tea daily before and after IUI (can continue into pregnancy).
- Mindfulness practice daily, two times per day,
- Low-intensity options as listed above if taking only oral medications. Exercise only on days 3 to 7 if you are doing injectables. After that, walk only.

When IVF Is the Way to Go

If any of the following circumstances apply to you, IVF is likely the way to go. Of course, there's always an upside in integrating East and West to improve your sense of well-being on the quest for baby.

1. MISSING, REMOVED, OR BLOCKED FALLOPIAN TUBES

There is no simple, holistic work-around for blocked fallopian tubes. In some mild cases when they are just in spasm or clogged with mucus, herbs and acupuncture can likely assist in relaxing and clearing them. Partial blockages might be opened when they push the dye through in an HSG. If your blockage is severe or your tubes aren't present, then fertilization of your egg is rather impossible without the intervention. Lucky for us, the IVF process of extracting your eggs, fertilizing them, and then "transferring" an embryo into your uterus provides a viable option to conceive.

2. HUMAN IMMUNODEFICIENCY VIRUS

If you or your partner has human immunodeficiency virus (HIV), IVF provides an option to avoid transmission. Interestingly, his sperm can be "washed" (i.e., extracted from HIV-infected seminal fluid). The sperm itself does not carry the virus and can safely fertilize your egg.

3. GENETIC DISORDERS

If you or your partner have or potentially carry a genetic disorder that could be passed on to your child, IVF provides options to reduce or eradicate that risk. A genetic test known as PGT allows the lab to perform a biopsy to discover which of your embryos carry the disorder, thereby ensuring that only the embryos that are not carriers will be transferred.

PHASE 1: PRECONCEPTION PLANNING

It's almost game time. This is your preparation period. It begins the moment you enter for a consultation and ends when you begin your IVF cycle. In these first few weeks, you will be preparing body and mind to undergo an intensive fertility process. Your fertility clinic will likely ask you to attend (virtually or in person) their IVF introductory session to help you prepare and feel informed. Next, you will order "pre-cycle" drugs to prime you for your IVF cycle. Some of the most common medications are Estrace (patch or pill), a birth control pill, or Lupron (injection). Estrace and Lupron are generally introduced if there is a case of low egg count or poor response to meds in a previous cycle. Birth control is used if you have a high FSH or cysts.

Once IVF begins, however, it's time to modify your diet and acupuncture protocol. These modifications are designed to not only optimize every phase but also make you feel better physically and mentally as you undergo the process of injections, appointments, and procedures. Make sure to slow down and engage in mindfulness practices to reduce the negative impact of stress on your efforts.

Sample Regimens for Phase 1

Preconception prep three to six months ahead of IVF:

- Do the Conception Cleanse followed by the 80/20 rule.
- Implement the Cycle Syncing Diet protocols.
- Start herb/supplement program.
- Get acupuncture once or twice per week.
- Meditate or unplug at least two times daily for five minutes or more.
- Exercise and eat to achieve a BMI between 20 and 25.

"Speedy" one-month plan:

- Do the condensed 10-day Conception Cleanse followed by the 80/20 rule.
- Implement Cycle Syncing Diet protocols.
- Start herb/supplement program.
- Get one to three acupuncture treatments per week.
- Meditate or unplug at least two times daily for five minutes or more.
- Engage in a mild to moderate exercise program.

Beginning IVF:

- Follow a clean diet (refer to the 80/20 rule in chapter 8) and incorporate healthy proteins and fats (chapter 9).
- Get acupuncture with electro-stimulation two to three times per week.
- Stick with a basic supplement program that will not interfere with medications such as NAC, magnesium, probiotics, omega-3, vitamin D, and a prenatal vitamin with high folate.
- Meditate or unplug at least two times daily for five minutes or more.
- Walk or do mild exercise (chapter 10).

Guide to Supplementation

There's currently a lot of buzz surrounding supplementation to assist ART/IVF outcomes, particularly those geared at improving egg quality. The following selection contains only those I've observed to integrate safely into medicated protocols.

COQ10/UBIQUINOL

CoQ10 works by enhancing the energy production of egg cells, resulting in better-quality embryos. The presence of CoQ10 in ovarian follicles has been linked to improved IVF outcomes. When ovarian follicles containing good-quality eggs were examined, researchers discovered higher levels of CoQ10 than in poor-quality follicles. Studies on mice have shown that your body's CoQ10 levels decrease with age, and treatment of mice with CoQ10 supplementation has led to larger litter sizes (Turi et al. 2011). Dose: 300 to 600 milligrams daily.

PROBIOTICS

Probiotics may help to create the ideal reproductive "microbiome" for optimal IVF outcomes. Studies have shown that when the transfer catheter is colonized with *Lactobacillus*, there's a much higher rate of implantation (Sirota, Zarek, and Segars 2014). Its positive effects are likely due to its ability to counteract bacteria known to contribute to failed IVF (Pelzer et al. 2013). Refer to appendix E for preferred probiotic brands.

ACAI

This antioxidant-rich berry is currently under clinical trial at CCRM of Colorado, the country's most prominent fertility center. High doses up to 1,800 milligrams daily are being used to improve egg quality.

OMEGA

Omega-3 fatty acids are some of the best and gentlest anti-inflammatory (and therefore "antiaging") supplements out there. They've shown promise in recent studies for treating egg quality of women of advanced maternal age. Omega-3s seem to slow the natural, age-related decline of reproductive function. I also use them to help build uterine lining and improve the odds of implantation. Caution on dosage for anyone on blood thinners like Lovenox, as they *also* thin the blood. Another consideration is to cease their use a few days before a procedure (egg retrieval, hysteroscopy, or laparoscopy) that could result in increased bleeding. Omega-3s are even great during pregnancy to support your nervous system, prevent prenatal and postnatal depression, and aid baby's development of IQ. Dose: 1,200 to 2,000 milligrams of EPA and DHA combined (Nehra et al. 2012).

(continued)

Guide to Supplementation (*continued*)

NAC

NAC is an amazing supplement for women who suffer from anxiety. It improves both your mood and the function of your liver to help "process" medications during an IVF or IUI cycle (Whitaker, Casey, and Taupier 2012). It may also help support egg development in conjunction with Clomid and other IVF medications for women with unexplained infertility, especially in cases where infertility is likely tied to insulin resistance (Bedaiwy, RezkH. Al Inany, and Falcone 2004). In a porcine study, an intake of 1,500 milligrams showed an increase in the amount of embryos that made it to the blastocyst stage. Dose: 1,000 to 1,500 milligrams (Whitaker, Casey, and Taupier 2012). I recommend 1,200 to 1,500 milligrams daily.

VITAMIN D

This fat-soluble, sunny nutrient packs a potent fertility boost. Several studies point to a link between vitamin D levels and IVF success ("Vitamin D Levels and IVF Success" 2022). More specifically, adequate vitamin D levels are correlated with a higher rate of pregnancies and live births. A study conducted at Columbia University/University of Southern California found that women with high vitamin D levels were 27 percent more likely to conceive than those with low levels (Ozkan et al. 2010). Supplementing higher levels of vitamin D has proved helpful in thickening the uterine lining of women with PCOS during an IVF cycle, combating the thinning effects of medications like Clomid (Lerchbaum and Rabe 2014). Dose: 2,000 to 5,000 IU daily.

VITAMIN E

This fat-soluble vitamin might well be a powerhouse for sperm, egg, and uterine lining. In one study, it showed promise if combined with other supplements and medications like L-arginine and sildenafil to build uterine lining (Takasaki et al. 2010). I recommend 400 IU daily. Beware of combining with blood-thinning medications.

MAGNESIUM

Sufficient magnesium ensures telomerase activity, which may assist healthy chromosomes and follicular growth (Stuefer, Moncayo, and Moncayo 2015). Magnesium levels decline as estrogen levels rise in the follicular (stim phase) of IVF. Larger (i.e., more mature) follicles had good levels of magnesium, implying that the eggs that develop well may in fact need the important mineral to thrive. Essentially, magnesium may assist in improved egg/embryo quality and improved IVF outcomes (Stuefer, Moncayo, and Moncayo 2015). In addition to its relevance to follicular growth, it helps to improve sleep cycles and calm anxiety. Last but not least, it promotes bowel regularity and helps with the bloat that accumulates with higher estrogen levels and with the retrieval. I recommend 250 to 400 milligrams either before bed or split between morning and evening.

PRENATAL/MULTIVITAMIN

Prenatal vitamins are presumed to be the catchall of supplements. The most common question I hear when I recommend individual supplements is "Don't I have those in my prenatal?" Yes, you do, but not in the therapeutic dosages required to get the desired results. That said, I still recommend a good multivitamin for microdoses of a myriad of nutrients. Prenatal multivitamins have improved pregnancy rates by as much as 33 percent in case studies (Westphal et al. 2004). Once you have your basics covered, you can add extra supplements specific to your needs. Look for prenatals that have a minimum of 800 micrograms of folate (or, better, 1,000 micrograms or more). If you suffer from constipation, then avoid prenatals with iron.

To make your search for the perfect prenatal supplement cocktail easier, appendix E has a list of recommended supplement brands. If you're looking for more information on where to find supplements, you can link here to our online dispensaries at https://us.fullscript.com/welcome/naturnalife or https://wellevate.me/naturnainstitute. If you need additional guidance, you can book a consultation with us or another qualified practitioner (see chapter 11).

Iron is an essential fertility nutrient, *but* it can easily cause constipation or systemic inflammation. As such, it is best sourced from foods or food supplements, such as liver pills or beet powder.

Pro Tip

For building uterine lining, use vitamin E, L-arginine, omega-3, raspberry leaf tincture, Wen Jing Tang Chinese herbal formula, and magnesium glycinate

Takasaki et al. (2010)

PHASE 2: STIMS

The real action starts on day 2 of your menses. Your practitioner will do an ultrasound (yes, on your period—ew, sorry) and take blood to check hormone levels (FSH, E2, progesterone [P4], and LH). Provided that your hormone levels look okay and you are free of hormone-producing cysts, you'll be ready to start "stims" (the medications that stimulate your ovaries) on the eve of day 2 or 3. Stims are typically administered via injections in your belly or thigh and include Follistim, Menopur, and Gonal-f. Oral medications such as Clomid and/or Letrozole might be paired with certain injectable medications depending on your fertility profile. This is becoming a more popular approach for women who have low ovarian reserve and/or those deemed "poor responders."

What's a Poor Responder?

Many women with low ovarian reserve or POF are dismayed when they produce very few eggs in an IVF cycle. Women with this profile often do best with an egg-banking approach, meaning multiple cycles but with potentially fewer medications.

Your prescription will vary depending on whether mini or conventional IVF is the most suitable approach for you (see the box "Mini versus Conventional IVF"). Expect to be on the meds for a period of eight to 12 days (shorter if your eggs grow fast, longer if they are slow to develop) until your eggs are mature enough to be retrieved and fertilized.

Are some of your eggs growing faster than others? If you have a "lead follicle," your doctor will likely introduce medications such as Ganorelix or Cetrotide to prevent you from ovulating prematurely.

Mini versus Conventional IVF

Conventional IVF, whereby higher dosages of follicle-stimulating medications are given, is still preferred by most fertility centers. That said, there are more clinics embracing this gentler approach to ovarian stimulation. Mini IVF uses low oral doses of meds like Clomid and letrozole in combination with Follistim and Menopur. This approach might be considered for women with a low ovarian reserve or those who produced very few eggs in a previous IVF cycle. Mini IVF may also work well for women with PCOS or a high AMH level in order to avoid ovarian hyperstimulation.

Although you'll likely feel okay when entering this phase, expect to close it out feeling bloated, tired, and grumpy. As your ovaries enlarge to accommodate multiple follicles, your estrogen will rise into the hundreds or thousands, depending on the number

Electroacupuncture significantly increases blood flow to the arteries of the uterus.

Stener-Victorin et al. (1996)

of eggs grown. The high estrogen, as well as the body's inability to fully metabolize the medications, results in fluid retention and fatigue. The added burden on your liver may also result in some not-so-pleasant mood changes.

Sample Regimen for Phase 2

Acupuncture plan:

- Get electroacupuncture with moxibustion two or three times per week.

Dietary plan:

- Follow the 80/20 rule on clean eating (chapter 8).
- Apply the Cycle Syncing Diet (chapter 9).
- Focus on foods rich in iron, vitamin C, omega-3s, omega-6s, and magnesium.
- Support natural estrogen with additional snacks like flaxseeds, pumpkin seeds, and nuts.

Mindfulness plan:

- Meditate or unplug twice daily for at least five to 10 minutes at a time.

Supplement plan:

- Licorice tablets by Metagenics (follicle growth), magnesium, NAC, omegas, vitamin D, CoQ10, acai, prenatal.

While these side effects aren't exactly enjoyable, they are thankfully not life threatening. Throughout this phase, allow yourself to feel empowered by the action you are taking to grow your family. And try not to pass judgment if your eggs aren't as plentiful as you'd hoped. It only takes one.

Try to get your BMI between 20 and 25 for best outcomes, especially if you've experienced implantation failure, miscarriage, or unexplained issues with egg or embryo quality.

Chang et al. (2013)

Thoughtful Exercise to Keep You Well and Sane

Gentle movement helps your mind process stress and helps your body eliminate toxins. Easygoing physical activity can mitigate the mood disturbances, lethargy, and bloat that come along with conventional fertility treatment. Keep in mind that it is essential to keep the forms of exercise low impact and short if you are taking medications to multiply your eggs. Ovarian torsion—a very painful and rather dangerous twisting of your ovary—can occur when the ovaries are enlarged. Think walking, low-resistance elliptical, and light weights for arms only.

PHASE 3: TRIGGER

The trigger shot sends the eggs into orbit. It is administered around 10 to 12 days of stims, when the eggs have grown to maturation. The trigger will release the eggs into a fluid-filled area where they hang out to be retrieved.

Side Effects of IVF

IVF medications are designed to coax your ovaries to produce multiple eggs. The enlarged ovaries are filled with fluid that can leak into the abdominal cavity after the eggs are retrieved. In some cases (i.e., when many eggs are retrieved), this leakage can cause ovarian hyperstimulation syndrome (OHSS). There are varying degrees of OHSS. In cases of mild to moderate OHSS, you'll experience symptoms such as uncomfortable distension and bloating in the abdomen, nausea, vomiting, diarrhea, rapid weight gain, and ovary tenderness. The more severe form, which requires hospitalization, may involve repeated vomiting, trouble breathing, and blood clotting. Since OHSS is most common in women who produce a lot of eggs, it's most often seen in younger women, especially those with PCOS. In recent years, the drug Lupron has also been successful in preventing OHSS, but acupuncture has also proved effective in several studies when used in place of the trigger shot (Cai 1997). Although Lupron is an effective option, natural methods such as acupuncture will help a great deal with the bloating and discomfort that come along with the trigger and retrieval. Why not do both?

My prescription for prevention and treatment of the symptoms of OHSS:

- Consume an electrolyte beverage daily, starting from the trigger shot to regulate your fluid balance. Try coconut water, maple water, electrolyte packets, or a pinch of salt and a few drops of maple syrup in your water.
- Get acupuncture leading up to and after the retrieval. Schedule for the day of the trigger shot, the day after retrieval, and every two to three days thereafter to help the body rid itself of extra fluids and calm inflammation.
- Prioritize foods high in I3C and calcium D-glucarate (broccoli, kale, brussels sprouts, etc.) to help the liver and colon process and eliminate excess estrogens.

Expect to feel bloated at this point in the cycle, particularly if you are a strong producer of eggs. The bloat that begins later in phase 2 is taken to all new levels after the trigger shot is administered.

Sample Regimen for Phase 3

Acupuncture plan:

- Schedule a session on the day of the trigger shot and the day after retrieval to reduce bloating, prevent OHSS, and assist your body in ridding the medications.

Dietary plan:

- Follow the 90/10 rule on clean eating.
- Apply Cycle Syncing nutrition (chapter 9).
- Add leafy greens and fiber like chia seeds to flush excess estrogen.
- Focus on foods containing I3C to detoxify estrogen mimickers. Eat two cups of cooked cruciferous vegetables—broccoli, cauliflower, brussels sprouts, cabbage, and collard greens—per day, totaling about 150 milligrams of I3C.
- Stay hydrated.
- Avoid raw foods.

Mindfulness plan:

- Meditate or unplug twice daily for at least five to 10 minutes at a time.

Supplement plan:

- Vitamin B6, NAC, magnesium, vitamin D, and probiotics.

PHASE 4: RETRIEVAL

In this phase, you start seeing the fruits of your labor. The retrieval of your eggs is scheduled roughly 34 to 36 hours after the trigger shot. The eggs are surgically extracted by your doctor while you're under anesthesia. That said, some centers administer only a local anesthetic, and you remain awake. Although I'm all for less medication, I've observed that the latter option can be dicey, as some women experience a lot of pain. Typically, extraction is done by inserting a needle through the vaginal wall to aspirate the eggs. It sounds awful, but most women experience only mild tenderness after the procedure. Once extracted, your eggs and your partner's sperm have a little mixer in a dish. If your partner's sperm is in good shape, the lab may leave the sperm to fertilize the eggs naturally. If there is concern of poor egg or sperm quality, they'll use ICSI to select the best sperm and insert a "superior" swimmer directly into each egg.

Typically, at this point, you'll feel elated that the heavy lifting is over, but you may have a bit of anxiety about the checkpoints you are about to undergo with fertilization and the anticipated progress reports on your embryos. Aside from dealing with a busy mind, you may experience some body symptoms, such as tenderness or bloat. The excess fluids and gas retained in your abdomen will give you a bit of a potbelly, and the anesthetic "hangover" may leave you groggy for a day or so.

À La Carte IVF Options

A complaint I often hear when a cycle fails is "Why didn't they offer me that test/procedure to begin with?!" Each doctor will have his or her own recommendations as to what tests and/or procedures are necessary in your case. It can be helpful to understand the options available to you in advance so that you can make informed decisions and minimize stress. Below are a few common "add-ons" to the standard IVF process for your consideration:

1. *ICSI.* This option selects the most viable male sperm to inject into the egg. It is thought to negate male factor infertility to a degree by making sure the egg is fertilized despite less-than-ideal sperm samples. One limitation is that ICSI-conceived children have a higher incidence of congenital defects and epigenetic syndromes (Alukal and Lamb 2008).

2. *PGT (formerly known as PGS).* This embryo biopsy may be used to determine whether chromosomal abnormalities could result in implantation failure, miscarriage, or a child with congenital or genetic defects. This testing does, however, have limitations. The cells analyzed in the tests are taken only from the outer layer of the blastocyst so as to not damage the part that turns into a fetus. The result is a tiny sample that may not even contain the correct tissues needed to determine a genetic issue. There is an approximate 10 percent chance that the sampled cells might not be indicative of the health of the embryo, meaning that the results might yield a false negative or false positive and that a perfectly viable embryo is thrown out (Brezina, Ke, and Kutteh 2013). That said, transfers of PGT tested embryos result in much higher pregnancy and live birth rates than untested embryos. That's enough for most people to opt in.

3. *Assisted hatching.* If you've experienced failed implantation during a previous IVF cycle, your doctor might recommend an added step to the IVF process called assisted hatching. A hole is poked in the egg membrane to help the embryo undergo the hatching process that occurs five to six days after fertilization. Hatching must occur for the egg to properly implant. It's been observed that embryos with thinner linings implant better, so the idea is that the outer layer gets in the way or is too thick to break through properly. It's also thought to be beneficial for eggs that have been preserved since the freezing process can potentially harden the membrane ("In Vitro Fertilization (IVF)" 2021).

4. *Endometrial receptivity assay (ERA).* The endometrial receptivity test, albeit controversial, may assist in properly timing your transfer for best outcomes. It is a biopsy of the lining of the uterus done to assess how long you need to be on progesterone prior to implantation to be the most "receptive."

5. *Receptiva.* Also a biopsy and often done in conjunction with the ERA, the Receptiva can detect inflammation in the endometrial lining due to endometriosis, bacteria, fungus, and so on. It is generally recommended when there has been implantation failure despite PGT-normal embryos.

The biggest physical strains on your body are behind you now. Phew! However, be aware that there are procedural checkpoints still to pass that may trigger pangs of anxiety. Note that you will see the "numbers" of eggs/embryos diminish throughout the checkpoints. Although it's scary, it's a good way to improve the odds that only strong, viable embryos are returned to your uterus, thus reducing your chances of failed implantation or miscarriage.

Here's what you can expect each step of the way:

1. *Retrieval quantity.* The number of eggs retrieved will not necessarily match the amount of follicles seen on an ultrasound. Some follicles may not actually contain eggs, so you may end up with fewer (or sometimes more) than expected.
2. *Fertilization.* On average, 50 to 70 percent of the eggs retrieved will fertilize. Fertilization rates depend on egg and sperm quality as well as the quality of the center's lab.
3. *Day 3 cell division.* Successfully fertilized eggs become embryos after three days. However, not all of the fertilized eggs will make it to this point.
4. *Day 5 cell division.* Many centers now push the embryos to day 5 (even day 6 or day 7 if they're progressing slower) so that they enter the blastocyst stage. Typically, around 30 percent of your original "catch" of eggs make it this far. It is at this point that the embryos can undergo PGT to determine which of them are most viable. There is a higher likelihood of a successful pregnancy when you wait until this stage. The PGT test often whittles your numbers down again to around 30 percent of those that made it to the blastocyst stage. Only the embryos that come back "normal" are returned to your uterus, though you can request your center to keep the abnormal embryos frozen until you decide what to do. Keep in mind the attrition at each stage so that your expectations are balanced.
5. *Transfer.* If you're doing what's called a fresh embryo transfer, one or more of the embryos are placed back in your uterus three to five days after fertilization (sometimes six or seven days). Progesterone suppositories or shots in your tush begin a few days before the transfer. If you're doing a frozen embryo transfer (FET), your embryos are frozen until your next cycle (a few days after your typical ovulation time frame) or as late as you want (there is no cap on how many years they can remain on ice). FET is very common today and will be the only option if you've opted for PGT testing.

Sample Regimen for Phase 4

Acupuncture plan:

- Schedule an acupuncture session the day after the retrieval (within two days is also acceptable) to reduce inflammation and help your liver metabolize extra medication. This is especially important if doing a fresh transfer.

Dietary plan:

- Continue all the recommendations from phase 3: hydration, fiber, B vitamins, and leafy greens.
- Integrate principles of the Cycle Syncing Diet in chapter 9 and focus on eating cooked, light, highly alkaline, and mostly plant-based foods.
- Avoid raw foods, caffeine, sugars (including excess fruits), fatty meats, and refined grains.
- If you are freezing your eggs/embyros, consider a 10-day detox diet.

Mindfulness plan:

- Meditate or unplug twice daily for at least five to 10 minutes at a time.

Supplement plan:

- Add vitamins C and E to phase 3 recommendations.
- Add I3C and calcium D-glucarate if you are freezing your eggs/embryos to help detox excess hormones.
- Add bromelain (500 milligrams with each meal), vitamin E (400 IU daily), and vitamin C (1,000 milligrams daily) if you are proceeding with a fresh embryo transfer.

PHASE 5: TRANSFER

This is it! You are finally putting the bun in the oven. This part of the process is a breeze compared to phase 4. It is performed three to five days after the retrieval of the eggs or around 17 days into your cycle if you're using a frozen embryo (see the box "Fresh versus Frozen Embryo Transfer"). You'll be awake, and you may get to watch a live video of your doctor placing the embryo strategically inside your uterus. A catheter is inserted with an attached syringe holding the embryo(s) to carefully place it in an ideal spot.

INTEGRATING EAST AND WEST 241

Three-Day versus Five-Day Embryo Transfer

The transfer of your fertilized embryos takes place either after three days or five to six days of incubation. Each window has its own pros and cons.

In a three-day transfer, you'll likely have more embryos intact than if you waited until day 5. If you have few eggs to begin with, this might be the way to go (more on that to come). That said, a day 3 embryo is less likely to result in a live pregnancy than a day 5, which is why many fertility centers and patients alike are leaning into day 5 as an option.

In a five-day transfer, the embryos are incubated until they become blastocysts. An embryo that makes it to day 5 is theoretically more likely to be stronger and more viable. It's also easier for the doctor to give the blastocysts an embryo morphology score that determines their likelihood to implant (Hatırnaz and Pektaş 2017). The real allure is that five-day transfers allow the option of PGT-A testing *and* have better success rates. The downside is that after sitting in a dish in a lab for five days, many embryos will stop developing despite science's best efforts. If the IVF procedure extracted only a small number of eggs, that makes waiting until day 5 riskier, as you could potentially lose most or all of them.

You'll be on far fewer medications in between the retrieval and the transfer—unless you have a blood-clotting issue or an immunological condition. In those cases, you'd be given a blood thinner or a mix of steroids or antibiotics and immunosuppressive drugs, respectively. More often, the cocktail is estrogen and progesterone to enhance your uterine lining and create an optimal hormonal environment for implantation.

Fresh versus Frozen Embryo Transfer

A fresh embryo transfer refers to placing the embryos in the uterus several days after they have been retrieved and fertilized. Depending on your practitioner's advice, your embryos will be left to incubate for either three or five days. This was once the favored route prior to the improvement in freezing techniques. A fresh transfer is still nice if you'd prefer not to wait around for another cycle. It's also a great option if you produced only a few eggs and intuit that they'd be better off in your uterus rather than the less natural lab environment.

In a frozen embryo transfer, your embryos go through the same retrieval and fertilization process, but when they reach the desired maturity, they are frozen until you are ready to use them. Embryos that undergo testing are frozen while you wait for the results. With a FET, you'll be given a likely date of transfer in advance (as long as your uterine lining is developing properly). It's a nice change from the suspense of the previous phases. This approach allows you a lot more recovery time to reduce inflammation and de-bloat after retrieval. This alone may account for its success rate. Women with pro-inflammatory conditions such as endometriosis and PCOS may want to consider this option.

This is one of the most critical times to take advantage of acupuncture's effects. Not only will it ease the side effects, but a meta-analysis of 23 separate trials involving a total of 5,598 patients showed a major increase in clinical pregnancy rates in groups that underwent frequent acupuncture around phase 5 (i.e., transfer) compared to all the control groups (Zheng et al. 2012).

Expect to feel a bit bloated and lethargic at this stage, and you may end up a little backed up. Synthetic progesterone is usually the culprit, as it can make you more prone to yeast infections, slow your bowels, and contribute to fatigue.

Sample Regimen for Phase 5

Acupuncture Plan:

- Schedule one acupuncture session before and one after transfer (for a total of two sessions in one day). This protocol is proven to improve pregnancy rates and increase the chances of live birth (Manheimer et al. 2008; Smith et al. 2019).

Dietary plan:

- Follow the 80/20 rule on clean eating.
- Integrate Cycle Syncing Diet and focus on calming and warming foods from chapter 9: slow-cooked foods (stews, soups) millet, green and root vegetables (spinach, Swiss chard, parsnip, squash), dark meat of chicken, lamb, sprouted sunflower seeds, and sesame seeds.
- Continue hydration and high fiber intake from previous phases.
- Avoid raw, cold foods.
- Limit intake of fruits and refined carbs.

Mindfulness plan:

- Meditate or unplug twice daily for at least five to 10 minutes at a time.

Supplement plan:

- Vitamins E and C, bromelain, magnesium, probiotics, omega-3, prenatal, vitamin D.

PHASE 6: THE WAITING GAME

The finish line is in sight! With the procedures behind you, phase 6 is an exciting time, but it's also nerve wracking. The anticipation makes it arguably the most difficult stage. You enter a 10- to 14-day waiting period to see if the embryo(s) implant(s). You notice every twinge or flutter and may also scour online chat rooms to take note of other women's experiences. It's natural to want to pee on a stick (or 10) as soon as Clear Blue tells you that you can, but I recommend you wait for the test at the fertility clinic. It's the most accurate assessment and cuts back on the anxiety and guesswork.

Expect to have a very busy mind during this phase, making mindfulness practice a must. You'll be tuned into every sensation in your body, trying your best to ascribe some meaning. If you are doing progesterone injections, your tush may start to develop hard and tender lumps.

Sample Regimen for Phase 6

Acupuncture plan:

- Schedule two sessions per week for implantation and sanity.

Additional holistic treatment:

- Get moxibustion on lower belly for implantation and on backside to relieve tenderness on progesterone lumps.

Dietary plan:

- Continue focus on hydration, monounsaturated fats (olive oil), and healthy, fiber-rich foods (butternut squash, delicate squash, millet, sprouted sesame seeds, etc.).
- Add luteal phase recommendations from the Cycle Syncing Diet in chapter 9.
- Avoid sugar, booze, caffeine, fried foods, gluten, dairy, and corn.

Mindfulness plan:

- Meditate twice daily for at least five to 10 minutes at a time.

Supplement plan:

- Continue the same supplementation recommendations from phase 5.

Sample Plans for IVF

Base plan (mini or conventional IVF), acupuncture:

- One or two times per week starting three to six months prior to cycle
- Two or three times per week of electroacupuncture in phase 1
- One session the day after retrieval
- Two times the day of transfer before and after embryo transfer
- One session within three to five days of transfer and two times per week until pregnancy test results

Also include the following:

- Cycle Syncing Diet (refer to chapter 9)
- Nettle and raspberry leaf tea daily (can mix together)
- Walking daily, 30 to 60 minutes
- Mindfulness practice twice daily

Establish Your Support System Early

If you're not already seeing a practitioner of natural medicine or therapist, there's no better time to reach out and make an appointment than right now. A qualified practitioner will be able to help you plan out your treatment schedule to best optimize the IVF and/or help you manage your mental health. If your fertility doctor is with you in the endeavor, then they might be able to recommend someone. Otherwise, a good source for qualified practitioners is the Acupuncture and TCM Board of Reproductive Medicine. Their website (ABORM.org) lists the practitioners in your area who have gone through specialized training to receive the accreditation. If you prefer to work with a naturopath, you can find qualified specialists in your area via the American Association of Naturopathic Physicians or the World Naturopathic Federation.

Keeping Your Options Open

If you're considering ways to pause the biological clock, egg preservation (aka egg freezing) has become widely available. It's a trending procedure, and companies are even paying for female employees to undergo the process so as to provide peace of mind for future family planning.

Although egg freezing is certainly on the rise, it's still difficult to fully assess success rates. I was surprised to learn that most women never follow through on using their frozen eggs. Some studies have shown that rates of usage for frozen eggs sit at only about 3 to 9 percent. Since so few women have yet to take the plunge to thaw, fertilize, and try for pregnancy, we are still lacking tangible numbers to have a high degree of confidence in the method. The data we do have suggest that the highest levels of success are found among women who freeze their eggs by the age of 35 (MacMillan 2019). As with many aspects of our fertility, age is a key factor in success. The other key factor is the number of eggs frozen. A bank of at least 10 to 20 eggs in healthy women under 35 years old is recommended to try to "guarantee" one baby. As your age goes up, you essentially want to freeze more for your baby "insurance policy."

The process to undergo egg preservation involves all stages of an IVF except the fertilization and transfer. As such, we don't get the data on fertilization and the progress of the embryos. A 2017 study suggested freezing 61 mature eggs if you are around 42 years old. The same study predicted that women aged 34 and 37 would have a 90 percent and a 75 percent chance of success, respectively, by freezing 20 mature eggs (Goldman et al. 2017). However, these were only predictions, based on statistics of how many eggs tend to fertilize and progress into healthy embryos in various age-groups. The truth of the matter is that there are no guarantees. The best way to guarantee a baby is to start trying *now*. If that isn't a possibility, then egg freezing could be a great plan B.

An Undesirable Solution

One wise doctor once suggested fertilizing part of a batch of eggs with donor sperm just to make sure they are viable. This is because good-quality eggs will fertilize and progress into embryos, and unhealthy or immature eggs are more likely to fail fertilization or arrest in their development. That said, most women doing egg freezing are holding out for Mr. Right and may not love the idea of fertilizing their hard-earned eggs with a stranger's sperm. If this idea doesn't sound awesome to you, then I'd suggest multiple retrieval cycles to try to get a lot of eggs (minimum 20). You'll have a better chance that at least one is ideal. Also, hold a very frank discussion with your doctor about statistics for your age and fertility profile to see what his or her opinion is on the viability of your eggs.

Natural medicine and the lifestyle techniques outlined in this book can help you prepare for egg freezing by optimizing your ovarian health and egg quality. Methods such as acupuncture, supplementation, and cleansing should ideally be started three or more months before your egg freezing cycle. If this isn't an option, use the advice laid out here and start *now*.

Signs That Integration Is Your Best Bet

Not quite sure natural medicine is right for you? An integrative approach, which incorporates natural methods with conventional medicine, is often preferable for women whose odds of pregnancy (according to their "fertility profile") are lower than average. The addition of alternative strategies to conventional technologies has the potential to sway the numbers further in your favor. While there are extra considerations of cost and time spent incorporating new strategies, there is huge upside with little to no downside. Let's explore some scenarios where evidence suggests an integrative approach is the ideal way to go.

TRYING FOR AN EXTENDED TIME

Even if you've been trying for only a couple months, it can feel like an eternity. In reality, women under the age of 35 are recommended to try for a year before seeking the advice of a fertility specialist. For women over 35, the time frame is six months. In many cases, however, you may have a gut feeling that something is off, and you want to do your due diligence to make sure everything is alright "down there." Our fertility sees a steep decline beginning in our early thirties and accelerating from age 35 onward. That being the case, a fertility assessment is often helpful in determining if your fertility numbers are in order. If the worry is getting the best of you, your gynecologist can help assess the situation by doing a baseline hormonal assessment. Seeing some data can be helpful in determining whether your clock is ticking faster or slower than you thought. If everything comes back normal, my recommendation is to follow the advice outlined in chapters 2 and 4 to 10 and give it another few months. Should you want a good catalyst, incorporate the help of an acupuncturist, naturopath, or other qualified natural medicine practitioner. If six months or more of incorporating these recommendations doesn't yield you the results you are looking for, it might be time to integrate.

Sample Integration Plan
for Extended Trying Time

Integrate the following into your fertility treatment plan:

- Conception Cleanse (chapter 8)
- Cycle Syncing Diet (chapter 9)
- Mindfulness practice twice daily
- Basic supplement program: vitamin D, prenatal, magnesium, omega-3
- Acupuncture one to three times weekly and/or the recommendations of a naturopath or herbal practitioner

---

OVULATORY ISSUES

Are your pee sticks not registering that smiley face that confirms ovulation? If this is the case and/or your periods are absent or irregular, it might be helpful to head into the gynecologist's office or fertility center for observation (monitoring). You can get a pretty good idea from charting your cycle (see chapter 2) at home, but to be 100 percent sure as to what's going on down under, blood tests and ultrasounds are an immense help. Natural medicine offers very effective solutions for ovulatory issues, but the caveat is they can take time (three to six months). If you are in a hurry, which I know many of you are, integration will sometimes provide a more expedient solution. Drugs like Clomid, for example, work well in conjunction with Chinese herbs and/or acupuncture to induce ovulation. Another important consideration is the underlying cause of the ovulatory issues and your age. Hypothalamic amenorrhea, PCOS, and mild hypothyroidism can be corrected with natural medicine, but it can take time. If you are over age 40 or have extremely low ovarian reserve, being under the care of a fertility doctor while integrating natural strategies will likely be your best bet.

> Diet modification alone has been shown to reduce the time to pregnancy by decreasing the chance of infertility due to ovulatory disorders by 66 percent.
>
> Panth et al. (2018)

Sample Integration Plan for Ovulatory Issues

Integrate the following into your fertility treatment plan:

- Stress reduction (chapter 6)
- Conception Cleanse (chapter 8)
- Cycle Syncing Diet (chapter 9)
- Mindfulness practice twice daily
- Acupuncture and moxibustion twice per week
- Supplement with myoinositol, NAC, magnesium, probiotics, omega-3s, and vitamin D

POOR EGG QUALITY

If you've been told your infertility stems from poor egg quality, you are in good company. Before jumping into suggestions, it's important to understand why egg quality is such an important factor in IVF success. Low quality egg generally leads to low fertilization rates and poor progression of the embryos. You'll essentially have weak embryos that are less likely to survive the division that occurs over the three- to seven-day period before implantation or freezing/preservation. These embryos may also be less likely to pass PGT testing. It boils down to a scenario wherein you may end up with nothing to put back in your uterus, and if you do, you'll be at higher risk for miscarriage, failed implantation, or a child with health issues.

There have been studies that suggest that the supplement CoQ10 in tandem with IVF can rejuvenate the eggs of older women or those with premature ovarian aging. Essentially, it jump-starts the mitochondria of the egg cells, improving their function for better egg formation (Ben-Meir et al. 2015). NAC has achieved similar results. Thanks to its enormous power to fight off oxidation and chromosomal damage, it can also prevent or delay ovarian aging and improve egg and embryo development. A study on pig embryos found that NAC reduced the amount of frag-

> Research suggests that myoinositol can potentially improve egg and embryo quality in women with PCOS (Ciotta et al. 2011). A 2002 study in Hong Kong linked it to better egg and embryo quality in non-PCOS sufferers, too.
>
> Chiu et al. (2002)

mented DNA and increased the percentage of embryos reaching the late blastocyst stage (Whitaker and Knight 2010). Omega-3, magnesium, and a variety of antioxidants also show promise.

Melatonin is another supplement with some good evidence to back it. As a potent antioxidant, adding three milligrams of melatonin before bed can potentially protect against oxidative stress and keep your eggs healthier. You produce melatonin on your own to get to sleep, but levels naturally decline with age. Mouse embryos grown in a lab with melatonin supplementation showed an increased rate of forming blastosis (advanced) stage embryos (Zhao et al. 2017). Another study demonstrated that taking a dose of three milligrams starting on day 5 of the cycle before IVF retrieval improved egg quality, fertilization rates, and pregnancy outcomes (Tamura et al. 2013). Although there is good evidence to back the use of melatonin, I recommend proceeding with caution due to its potential to affect thyroid and reproductive hormone levels.

Chinese Herbs for Improved IVF Outcomes

Chinese herbal medicine shows promise for issues pertaining to egg quality. In one study, a modern formulation called "macrophage-activating Chinese mixed herbs" (MACH) used a blend of pumpkin seed, plantago seed, Japanese honeysuckle flower buds, and safflower flower, mixed with *Bifidobacterium* probiotic powder, and resulted in improved embryo quality and increased blastocyst development in 90 percent of cases. Women who had multiple ART failures in the past produced viable, early stage embryos by integrating this herbal mixture.

Ushiroyama et al. (2012)

Clinically, I've observed improvement in embryo quality with the introduction of acupuncture before and during an IVF cycle. Its positive effects are likely due at least in part to its ability to increase circulation and reduce inflammation and its associated free radical damage, which is a major causative factor of egg degradation. Patients have duly noted that after several months of acupuncture, the cycle outcomes often improve markedly in some cases.

Sample Integration Plan for General Poor Egg Quality

Integrate the following into your fertility treatment plan:

- Stress reduction (chapter 6)
- Conception Cleanse (chapter 8)
- Cycle Syncing Diet (chapter 9)
- Mindfulness practice twice daily
- Acupuncture and moxibustion twice per week
- Supplement with omega-3s, vitamin D, ubiquinol, NAC, melatonin, acai, and resveratrol

Male Factor Infertility

Your partner's reproductive health matters; it needn't all rest on your shoulders. If his sperm is less than ideal, you may encounter poor embryo development. The amount of DNA fragmentation present also plays a role in whether the sperm will produce a viable embryo. This is an area that unfortunately gets very little attention, with most of the focus placed on egg quality. In the United Kingdom, 30 percent of infertility cases can be attributed to a male factor. In the United States, it's similarly one-third of cases (West 2010). That said, specialists say that only 10 percent of embryo quality is attributed to the male.

Male fertility is negatively influenced by hormonal imbalance, overexposure to free radicals, toxins, infection or other immune issues, and structural issues like varicoceles (basically a varicose vein in the testicle). Diabetes is also a factor that could greatly influence sperm quality.

Fortunately, there are supplements and lifestyle changes he can put into play. Start by getting him on a good multivitamin. If you can nudge him a tad further, then add a potent fish oil, some extra minerals, and antioxidants. Vitamin E and selenium, for example, have been shown in research to improve sperm quality by reducing oxidative stress (Keskes-Ammar et al. 2003). Similarly, CoQ10 has been successful in improving sperm motility and seminal concentration (Lafuente et al. 2013). He would also benefit from following the low-inflammation, insulin-balancing, and detox diet tips suggested for you in chapters 4 through 8. Having each other for motivation and solidarity makes the journey more bearable for both. You might even have some fun keeping each other accountable. Finally, acupuncture, especially electroacupuncture, two times per week for eight weeks increases circulation in the testicles to boost sperm quality. One study led to a 26 percent increase in viable embryos when the men underwent this acupuncture regime (Mingmin et al. 2002).

If your partner is resistant, then keep focusing on you. The hope is that he sees the many positive changes in you and decides to hop on board. For more information on improving the male factor, you can look back at the supplements guide in chapter 11.

POOR RESPONDER

Not everyone's body has an ideal response to the fertility medications. This is often the case for women with very low ovarian reserve (AMH under 0.5 and/or low AFC) and/or POF (high FSH). Women with this profile may not render many eggs from IVF with either high or low dosages of medications. In some cases, your ovaries might protest by halting egg growth altogether or having one speed ahead and develop much faster than the others (aka a lead follicle). The development of cysts is also a common by-product of a poor response to meds.

What Halts an IVF Cycle?

If your doctor's blood test and ultrasound results show any of the following issues, IVF may be on pause until they are resolved since they can potentially render IVF ineffective:

1. High estrogen levels may suggest the presence of a lurking cyst. Cysts can interfere with the signaling from your brain to your ovaries. Essentially, they scramble what the medications are trying to accomplish.
2. High FSH levels are an indication that you likely won't produce eggs well in that cycle and/or that they might be poor quality.
3. High LH is similar to high FSH in that it could indicate that any eggs produced this cycle will be of poor quality.
4. Few or no antral follicles (found via the ultrasound) means the IVF drugs won't have much to work with.

A study on women with PCOS showed that electroacupuncture during IVF reduces the amount of medication required (Yang, Cui, and Li 2015). Those doing electroacupuncture also had a tendency to produce a higher quantity of good-quality embryos. In another study, women who received acupuncture at the time of IVF egg retrieval showed increased pregnancy rates.

Paulus et al. (2002)

Myoinositol (two grams daily) may improve IVF outcomes for poor responders. It can lead to a higher proportion of mature eggs retrieved and may improve the quality of the embryos (Pacchiarotti et al. 2015). Last but not least, it seems to reduce the amount of medication required, making it less taxing on your body and your bank account!

Laganà et al. (2018)

Within the past decade, DHEA has grown more popular with fertility clinics as a way to improve IVF outcomes for women with diminished ovarian reserve (DOR). Limited evidence suggests that it can raise AMH levels and increase chances of pregnancy for poor IVF responders (Fouany and Sharara 2013; Kachhawa et al. 2015). Large-scale, double-blind studies are lacking, but with a lack of other solutions for low egg reserve, it might be worth a try. DHEA should not be taken by women with PCOS or testosterone excess.

Sample Integration Plan for Poor Responders

Apply the following alternative action items to your ART program:

- Acupuncture and moxibustion two times per week to improve ovarian responsiveness and bolster follicular development
- Conception Cleanse (chapter 8)
- Cycle Syncing Diet with a focus on folic acid (chapter 9)
- Supplement with omega-3s, vitamin D, ubiquinol, NAC, myoinositol
- Start a customized Chinese herbal remedy (prescribed by a certified herbalist)

POOR GROWTH OF UTERINE LINING

With few effective options available in Western medicine, this is an area where integrative approaches shine. Poor development of uterine lining is an issue that prompts many fertility doctors to refer patients my way. If your lining won't thicken and remains at a width less than seven millimeters, your embryo(s) may not have enough nourishing tissue to implant. The reasons behind an underdeveloped endometrium vary widely. The most common causes I see are PCOS, amenorrhea, fertility medications (Clomid), infection, or scarring. Women with a history of PID or other causes of uterine scarring have a trickier time combating this issue, but I still see the most clinical success with integrative methods outlined later in this chapter.

The conventional medical approach to thickening lining is the use of Estrace and, in some cases, sildenafil, also known as Viagra (the little blue pill). Some women, however, don't respond to this protocol and stay on estrogen (Estrace) for weeks or even months to no avail. Side effects are bloating, irritability, weight gain, and feeling rotten overall. This was the case for my patient Lauren. She was in her early thirties and did not ovulate due to her PCOS. IVF seemed like the best bet since women with PCOS often produce a lot of eggs. Although she did in fact produce an abundance of eggs and embryos, her lining wouldn't thicken despite two months of Estrace and sildenafil. Her doctor was at his wits' end, and Lauren was in despair. To add insult to injury, the estrogen had made her pack on 20 pounds, and her lining still wouldn't budge! I put Lauren on an anti-inflammatory diet with supplementation of omega-3, raspberry leaf, an herbal formula called Wen Jing Tang, and vitamin E. We did two acupuncture sessions per week with the addition of electro-stimulation. Within two weeks of this beginning regime, her lining was 11 millimeters, and her doctor was very pleased. They transferred the embryo back to her uterus, but, unfortunately, it did not implant. I surmised that her body had become too inflamed from the excess estrogens. After the failed cycle, I placed Lauren on a cleanse. She followed the protocol for three weeks and then got her period on her own. That next cycle, she postponed the IVF for two months to enjoy her newfound health. It turns out that she didn't need that next IVF cycle anyway because she got pregnant during her "time-out."

Want a protocol like Lauren's? The basics of Lauren's program were supplements that thin the blood and reduce inflammation (omega-3 fatty acids and vitamin E), invigorating supplements (CoQ10), and herbal uterine tonics (raspberry leaf tincture and the Chinese herbal formula "Warm the Valley," or Wen Jing Tang) that increase circulation in the uterus. Studies have shown that herbal mixtures, such as the formulas Shao Fu Zhu Yu Tang, Yi Shen Tiao Xue Tang, Shu Gan Huo Xue Tang, and Wen Yang Yi Shen Tang, are also effective in both thickening the lining and improving overall conception rates in women with PCOS (Jian-jun 2007). Teas such as raspberry leaf, nettle, and red clover are also helpful.

Combine a protocol like Lauren's with the standard conventional treatment, and the results are impressive. For example, one study showed incredible endometrial thickening through the combination of sildenafil and five acupuncture sessions. All of the patients achieved a lining thickness of 10 millimeters or more, including a woman who began with a thickness of only five millimeters. Another had used

Expert Tip

You can also do a "mock" cycle with acupuncture and get monitored by your doctor to watch the uterine lining build. That way, you'll know in advance what can be achieved, and, equally as important, your doctor will know, too.

only sildenafil in a previous IVF cycle and failed to achieve proper thickness but then succeeded with the aid of acupuncture (Yu et al. 2007). That's integrative medicine at its finest.

Sample Integration Plan for a Thin Uterine Lining

Apply the following alternative action items to your ART program:

- Acupuncture with electro-stimulation with moxibustion two or three times per week for two to three weeks prior to your transfer
- High-protein, low-carb, low-inflammatory diet
- 20 to 30 minutes of mild to moderate daily exercise
- Mindfulness twice daily
- Two cups of raspberry leaf tea or 50 drops of Rubus gemmotherapy tincture three times daily
- Supplement with omega-3, CoQ10, vitamin E, magnesium, probiotics, and vitamin D
- Customized Chinese herbal remedy (prescribed by a certified herbalist), such as Wen Jing Tang, Tao Hong Si Wu Tang, or Si Wu Tang

IMPLANTATION FAILURE

The frustrating complexity of this issue makes it the poster child for integrative approaches. The reality is that even a healthy embryo can fail to implant for unknown reasons. Sometimes there are issues with building the uterine lining, but that is less often a factor, as it is measurable in advance via ultrasound. From what I've observed over the years, there is often a subtle interplay of factors that make the uterus less receptive (i.e., the Big Four). Much like in the case of a thin uterine lining, natural and integrative approaches are the way to go in this murky arena.

> Insulin resistance is often a culprit behind failed implantation (Chang et al. 2013), so eliminating alcohol, sugar, and refined carb intake is a big help.

Phoebe was one of these women. She was only 28 and described herself as a happy and healthy person before starting her fertility journey. Phoebe had the very frustrating "unexplained infertility" diagnosis. She had the significant advantage of being able to produce high-quality, chromosomally normal embryos. But despite the high success rates for this type of embryo, she'd undergone four failed transfers! Furthermore, she had been visiting an acupuncturist for months to no avail. She finally asked her fertility doctor if there was anything else she could do, and he sent her my way. Her next transfer was two weeks away, so it was crunch time. I dissected her diet and found that she was consuming tons of inflammatory foods. She was a vegetarian and a sugar and carb monster. Wine was also making a regular appearance (more sugar!). I took her off all inflammatory foods immediately (gluten, dairy, sugar, booze, caffeine, soy, corn, and so on) and had her eating lots of cooked leafy greens and plenty of sprouted seeds. I encouraged her to upgrade her water filter to one that filtered all heavy metals, bacteria, and fluoride so that we got rid of hormone-disrupting toxins. I suggested she needed to increase her acupuncture to two sessions per week, with the addition of moxibustion and herbs. At the time of this writing, Phoebe just gave birth to baby number 2! After the success of the last round, she repeated the same protocol and successfully conceived her second child on the first try.

Sample Integration Plan for Implantation Failure

Apply the following alternative action items to your ART program:

- Acupuncture and moxibustion two times per week for at least four to six weeks leading up to transfer to reduce inflammation, stress, and immune factors
- On day of transfer, schedule two acupuncture sessions before and after embryo transfer
- Conception Cleanse followed by Cycle Syncing Diet and a low glycemic, low-inflammatory diet
- 20 to 30 minutes of mild to moderate daily exercise during the four days leading to transfer
- 30- to 60-minute walks daily after transfer
- Mindfulness twice daily
- Supplement with probiotics, omega-3s, vitamin D, bromelain (for 10 days starting with day of transfer), and magnesium
- Customized Chinese herbal remedy (prescribed by a certified herbalist)

PRO TIP

Adding a few extra acupuncture sessions in your luteal phase (the part between transfer and the pregnancy test) can produce positive results. In one study, 225 infertile people were broken into two groups (Dieterle et al. 2006). One hundred and sixteen of them received luteal phase acupuncture, focused on improving circulation, during an IVF/ICSI cycle. The other group was given placebo acupuncture. The pregnancy rates of the people who received the real acupuncture were more than two times higher.

MISCARRIAGE

The pain of loss is a pain like no other. It can lead you to mistrust your body and lose faith in your ability to carry a pregnancy to term. Even when you do conceive again, instead of elation and joy, you are fraught with the anxiety of another potential loss.

Miscarriages can be caused by immune issues, blood-clotting factors, and thyroid or other hormonal imbalances but are most often caused by chromosomal abnormalities. Since chromosomal issues account for up to 70 percent of miscarriages, it can be somewhat mitigated by doing PGT screening. For women with a history of miscarriage, this testing is a logical next step. If miscarriages persist despite good-quality embryos, then it warrants a look at the Big Four and the possibility of immune or blood-clotting factors.

Did You Know?

One meta-analysis in 2012 showed that Chinese herbal medicine increased chances of sustaining pregnancy past 28 weeks' gestation by 94 percent, while Western medicine techniques showed 73 percent.

Li et al. (2010)

Immunological Treatment for Failed Implantation or Recurrent Miscarriage

Do you have a hunch that an autoimmune condition may be thwarting your baby-making efforts? When your immune system starts attacking your fertility, reproductive immunology provides options such as steroids, immune-modulating intravenous (IV) drips, antibiotics, and more. Still, many fertility doctors disregard these types of treatment, believing they are unproven and/or detrimental to your health. While this may be true, I've seen that in select cases, certain patients who weren't otherwise able to conceive achieved pregnancy through these methods. You have a say in your treatment, and the following are a few resources to aid in your knowledge of implantation failure or recurrent miscarriage. For a comprehensive review, I recommend Dr. Jonathon Scher's book *Preventing Miscarriage*. He is quite literally the "father of reproductive immunology" in New York City and a lovely, caring doctor to boot. It is my firm opinion that addressing the Big Four through lifestyle and natural medicine is an effective way to combat much of the immune dysregulation faced by women struggling with infertility. All said, I want you to know all your options, so here you go!

- *Antibiotics.* Kill bacteria that may cause inflammation of the uterine lining, prevent implantation, or cause miscarriage
- *Prednisone.* Suppresses inflammation and immune overactivity
- *Intravenous immunoglobulin (IVIG).* Treats elevated APA and natural killer (NK) cells
- *Intralipids.* A soy infusion used to suppress NK cells
- *Neupogen.* Administered as a wash or injection, causes the body to generate neutrophils and can help in cases of failed implantation and recurrent miscarriage

Conventional Treatment of Recurrent Miscarriage Due to Clotting

The genetic predisposition toward clotting factors mentioned in chapter 3, such as Factor Leiden and MTHFR, may interfere with your ability to nurture and hold pregnancy. While I find that acupuncture, a clean diet, and supplementation are an effective approach, conventional medicine offers the options below:

- *Lovenox.* An injectable medication that thins the blood to prevent clotting issues that might result in failed implantation or miscarriage
- *Aspirin.* A common oral medication that serves as a milder option in place of Lovenox to thin the blood and mildly suppress inflammation

The Big Four can cause underlying immune, genetic, and clotting factors to get out of hand. If your body is not accepting or retaining a pregnancy, it signifies that something requires thoughtful attention. I see many women get pregnant after homing in and changing their lifestyles.

Did You Know?

CHM has also been shown to improve the maturation of dominant follicles, even in older women, helping to produce a more viable embryo and reducing the chance of miscarriage due to progesterone deficiency in the first 10 weeks of pregnancy.

Heese (2006)

Sample Integration Plan for Miscarriage

Apply the following alternative action items to your ART program:

- Acupuncture and moxibustion two times per week for at least four to six weeks in preparation for next cycle
- Cycle Syncing Diet (chapter 9)
- Eat cooked foods and small amounts of dark meat protein (dark meat chicken, venison, turkey, etc.)
- Mindfulness practice and movement daily
- Supplement with probiotics, omega-3s, vitamin D, magnesium, iron (in the form of liver pills or plant sources such as beet powder), vitamin C, and methylfolate with vitamins B6 and B12
- Customized Chinese herbal remedy (prescribed by a certified herbalist)

Accessing Your Inner Calm

Fertility treatment can be a disillusioning process that may at times challenge your resolve. With all the poking, prodding, and doctor visits, you start to feel like a lab rat. One study observed how women felt during and after IVF treatment and found that 37 percent showed occasional or chronic emotional distress throughout the duration of their treatment and beyond (Gameiro et al. 2016). Honestly, that number seems very low to me. I'd say more like 99 percent of women feel insane throughout this process. The type A brain, in particular, has the tendency to obsess over details in the quest for a viable solution *now*, hence falling into the black hole of online chat rooms, where much of the information doesn't apply to you (yet you can't help but keep reading).

The fertility process can be extremely isolating. Anxiety, depression, guilt, and extreme loneliness commonly accompany the process. When pursuing any kind of fertility treatment, integrating East and West can both improve outcomes *and* safeguard your sanity. Need help calming your mind? Acupuncture basically simulates a meditative state by prompting your brain to release dopamine, serotonin, and other endorphins that make you feel upbeat, relaxed, and peaceful. Patients experiencing anxiety over upcoming IVF cycles show overwhelming improvement with acupuncture, reporting relief from mental and physical anxieties (de Lacey, Smith, and Paterson 2009; Isoyama et al. 2012). It's no wonder it's been linked to higher IVF conception rates (Balk et al. 2010). If acupuncture doesn't appeal to you, then try accessing your inner calm via practices such as meditation, breathing, unplugging, or yoga. Even five minutes of any of these daily can change your life.

What to Avoid during IVF

- *Toxins.* Switch to nontoxic everything. Salons are full of toxic fumes from hair bleach, dyes, and nail polish. Cleaning products aren't much better. A 2001 study in Sweden (Wennborg 2001) linked organic solvents containing benzene, alcohols, and acetone to reduced pregnancy outcomes in women, and common phthalates have been linked to abnormal embryo growth ("Cheatsheet: Phthalates" 2008), not to mention the heavy metals in our drinking water. Refer to chapter 7 for a refresher.

- *Inflammatory foods.* Eat clean! Sugar, refined carbs, conventional dairy, and the other foods mentioned in chapter 4 skyrocket your glucose and insulin levels and spur an inflammatory response. In such an environment, your eggs and uterine environment will be subject to a lot of oxidative stress. Keep it clean to get baby on board!

- *Booze.* Seems like it's a fine idea to relax with a glass of wine amidst the stress of an IVF cycle? Think again. In one study, women who drank regularly in the year prior to the procedure were 13 percent less likely to have a successful retrieval of their eggs (Klonoff-Cohen, Lam-Kruglick, and Gonzalez 2003). Women who drank a week or even a month prior to the procedure were almost three times less likely to conceive and twice as likely to miscarry as women who didn't drink. Their partners were also evaluated in the same study, and men who drank regularly one month prior to IVF increased the chances of miscarriage by approximately three to 38 times!

- *Caffeine.* Studies have linked caffeine to increased risk of miscarriage. One study found that a single cup of coffee, or less than 50 milligrams of caffeine, per day decreased the chances of live birth (Hornstein 2016). Another linked daily consumption to fewer eggs retrieved during an IVF cycle. For some women, it might be fine, but in others, it kicks up their stress response to another level. In my opinion, it's just not worth it.

You've Got This

An integrative approach to fertility care can be the ultimate leg up for those of you pursuing conventional treatment. If you've been at this for a while, those failed attempts are calling to you to bring in some help. Consider integration to be essential in planning your next move. Use this chapter to craft an integrated plan to boost your odds. Your next cycle will be a completely different experience and, hopefully, the last one you'll undergo.

CHAPTER 13

Different Path, Same Destination

Careful attention and introspection are required to survive the fertility process. When your expectations aren't met, fear and anxiety set in, and the mental chatter is agonizing. You feel like you are chasing the clock, and pausing will set your time line back even farther. A doctor bewildered at how to help us doesn't exactly bring on a feeling of peace either. It can be difficult to acknowledge the reality that there still may be quite a road ahead. Are you prepared to take it on? If so, keep going. I've witnessed enough miracles to know it's worth the fight. But if you feel you can't take more beatings physically, emotionally or financially, might you consider an option that could get you your baby quicker and, hopefully, with a greater sense of ease? The journey you take doesn't have to play out exactly the way you pictured it as long as you keep moving forward.

Roads Less Traveled

Plans fall through, but the dream doesn't have to. If hope of having a baby the old-fashioned way has fled, it could be time to regroup and explore another path. The beauty of the modern world is that you have many alternative routes to motherhood available to you. You may find that a weight lifts when you open your heart and mind to the options available.

THE DONOR ROUTE

The donor route involves the purchase of a group of eggs (fresh or frozen) from a donor who has been carefully screened to have a high potential for quality eggs. The eggs would then be fertilized with the sperm of choice (your partner, a friend, or a donor), and you would receive the transfer of the embryo into your uterus. Egg donation can be a great option for women and couples who have had challenges acquiring quality eggs and/or viable embryos. In many cases, you can find a "proven" donor: a woman whose eggs have previously made babies. At the very least, you'd have info on their egg reserve and the likelihood that they would be a good "producer." Many donors have also done previous cycles so that you can see data on how they've fared.

Initially, many of you ladies and/or your partner may have a resistance to using someone else's eggs. There is concern that the baby is somehow "not yours" because it lacks your DNA. While I understand this concern, I prefer to view the journey to conception through a metaphysical rather than biological lens. It's the "soul" that you are inviting into your world, not just an embryo. DNA isn't even half the magic.

The field of epigenetics can also be helpful in this arena. Epigenetics is a complex study, but essentially, it examines why and how our genes switch on and off. Epigenetic changes to cells is a natural occurrence that can be influenced by age, our environment, and our everyday lifestyle. What I'm getting at is that the mother who carries the baby has a great deal of influence on the development of her child regardless of where the egg came from. According to research, the most fundamental impact of the genes occurs in utero. As such, the environment and the mother's lifestyle choices (even before conception) play a critical role in the child's overall health. The physical appearance of every child is influenced by an entire gene pool of parents, grandparents, and so on. According to epigenetic study, after a baby comes into this world, those genetics will continue to modify, switching on and off, and cells will continue to change. In essence, even if the baby does not resemble you at first, there's still a good chance the child could develop your features as he or she gets older. My patients with donor children consistently tell me that everyone comments on how much their children resemble them. From what I've seen, I'd have to agree! In any case, you'll be able to peruse donor catalogs to find the right fit for your family. You can choose someone with the same height, eye, and hair color. You'll have access to information on her education, interests, and health so that you can make an informed decision. Believe it or not, this part of the process is usually very enjoyable. I've had a great time being the sounding board for my patients as they narrow down their choices to select their ideal donor.

Another positive aspect that many women don't initially consider is that using donor eggs can provide significant stress relief, lifting much of the pressure off of *you*. You have handled your fertility journey with utter grace, but it's a heavy load for anyone to carry. Donor eggs are a way to escape the exhaustion and emotional turmoil of undergoing 20 or more IVF cycles to find one good egg.

Ask an Expert—Epigenetics

The epigenetic influence is pretty mind-boggling but too remarkable to leave out of our discussion. To explore the topic a little deeper and get a clearer perspective, I asked my longtime colleague, Dr. Briana Rudick, director of the Third Party Reproduction Program of Columbia Fertility, to shed some more light on epigenetic magic as it pertains to using donor eggs. Here's what she had to say.

"Perhaps the biggest bump that women face when considering a donor egg is the loss of genetic identity. A lot of this has to do with preconceived notions of 'nature' versus 'nurture.' What we have learned over many years is that it isn't just 'nature' or just 'nurture'; it really is a combination of both. How healthy a woman is when she carries, her ability to breastfeed, and her ability to bond with her infant and later her toddler leaves a very long-lasting fingerprint upon the health of the child physically, mentally, and emotionally.

"Because she carries, she is the biological mother, and being the biological mother has many benefits, such as breastfeeding and the ability to bond with her baby. She will experience all of the many ups and downs that go along with pregnancy and the postpartum period.

"Epigenetic influences do, in fact, impact gene expression. So I tell patients that the DNA of any individual is like the blueprint of a house. Not all the sketched rooms actually get built, however, the same way that not all genes are expressed. Much of what determines gene expression is determined by the in utero environment, a lot of which we still don't understand. But your physical and mental health during this journey does impact your baby."

An intriguing observation I've made in my own practice is that in some cases, women who had their first baby via donor conceived their second naturally. It seems backward, but sometimes our body needs guidance on what to do and then figures it out from there. There are no guarantees this will occur, but crazier things have happened.

Donor Eggs in a Nutshell

The advantages:

- Increased chance of pregnancy and live birth for those with egg quality issues
- Less intensive IVF process (no stims, retrieval, and so on)
- Epigenetic influences

The cautions:

- Concern about a lesser chance of family resemblance and how to tell your child when grown
- Costs
- Donor eggs still no guarantee of success

GESTATIONAL CARRIER

If you were able to produce good-quality embryos but struggled to achieve successful implantation or hold a pregnancy, a gestational carrier may be your best route. I've had patients with recurrent miscarriage or pregnancy loss who found salvation in this option. This is also the safest option for you and baby if you've been told that "carrying" may be dangerous due to large fibroids, severe endometriosis, extensive scarring, structural abnormalities, immune challenges, or uterine malformations. As with an egg donor, you'll need to "match" with a gestational carrier via your fertility clinic or an agency. You may want to choose a "proven" carrier who has had her own children or carried for other mothers to be. As with donor eggs, you'll be able to view the profile of the woman and gain insight

> What's the difference between a gestational carrier and a surrogate? The terms are often used interchangeably in movies and TV, but they're quite different! In the case of a gestational carrier, your eggs and your partner's sperm are fertilized to create the embryo, which is then implanted in the carrier's uterus. With a surrogate, on the other hand, your partner's sperm is used to fertilize the surrogate's eggs, and she carries the pregnancy.

as to her health history and work and lifestyle habits to make sure you are comfortable. The process involves the first four phases of an IVF cycle to stimulate, retrieve, and fertilize your eggs. The difference is that your fertilized embryo is then transferred to the gestational carrier. You'll want to make sure gestational surrogacy is available where you live. In New York, for example, it was only more recently legalized.

Gestational Carrier in a Nutshell

The advantages:

- Higher chance of implantation and live birth for women with a history of failed implantation, miscarriage, or pregnancy loss
- Mitigates risk of complications for women with uterine scarring, severe fibroids, and structural abnormalities

The cautions:

- Expect a longer "match" period
- Illegal in some states, in which case you will need to find an agency to help you in a neighboring state where it is legal
- Expensive
- No guarantees

ADOPT YOUR ANGEL

Adoption is—and always has been—a dream of mine. I know there is a child out there who is meant to join my family, and I dream of the day I find them. I view it much like the quest for the Dalai Lama. In the Tibetan Buddhist tradition, when the time is right and the next descendant leader is needed, the men venture from village to village seeking the perfect person who's already out there waiting for them. It's a beautiful thing to give a child a home, and watching yourself transform into a mother throughout that process is equally inspiring.

Typically, adoption is mediated through an agency, though I've had patients do it as individuals, with or without a lawyer. Before you begin searching, you may want to decide whether you'd prefer a closed or an open adoption. If you are open to either, then great, but you will need to know in advance.

Open versus Closed Adoption

An open adoption means you remain in contact with the child's birth parent(s), sending them updates and perhaps even allowing them to visit your child. A closed adoption cuts all ties with the birth parent(s) the moment all the paperwork is signed.

Adoption can be tricky in ways and isn't always straightforward. Sometimes the birth mother backs out at the last minute or even after you have taken the baby home (adoption revocation laws and time frames vary by state). It can also be pricey thanks to agency fees and the like. That said, there are agencies that offer sliding scales, and there are grants available for those who seek them out.

I interviewed a woman on my podcast, Fertility in Focus, about her journey to adoption. She said there were two things that led her to adopt. The first was the strain financially. She just couldn't afford more IVF, especially given that there was no guarantee of a baby even if she did continue. The second was that the desire to become a mother began to outweigh how she got there. Amen.

Adoption in a Nutshell

The advantages:

- One of the only routes that guarantees you a child
- A child is given a loving home
- Eliminates the physical and emotional stress of fertility treatment
- Safer for women with underlying health conditions like severe endometriosis, fibroids, or uterine malformations

The cautions:

- Can be expensive
- The risk and heartbreak of having a parent back out of the adoption process
- Can be time consuming

FOSTERING A CHILD

Fostering is an incredible act of service and an amazing opportunity for you to open your heart and your home to a special someone. In this scenario, you may encounter some legal red tape, but the payoff is well worth it. Foster children may be orphans, but in many cases, they have been extracted from a dangerous or neglectful home. They are dependents of children's court, and many are still the subject of legal battles between the parents and the state.

Because of the likelihood of ongoing court proceedings, fostering or adopting from foster care is a lot more involved than adopting directly from the child's birth parent(s). It's thought to be intended as a temporary arrangement that can eventually lead to adoption, though that's not guaranteed. Qualification requirements include obtaining a foster parent license with your state and passing a "home study" on your residence. Then you'll be registered as a foster parent and matched with a child who will be placed in your care. If the child you foster is still in the "reunification" process, their birth family still has parental rights. As the foster parent, you are expected to participate in that process until a verdict has been reached regarding whether the child will be removed from foster care and returned. You will bring them to court dates, and social workers will check in on the child regularly.

In some cases, since foster children are often taken from abusive or neglectful homes, they may have more challenging care needs, both physical and emotional. This is not to say foster children are more "unstable" or undisciplined but rather that they may initially struggle to trust and connect with you. It's important that you are prepared to help the child through these struggles. This is, of course, not the case for all foster children; I've seen many slide joyfully into the routine and care of their new family. The nature of fostering also means the child will likely be older or at least a toddler.

Fostering requires you to both persevere *and* surrender simultaneously, much like trying to get pregnant yourself. You could put in months or even years of careful, loving effort only for your hopes and expectations to fall through. It is not for the faint of heart, but I will tell you that my patients who chose this option learned and loved so deeply that they were at peace if the child returned to his or her biological parent(s). An open mind, tenacity, and flexibility make undertaking this path easier.

Fostering in a Nutshell

The advantages:

- You give a child a loving home, even if only for a short period.
- It is possible to adopt a foster child.
- You can help a child through a difficult stage in their life.

The cautions:

- Fostering and adopting a foster child involves more legal red tape than other avenues.
- Adoption is not guaranteed.
- A foster child may struggle to adjust, trust, and connect.

Sometimes even the best-laid plans are imperfect. Most of the time, it's our expectations that get the best of us. We so desire for it to happen just the way we pictured it. But without flexibility, we may block ourselves from our true destiny. The unexpected path may even hold richer meaning and rewards thanks to the adventure it took to get you there. My patients who journeyed along less conventional routes to become parents never regretted it.

Outro

MIND, BODY, AND FERTILITY

Before I leave you, I want to impart some thoughts and solutions regarding emotional wellness and its ties to the quest for baby. The emotional exhaustion of infertility can lead many women to develop an apathetic or negative attitude toward fertility efforts. When infertility steals your sense of control, it's natural to experience negative emotions like grief, sadness, worry, and self-doubt. Many of my type A patients have said some version of the following to me: "Things have most always gone my way. I'm having so much trouble accepting that having a baby isn't following the same trajectory!"

Conception and motherhood are very important milestones in many women's lives, but *many* does not mean *everybody*. Many women and couples lead very happy lives without the addition of little ones. For those of you with hearts and minds set on a baby, however, the fertility struggle is a very *real* and even torturous emotional whirlwind. Quite understandably, you want to conceive *now*, without a hitch, because you decided now is the time. Unfortunately, for many of us, the body and spirit don't necessarily align with the expectations and time lines we carefully crafted in our minds.

Fertility Blocks You Might Not Consider

In Chinese medicine, it is believed that negative emotions block the flow of vital energy through the body, including its reproductive organs. An energy blockage can translate to poor circulation and organ function (i.e., the liver is the seat of emotions, and its function can be affected by unresolved stress and resentment). Healthy emotions create healthy energy flow that helps remove undetected obstacles to baby.

My Journey

My teens and twenties were characterized by a plethora of hormonal troubles (think everything from cysts and painful periods to hormonal acne, mood issues, and absent periods). I chipped away at these things with natural medicine and nutrition over time and got to a point where my PCOS was in remission, my skin was clear, and periods and ovulation were in a predictable 27- to 28-day cycle.

In my mid-thirties, I decided it was time to have a baby. The desire had been there for a while, but now, with my career in a good place and a heightened awareness of my clock ticking, the time seemed right. I had been a fertility and women's health specialist for many years at that point. I helped patients with my "fertility profile" (PCOS and/or low ovarian reserve) on a regular basis, so I knew there might be challenges along the way. Imagine my surprise when I got pregnant on my honeymoon. First try, baby! I was thrilled. I heard the heartbeat at my eight-week checkup. I felt like I was going to hurl at the slightest provocation. Everything was progressing well. Then came the 10-week scan. The doctor ran the ultrasound over my belly several times, but it was soon clear that she wasn't able to pick up a heartbeat. I had miscarried. Despite knowing so many women who had endured this same experience, I could not have fully prepared myself for the pain. Amid the sorrow and profound sense of loss, I wanted answers. I needed a "why." I scheduled a dilation and curettage (D&C) for the following week to test the embryo for abnormalities. I recall feeling like I was in a bad dream in the hospital waiting room. After the procedure, I left the hospital in a daze, one that didn't immediately lift. Looking back, I think I was quite depressed for a time. I followed the advice I'd given many others and took the next few months to heal and reset.

A couple months later, feeling more like myself again, my husband and I gave it another go. It turned out the loss had been due to a chromosomal defect, as most miscarriages were. At the very least, I had an answer as to why I had miscarried. Because the first pregnancy happened so easily, I just followed the basics, charting my fertility signs to time for ovulation. My period kept coming, month after month, then one day I peed on yet another stick. Positive! I stood there in the bathroom, staring at it. The damn pink line wasn't darkening. It was a faded pastel even though my period was already past due. I suspected it was a chemical pregnancy; I'd seen many of them before. My gynecologist confirmed that this was indeed a "blighted ovum." That means I had a gestation sac (i.e., the fluid-filled cavity that's supposed to form around an embryo), but the embryo wasn't developing inside. I would miscarry again. It took only a couple weeks, and it was so early that there would have been nothing to biopsy. I progressed through what I refer to as a "mini" miscarriage—perhaps a bit worse than a period but nothing major. I wasn't quite as devastated; I was more annoyed.

I was able to resume trying after another month or so. My head wasn't in the greatest place over the next few months, as more time passed with no pregnancy. I lamented every beer my husband drank and cursed my age, PCOS, and low ovarian reserve. I reflected on what could be getting in my way and tuned into the fact that I hadn't thoroughly addressed all the aspects of my lifestyle. "What would I tell a patient right now?" I followed my own advice and looked inward. Up to this point, I'd done acupuncture, was taking a few supplements, and was eating clean, but I had not addressed my stress levels or tried taking herbs. My gynecologist had suggested that I see a fertility doctor and pursue IVF given my low ovarian reserve and advanced age (35 years old). I wanted to give it one more chance before I sought intervention. I still hadn't employed all of my techniques, and it was time to get busy.

As my grief dissipated and I began thinking clearly again, I realized I needed to lay out a new plan, based on my experience, and take action. I started taking herbs, modified my work schedule, reduced the intensity of my exercise, and focused on getting more rest. I homed in on a herbal and supplement regime to improve my egg quality and was conscious of how much stress and strain I placed on myself. Last but not least, I took five days off work and traveled to a warm place where I unplugged completely. Those five days were spent dancing, doing yoga and art, and enjoying people and nature. Not long after implementing my new regimen, that pink positive line appeared again, clear as day this time. My daughter, MP, is now five years old.

My fertility journey was rocky but nothing compared to the challenges many women face. It was the stories of these women that gave me strength in the process. Trash bins of negative pregnancy tests, miscarriages, and the sheer disappointment of unfulfilled desires can leave emotional scars. Even after MP was born, I never forgot the pain and frustration of that time. I'm grateful, however, that I can use my understanding of those circumstances to connect on a deeper level with the women who visit my center. No one understands the way that another woman can. The pain, loss, and perseverance unite us all.

Necessary Shifts

While meditation and other mindfulness practices are effective means of healing your heart and mind after past miscarriages, abortions, abuse, mistrust, and unconscious fears of parenthood, you may feel you still need some outside guidance to help you gain perspective. Therapy is always a viable option, but if you're looking for an alternative to the normal talk therapy, I personally have found success with coaching. It is an ideal approach for type A women because our focus is on moving forward rather than looking back (other than to learn, of course). In coaching, you have someone help you grow awareness about the things that are affecting you, one who can then help direct you in how to reframe your outlook in order to get "unstuck." Instead of spending a ton of time unpacking your childhood or past negative experiences, you learn to reshape your view of your current personal challenges and obstacles, perhaps even coming to view them as opportunities. I offer free coaching and information through my podcast, Fertility in Focus, but if you are looking for something more tailored, I suggest you seek out a coach or therapist who knows the realm of infertility. We also offer in-person and remote fertility coaching through my fertility wellness center, the Naturna Institute, in New York City or via my website: christinaburns.com.

Believe, Conceive

In writing this book, I hope to have provided you with guidance needed for you to feel empowered. Our thoughts and beliefs have an incredible impact on our outcomes, and, as such, I want you to be telling yourself that you can do this—*you can have your baby.*

Now that you've taken the reins, you've likely already begun to experience a certain level of physical, emotional, and spiritual transformation. No baby yet? Keep the faith. In some cases, women get pregnant on this program within the first few weeks, but in all honesty, quick, easy fixes are not the name of the game. Modern stressors have likely been kicking your butt for years and it can take time for your body and mind to assimilate the benefits of the positive changes you are making. Part of that process may also result in the clarity and acceptance needed to pursue an alternative path to motherhood.

Whether you choose an alternate route, natural medicine, or integration, I hope your chosen path feels right because it was crafted just for you. Taking charge of your physical and emotional health isn't just about making babies. It's a reset. Maybe you wanted to make some changes but just weren't getting around to it. You needed a reason—a really good one. The desire for a baby got you there.

Appendix A
GUIDE TO AVOIDING TOXINS

Environmental Toxins and the Sources in Which They Can Be Found

Heavy metals: Some fish and unfiltered water
DEA (Diethanolamine): Facial cleansers, oil controllers
MEA (Monoethanolamine): Hair dye, shampoo
TEA (Triethanolamine): Moisturizers, eye creams
Phthalates and parabens: Plastics
FD and C color pigments: Cosmetics (mainly eye shadow), shampoo
Fragrance: Perfume, eau de toilet, scented moisturizer
Imidazolidinyl (Urea and DMDM): Body wash, moisturizers
Potassium bromate, bromated flours: All bread products
Quaternium 15: Makeup, skin creams
Isopropyl alcohol: Astringents and skin care products
Mineral oil: Most conventional makeup brands
PEG (polyethylene glycol): Internal analgesic, oral gel, shaving cream, over-the-counter painkillers
Propylene glycol: Makeup products
Sodium lauryl sulfate: Shampoo, toothpaste, detergent
Tricolsan: Antibacterial soaps, detergents, toys, products labeled "odor fighting," "freshening," or "long lasting"
Talc: Cosmetics, powder, household paint supplies
Petrolatum: Creams, cosmetics

Avoidance and Modification Cheat Sheet

The following tables are recommendations of things to avoid and healthier alternatives. For more extensive lists, visit the website of the Environmental Working Group (EWG) at https://www.ewg.org.

Food and Water

Avoid	Add or Supplement With
Tap water or water filtered through a plastic filter	Drink filtered water like Essentia Water and Smartwater or filter your own with a carbon filter: Berkey filters and the Propur water filters are recommended. Obtain a water quality report from the Environmental Working Group (EWG) National Drinking Water Database (https://www.ewg.org). Consider getting your water tested for lead.
Nonorganic produce	Eat organic and local food whenever possible. Think about joining a local CSA (Community Supported Agriculture) or doing your shopping at the local farmers market when the weather is appropriate. To help with your produce shopping, reference this site to discover which crops are most often GMO contaminated: https://www.ams.usda.gov /rules-regulations/be/bioengineered-foods-list. You can also refer to the Clean 15 and Dirty Dozen using this link: https://www.ewg.org/foodnews /dirty-dozen.php.
Nonorganic eggs and meats	Eat organic or pasture-raised eggs. Choose higher-quality meat and eat less of it. Look for grass-fed beef.
Fish with high mercury content, like king mackerel, shark, swordfish, tuna, and tilefish	Consume wild-caught fish. Choose seafood with a lower mercury content, like anchovies, catfish, clams, cods, lobster, scallops, and tilapia. This is a great website for getting sustainable fish: https:// www.vitalchoice.com. For more information concerning the mercury concentration in fish, check out the FDA's list of mercury levels in commercial fish and shellfish: https://www.fda.gov.
Microwaving and storing food in plastic	Switch to glass, stainless-steel, ceramic, or wood containers.
Processed and canned food	Try meal prepping or buying food packaged in glass or paper.
Drinking from plastic water bottles	Drink from BPA free or stainless-steel containers.

Avoid	Add or Supplement With
Plastics marked 3 (PVC or vinyl), 6 (polystyrene foam), or 7 (can contain BPA)	Choose plastics marked 1, 2, 4, or 5. Eco-kids, Green Toys, and Apple Park are recommended nontoxic toy brands.
Bromated flour	Check your local farmers market for bread choices. Bread Alone brand is safe.

Household Cleaning

Avoid	Add or Supplement With
Cleaners with ammonia or chlorine bleach, toilet cleaners, oven cleaners, or heavy-duty degreasers with hydrochloric acid, phosphoric acid, sodium, potassium hydroxide, or ethanolamines	Choose products that say "nontoxic," "biodegradable," "chlorine free," "phosphate free," "fragrance free," and "no dyes." Healthy brands include Love Home and Planet and GreenShield Organic. Recommended detergents brands include GreenShield Organic by Free and Clear, Dr. Bronner's, and Seventh Generation. Cleanwell antibacterial soap is nontoxic. Or make your own environmentally friendly cleaning products. Check out this link with plenty of do-it-yourself cleaning product ideas: https://greatist.com.
Dust and dirty fabrics	Clean often. Fabrics are a host for allergens, like mold, pollen, and dust mites. Use a HEPA filter in your home and bedroom.
Wearing shoes in the house, which tracks in dust and allergens	Go barefoot or get a pair of house slippers
Air fresheners and scented products that don't disclose the ingredients in their fragrances. Often these products contain endocrine disruptors, such as phthalates and synthetic musks.	Open your windows to promote ventilation and circulation of air. Turn on a fan or HVAC system to increase the movement of fresh air.
Avoid cat litter and contact with rodents (including pets). Rodents carry viruses that can be harmful and even deadly to an unborn baby.	

Beauty Products and Clothing

Avoid	Add or Supplement With
Products with ingredients you can't pronounce. Cut out nonessential personal care products like perfume.	Check out the EWG Skin Deep cosmetics online database at https://www.cosmetics database.com. Type in a product or an ingredient to find if there is a known toxic effect on the body. Natural makeup brands include First Aid Beauty, Fresh, Burt's Bees, Lush cosmetics, Obsessive Compulsive Cosmetics, Doctor Hauschka, and Clarins. You can refer to this list for more recommended brands: https://www.thegoodtrade.com. Recommended brands for moisturizers and eye creams include Osea, Ren, Pangea Organics, Kosmatology, Healthy Body Investment, Epilynx, Madeon Skin. If you're looking for natural and healthy face washes, refer to this list: https://www.thegoodtrade.com. Natural alternatives to astringents and skin care products are Witch hazel, tea tree oil, and lavender. Brands like 100% Pure and Juice Beauty can often be found at Whole Foods.
Nail polishes containing the "toxic trio": formaldehyde, toluene, and debuted phthalate (CBP). They can cause skin irritation and birth defects.	While no nail polish is completely natural, the following are some healthier alternatives: Zoya, Suncoat, Piggy Paint, Honeybee Gardens, RGB, Sheswai.
Hair Products, Brazilian blowouts, other hair straightening treatments, hair coloring, and perms	Recommended brands are Zalik Naturals, Grown Alchemist, Innersense Organic Beauty, Viori, Prose, John Masters Organics, Alaffia, Devachan, Wen Healthy Hair, Shea Moisture, and Oribe. Refer to this list of natural hair products for further brand recommendations: https://www.thegoodtrade.com.

Avoid	Add or Supplement With
Wearing dirty clothing	Wash clothes before wearing them. Some of the safest laundry detergents include Sun and Earth Laundry Detergent, Seventh Generation, Planet Ultra, Molly's Suds, and Dr. Bronner's.
Conventional dry cleaners. Most dry-cleaning systems use a chemical called perchloroethylene (PERC), which can pollute the air in your house.	If you must use dry cleaning, air the clothes (with bags off) outside or in the basement for two to three days prior to transferring them into your closet.
Oral gel, shaving cream, and toothpastes with PEG (polyethylene glycol) or sodium lauryl sulfate	Clean brands include CheapDEO, Himalaya, Tom's of Maine, and Auromere.

Air Quality

Avoid	Add or Supplement With
Smoking	If you're trying to quit, here is a website with some helpful resources: https://smokefree.gov.
Gas fumes	Have someone else pump your gas if possible.
Air fresheners	Open your windows and buy plants to filter air. Good options are gerbera daisies, chrysanthemums, English ivy, spider plants, and bamboo. Opt for beeswax or soy candles, simmer pots, and homemade air fresheners. Here's a link for do-it-yourself air fresheners: https://www.theprairiehomestead.com.
Air filters that produce ozone	Buy a HEPA air purifier. Here's a helpful link if you're shopping for an air purifier: https://www.apartment therapy.com.
High levels of humidity, which attract dust mites and mold	Buy a dehumidifier. Aim to keep humidity at about 30 to 50 percent.

Home Improvements

Avoid	Add or Supplement With
Paints, glues, and flooring materials labeled "antifungal" or containing formaldehyde-releasing preservatives	Some trusted brands for home improvement products: Forest Stewardship Council (FSC), Global Organic Textile Standard (GOTS), Oeko-Tex Standard 100, Greenguard When buying paints, look for these labels: Green Seal-11 certified, milk paints (healthier alternative to water-based latex or oil-based paints), low or no VOC (less than 50 g VOCs per liter). Always work in well-ventilated areas.
Any home built before 1978 may have lead in it. Never sand or remove paint yourself.	Hire a contractor who is certified in lead removal.
Pesticides in your lawns and gardens	Use organic or integrated pest management techniques. Here's a link with some options for organic gardening: https://www.gardeningchannel.com.

Electronics

Avoid	Add or Supplement With
Excessive electromagnetic field (EMF) exposure	Reduce your use of microwaves, computers, and cell phones. Especially take care to keep phones away from the genitals and head. Don't put your phone in your pockets or under your pillow. Laptops should be used on a desk rather than your lap. For more on EMFs and their possible link to health, check out this World Health Organization article: https://www.who.int.
Leaving your internet on all night	Use a timer plug to turn off your internet router in the evening. Choose times based on your schedule or try turning it off from 11 p.m. to 6 a.m. Turning your internet off at night significantly lessens the time you're exposed to Wi-Fi signals.
Leaving your phone on all night	Switch your phone to airplane mode at night, especially if you keep it in your room or use it as an alarm clock.

Workplace Exposures

Avoid	Add or Supplement With
If you are exposed to chemicals or toxins, request a change in duties prior to getting pregnant.	Get information and training about hazardous substances in your workplace. Follow guidelines to avoid exposure (use protective gear, ask your employer for substitutes for toxic substances, and so on). If you live with someone who works with toxic chemicals, have the person change and shower before coming home. They should keep their tools and clothing away from other people in the household. Work clothes should be washed separately if the person is exposed to chemicals or toxins on the job.

Source: "EWG's Guide to Triclosan." Environmental Working Group. Accessed January 22, 2022. https://www.ewg.org/research/ewgs-guide-triclosan.

Appendix B
GUIDE TO CASTOR OIL PACKS

I frequently recommend at-home castor oil packs as a form of self-treatment. The following are the items needed to make your own pack and easy use instructions.

Items Needed to Make Your Own Pack

1. A piece of thick cloth (flannel, wool, or cotton works well) about the size of a dish towel
2. Castor oil
3. A bowl
4. A hot water bottle or heating pad
5. A large plastic storage bag

How to Use the Pack

1. Place the cloth in your bowl and pour castor oil over it until it is saturated.
2. Apply the cloth to the lower right side of your abdomen.
3. Cover with the plastic bag, then place a heating pad or hot water bottle on top of that.
4. Meditate, read a book, watch a movie, or just rest for about 45 minutes until the castor oil soaks in completely.
5. When you are finished, take off the pack and wipe off any excess oil on your skin with a clean towel.
6. You can keep the pack in a plastic bag in a cool place or the refrigerator. Just add another tablespoon of castor oil for the next session.
7. With use, the pack gradually absorbs toxins. Discard the pack and make a new one after 10 uses.
8. Keep in mind that the castor oil stains fabric, so wear clothing you don't mind getting messy.

Appendix C

CONCEPTION CLEANSE–FRIENDLY RECIPES

For additional guidance on nutrition, my Eating for Optimal Fertility course is available through christinaburns.com and https://naturnalife.com.

Breakfast

CHIA COCONUT PUDDING

Directions:

Place ½ cup of chia seeds in a bowl. Whisk 2 cups coconut milk, ½ tsp. vanilla extract, ¼ tsp. cinnamon, and a pinch of salt together in a bowl; pour over chia seeds and stir well. Allow coconut milk–chia seed mixture to soak until thickened, at least 20 minutes, or cover bowl with plastic wrap and refrigerate overnight. Stir pudding and top with ½ cup of berries of your choice (strawberries, blueberries, or raspberries). For extra crunch, add chopped nuts.

SWEET POTATO TOAST

Directions:

Cut sweet potato into thin slices, about ¼ inch thick. Place in toaster oven and set it to the maximum cook time. When it pops, flip the slices and toast one more time. Depending on the strength of your toaster oven and your preferences, you may need to toast it once more after. Remove from toaster and let cool. Top with any of the following:

1. tahini + sesame seeds + goji berries
2. egg + sea salt + freshly ground black pepper
3. mashed avocado + sea salt + red pepper flakes
4. crunchy almond butter + cardamom
5. almond butter + blueberries + cinnamon
6. Dijon mustard + smoked salmon + black pepper + parsley

GRAIN-FREE OATMEAL

Ingredients:

- 2 cups shredded coconut
- ½–1 cup hemp seeds (less if you choose to add dried fruit to your base mix)
- ½ cup chia seed
- ½ cup whole or coarsely ground flaxseeds
- ¼ tsp. sea salt

Optional:

- ½ cup chopped fruit
- ¼–½ tsp. various spices. My favorite flavor combos are (1) cinnamon, cardamom, and ginger; (2) cinnamon, cumin, cardamom, black pepper, and coriander; and (3) cloves, allspice, nutmeg, ginger, and cinnamon

Directions:

1. Combine all ingredients in a bowl and stir together thoroughly.
2. Include any optional ingredients you like.
3. Transfer to a wide-mouth quart jar to store in the refrigerator.
4. To prepare 1 serving of oatmeal, place ½ cup of dry mix in a bowl and add 1–1½ cups very hot water (just shy of boiling).
5. Stir well and allow to sit for 3–5 minutes.
6. Add fresh fruits, nuts, unsweetened chocolate, bacon crumbles, chicken or turkey sausage, coconut or almond milk, honey, coconut oil, or grass-fed butter to make it exciting.

PROTEIN GRAINS BOWL

Ingredients:

- 1 cup uncooked white quinoa
- 1 cup unsweetened hemp seed milk, plus more for serving
- 1 cup coconut milk (light canned or the beverage in a carton)
- Pinch of sea salt
- 2–3 tbsp. (30–45 ml) maple syrup or coconut sugar
- ½ tsp. pure vanilla extract
- ¼ tsp. cinnamon

For Serving (Optional):

- Mixed berries
- Hemp seeds or chia seeds
- Dried coconut flakes

Directions:

1. Thoroughly rinse quinoa in a fine mesh strainer for 2 minutes, using your hands to sort through and pick out any discolored pieces or pebbles that may remain.
2. Heat a small saucepan over medium heat. Once hot, add rinsed, drained quinoa and toast for 3 minutes, stirring frequently, to dry up water and slightly toast.
3. Add hemp milk, coconut milk, and a pinch of salt and stir. Bring to a boil over high heat, then reduce heat to low and cook for 20–25 minutes, uncovered, stirring occasionally. If it stops simmering, increase heat to medium-low. You're looking for a slight simmer throughout the cooking time.
4. Once the liquid is absorbed and the quinoa is tender, remove from heat and add cinnamon and vanilla (optional). Stir to combine.
5. Taste and adjust flavor as needed. Add a bit more coconut or hemp seed milk if you prefer the texture thinner.
6. Serve each bowl of quinoa with any other desired toppings (listed above).
7. Best when fresh, though leftovers will keep covered in the refrigerator for 2–3 days. Reheat in the microwave or in a small saucepan with additional milk to add moisture back in.

BREAKFAST SMOOTHIE

Ingredients:

- 1 cup hemp milk or almond milk (room temperature)
- ½ cup fresh blueberries and ½ cup fresh papaya
- 1–2 scoops hemp protein, flax, or chia powder or other fiber/approved protein powder if desired
- ⅓ avocado for creaminess

Directions:
Put everything into the blender, process, and sip!

GREEN SMOOTHIE

Ingredients:

- 1 scoop protein powder
- ½ cup coconut milk, almond milk, or water
- 1 cup zucchini, chopped (steamed)
- ½ avocado
- 1 handful baby spinach (steamed)

Lunch/Dinner

SAUTÉED GREEN VEGGIES

Directions:

1. Use any combination of the following: spinach, kale, Swiss chard, mustard greens, snap peas, and green beans.
2. Place olive oil in a frying pan and heat to medium.
3. Add garlic, ginger, and onion (any combination or none) for 30 seconds.
4. Add green vegetables (peas and beans earlier than leafy greens), coat in oil, and then add ¼ cup water and turn to high heat. You can put a top over them or just stir with a wooden spoon until wilted and bright green.
5. Optional: sprinkle sea salt, coconut aminos, lemon juice, sesame oil, or gomasio after the cooking is finished to reduce salt content and amplify flavor.

RED LENTIL COCONUT SOUP

Ingredients:

- 1 cup filtered water
- ½ cup stock (either from Essence soup video or ½ bouillon cube with ½ cup warm water)
- ¼ tsp. sea salt
- 2- by-2-inch piece of kombu
- ½ cup red lentil
- 1 medium tomato
- 1 cup coconut milk, full fat
- ½ tsp. caraway seed
- ½ tsp. cumin seed
- ¼ tsp. coriander powder

Directions:

1. In pot, add water, stock, salt, kombu, and lentils.
2. Bring to a boil. Turn down to a simmer and put the lid on. Cook for 10 minutes on low simmer. Dice tomato.
3. Add to pot all of the rest of the ingredients: tomato, coconut milk, and spices.
4. Blend using a hand mixer or any other mixing device accessible. (If you do not have a blender, you can use a fork to mash tomatoes, or you can sauté in a pan with a small amount of coconut oil prior to adding to soup, which will turn them into a tomato sauce.)
5. Cook for 3 minutes to incorporate flavors.

Options:

Add any other herb or spice desired (fresh basil, parsley, ginger, turmeric, and cinnamon).

Tips:

Adding in kombu helps with digestibility of legumes.
Kombu is rich in iodine and chlorophyll.
Coconut milk is a great replacement for dairy and is high in fiber; vitamins C, E, and B; iron; selenium; calcium; magnesium; and phosphorus. When using any canned products, be sure to check that the can is not lined with BPA.

CLEANSING VEGETABLE SOUP

Ingredients:

- 1 large onion, chopped
- 2 cloves garlic, minced (add to taste)
- 1 cube ginger root, chopped
- 2–3 carrots, sliced
- 2 stalks celery, sliced
- 1 medium zucchini, chopped
- 2 Roma (or other) tomatoes
- Basil to taste
- Parsley to taste
- 2 tbsp. chickpea miso
- Add other vegetables of your choice. Green beans, kale, and chard are very tasty and can be added at the end.

Directions:

1. In a large pot over medium heat, cook onion, ginger, and garlic in water until tender.
2. Add carrots, celery, and miso. Add more water as needed and simmer for 10 minutes.
3. Add tomatoes, zucchini, basil, and parsley, and more water, if needed, to achieve the consistency you like.

GRILLED VEGGIES

Directions:

1. Use any combination of the following vegetables, unpeeled, washed, and cut into 1-inch cubes or pieces:

    - Mushrooms
    - Broccoli
    - Red onion
    - Asparagus
    - Cherry tomatoes
    - Peppers
    - Eggplant
    - Zucchini

2. Toss with olive oil and balsamic vinegar and sprinkle with Italian herbs or just some pepper to taste.
3. Spread in roasting pan in single layers and roast approximately 20–25 minutes at 400°F until veggies are tender and slightly brown, stirring occasionally. The amount of time needed depends on the size of the veggie.
4. Use Celtic or Himalayan salt sparingly and pepper to taste. Serve while warm or use cold leftovers in salad.

BAKED SWEET POTATOES

Directions:

1. Preheat oven to 375°F.
2. Put 3–4 washed, peeled, and diced sweet potatoes on a cookie sheet.
3. Bake for 20–40 minutes.

ROASTED CAULIFLOWER SOUP

Ingredients:

- 2 tbsp. olive oil
- 1 onion, finely chopped
- 1 cauliflower, broken into pieces
- 3 cups chicken stock
- 1 cup coconut cream
- Salt and pepper

Directions:

1. Preheat oven to 380°F.
2. Place onion and cauliflower in a large ovenproof dish and drizzle with olive oil.
3. Sprinkle with some salt and pepper.
4. Roast until golden.
5. Place the cauliflower and onions in a large pot and add stock.
6. Bring to a boil.
7. Let it boil 5 minutes, add coconut cream, and season with salt and pepper.
8. Puree in a blender and serve with a little olive oil and some pepper.

TURKEY THIGHS

Directions:

1. Purchase 2 or 3 turkey thighs from a farmer's market or use organic/antibiotic-free thighs from a health food store.
2. Fill large pot of water so it covers all of the meat.
3. Add chopped (abundant) carrots, celery, and onion.
4. Add ½ tsp. Celtic salt and cayenne pepper or black pepper to preference. (If you are feeling adventurous, use fennel seeds or Italian herbs and seasonings.)
5. Cook on low for 2–3 hours and add additional liquid if it cooks down too low.
6. Serve or save for later!

BOILED CHICKEN THIGHS

Directions:

1. Purchase 4–6 chicken thighs from a farmer's market or use organic/antibiotic-free thighs from a health food store.
2. Fill large pot of water so it covers all of the meat.
3. Add ½ tsp. Celtic salt and cayenne pepper or black pepper to preference. (If you are feeling adventurous, use fennel seeds or Italian herbs and seasonings.)
4. Cook on low for 2–3 hours and add additional liquid if it cooks down too low.
5. Serve or save for later!

SALMON OR COD IN CARTOCCIO

Directions:

1. Preheat oven to 350°F.
2. Put 1–1.5 pounds of wild-caught salmon or cod on a large piece of tinfoil.
3. Garnish with capers, lemon, black pepper, and 1 tbsp. olive oil.
4. Fold tinfoil into a package, folding all four edges together on the top, containing the salmon in the pouch.
5. Put package in oven on a cookie sheet or in Pyrex for 20 minutes and check for desired doneness.
6. Remove and serve immediately or cool and serve at room temperature.

SOLE AND ASPARAGUS DINNER

Ingredients:

- .4 pounds of sole per person
- One fistful of asparagus per person
- Olive oil
- Sea salt and pepper
- Lemon
- Ghee

Directions:

1. Preheat oven to 375°F.
2. Bake asparagus for 15 minutes in flat Pyrex pan in an inch water before you add a few sole filets, lemon, 1 tbsp. of ghee, and a pinch of sea salt and pepper to taste.
3. Bake for 10 minutes uncovered (add more time if still undercooked).

ANCHOVY HOT BROCCOLI

Ingredients:

- 1 pound broccoli
- 1 small can anchovies
- Olive oil to taste
- Red pepper flakes

Directions:

1. Steam broccoli until soft.
2. Mash one small can of anchovies with some additional olive oil in a pan.
3. Add broccoli and stir/mash all together with a wooden spoon.
4. Add red pepper flakes if you like it hot.
5. *Do not* add any salt!
6. If it seems a bit intense this time, add more broccoli next batch.

COOKED SALAD WITH LEFTOVER INGREDIENTS

Directions:

Mix together the following in a bowl: baked sweet potatoes (fist-size serving), some leftover turkey leg or any protein you choose, leftover cooked (or raw if needed) spinach, optional fistful of arugula; add 2 tbsp. vinaigrette. Warm to taste. Add lemon juice for flavor if desired.

FISH WITH ZUCCHINI NOODLES

Ingredients:

- 2 large zucchini (about 1½ pounds)
- 1½ tsp. ground cumin
- ¾ tsp. salt, divided
- ½ tsp. smoked paprika
- ½ tsp. pepper
- 4 tilapia fillets (6 oz. each)
- 2 tsp. avocado oil

Directions:

1. Trim ends of zucchini. Using a spiralizer, cut zucchini into thin strands.
2. Mix cumin, ½ tsp. salt, smoked paprika, and pepper. Sprinkle generously onto both sides of tilapia.
3. In a large nonstick skillet, heat avocado oil over medium-high heat.
4. In batches, cook tilapia until fish just begins to flake easily with a fork, 2–3 minutes per side. Remove from pan and keep warm.
5. In the same pan, cook zucchini over medium-high heat until slightly softened, 1–2 minutes, tossing constantly with tongs (do not overcook). Sprinkle with remaining salt. Serve with tilapia.

TURKEY STUFFED BELL PEPPERS

Ingredients:

- 4 large bell peppers of your choice, stem and seeds removed, sliced in half lengthwise
- ½ cup sprouted brown rice, cooked
- 1 tbsp. avocado oil
- 1 pound ground turkey
- 2–3 garlic cloves, minced
- ¼ red onion, minced
- ¼ cup parsley, chopped
- ½ teaspoon salt
- ½ teaspoon pepper
- 1 cup marinara
- Shredded goat or vegan cheese

Directions:

1. Preheat the oven to 375°F.
2. In a large skillet over medium heat, add the avocado oil.

3. Add in the turkey and cook halfway (where it's still pink), about 3 minutes.
4. Add in the garlic, onion, parsley, salt, and pepper.
5. Stir and cook until the turkey is done, about 3–5 minutes.
6. Remove from heat and add marinara sauce and rice.
7. In an 8- by 8-inch baking dish, greased or lined with parchment paper, add the bell peppers and fill them with the turkey mixture.
8. Sprinkle with goat cheese and bake for 45 minutes.

LAMB STEW

Ingredients:

- 4 cups lamb or chicken broth
- 4 cups water
- One 32-oz. can crushed tomatoes, BPA free
- Bouquet garnish of thyme, oregano, parsley, and bay leaf
- 1 large red onion, diced
- 1 tbsp. coconut oil
- 3 lamb shanks
- 1 lemon, halved and seeded
- 1 cup Niçoise olives, pitted

Directions:

1. In a large pot over medium-high heat, combine the broth, water, tomatoes, bouquet garnish, and onion and cover.
2. Heat the coconut oil in a large skillet over medium-high heat until simmering. Add the lamb shanks and sear for 3 minutes on each side.
3. Add the seared lamb to the pot and bring almost to a boil. Reduce heat to medium-low and simmer gently for 2 hours.
4. Squeeze the juice from both lemon halves into the pot and then add the rest of the lemon along with the olives. Cook for 15 minutes more, uncovered.
5. Remove from the heat and allow the stew to rest for 15 minutes.
6. Remove the bouquet garnish and discard. Pull the meat apart and discard bones (or save for making stock).
7. Alternatively, put these ingredients into a slow cooker on low, add the lamb after searing it, and cook covered for 8 hours. Add the lemon and olives, cover, turn off the heat, remove the bouquet garnish, and pull apart the meat before serving.

Appendix D
HEALTHY SNACK IDEAS

Chia coconut pudding (see appendix C for recipe)
Raw, sprouted pumpkin seeds, sunflower seeds, almonds
Gopal's snack brand
Healing Home Foods crackers
Go Raw snacks
Seaweed snacks
Seed and nut butters
Smoothies (see appendix C for various recipes)
One piece of fruit
Leftovers from a meal

Appendix E
CHRISTINA'S BRAND RECOMMENDATIONS

Detox Smoothie Powders

Apex Energetics Clearvite

Supplements

Thorne
Douglas Labs
Protocol for Life Balance
Klaire Labs
Genestra
Seroyal
Pure Encapsulations
Integrative Therapeutic
Orthomolecular
Apex Energetics

Probiotics

Klaire Labs
Genestra/Seroyal
Silver Fern

Appendix F
TESTS TO ASSESS AUTOIMMUNE FERTILITY CHALLENGES

The following tests can determine whether your immune system can interfere with fertility:

Hashimoto's thyroiditis/antithyroid antibodies (ATA)
Antiphospholipid antibody test (APA)
Antinuclear antibody test (ANA)
Reproductive immunophenotype
Lupus anticoagulant (ETA)
RH factor
Natural killer cells assay
MTHFR
Factor Leiden
Prothrombin
IGG antibody
IGM antibody

These tests can be requested from your fertility doctor. If they all come back normal and you would like to do more in-depth testing into things (i.e., foods, pesticides, toxins, and molds) in your diet and environment that could be causing inflammation and immune flare-ups, you can explore the ALCAT test or other functional medicine tests, which you can order through my practice, Naturna. For a more in-depth study of these topics, I recommend *Preventing Miscarriage* by Dr. Jonathan Scher.

Bibliography

"A Basic Intro to Alternate Nostril Breathing." DoYou, January 8, 2015. https://www
.doyouyoga.com/a-basic-intro-to-alternate-nostril-breathing.

"Abdominal Fat and What to Do about It." Harvard Health, June 25, 2019. https://
www.health.harvard.edu/staying-healthy/abdominal-fat-and-what-to-do-about-it.

"Adoption Consent Laws by State: Adoption Network." Adoption Network, November 4,
2021. https://adoptionnetwork.com/adoptee-resources/adoption-consent-laws-by-state.

"Adoption Myths and Facts—Resolve: The National Infertility Association." Resolve,
September 13, 2019. https://resolve.org/what-are-my-options/adoption/adoption
-myths facts.

"Amount of Zinc in Lamb." Diet and Fitness. Accessed February 3, 2022. http://www
.dietandfitnesstoday.com/zinc-in-lamb.php.

"Ayurveda Treatments and Lifestyle Consultations for Better Health: Art of Living Retreat Center." Art of Living Retreat Center, December 16, 2021. https://artofliving
retreatcenter.org/event/ayurveda/treatments.

"Beans, White, Mature Seeds, Canned Nutrition Facts." Nutritiondata. Accessed
February 4, 2022. https://nutritiondata.self.com/facts/legumes-and-legume-products
/4320/2.

"Biotherapeutic Drainage™." Seroyal. Accessed February 5, 2022. https://www.seroyal
.com/biotherapeutic-drainage.

"Bisphenol A (BPA)." National Institute of Environmental Health Sciences. U.S. Department of Health and Human Services. Accessed February 3, 2022. https://www
.niehs.nih.gov/health/topics/agents/sya-bpa/index.cfm.

"Cheatsheet: Phthalates." Environmental Working Group, May 5, 2008. https://www
.ewg.org/enviroblog/2008/05/cheatsheet-phthalates.

"Dioxins and Their Effects on Human Health." World Health Organization, October
4, 2016. https://www.who.int/news-room/fact-sheets/detail/dioxins-and-their-effects
-on-human health.

"Endocrine Disruptors." National Institute of Environmental Health Sciences, U.S.
Department of Health and Human Services. Accessed February 3, 2022. https://www
.niehs.nih.gov/health/topics/agents/endocrine/index.cfm.

"Exposure to Phthalates May Raise Risk of Pregnancy Loss, Gestational Diabetes." Harvard School of Public Health, November 8, 2016. https://www.hsph.harvard.edu /news/features/phthalates-exposure-pregnancy-loss-gestational-diabetes.

"The Female Athlete: Looking after Your Hormones while Training." TrainingPeaks, December 3, 2021. https://www.trainingpeaks.com/blog/the-female-athlete-looking -after-your hormones-while-training.

"The Health Benefits of Tai Chi." Harvard Health, August 20, 2019. https://www .health.harvard.edu/staying-healthy/the-health-benefits-of-tai-chi.

"Hormones Explained (FSH, Progesterone)." Fertility Associates. Accessed February 3, 2022. https://www.fertilityassociates.co.nz/info-for-gps/hormones-explained-fsh -progesterone.

"Immunological Testing." Infertilitylab. Accessed February 4, 2022. https://www.infer tilitylab.com/immunological-testing.

"In Need of Some Deep Breaths? Try These Pranayama Breathing Practices." Yoga Journal, December 8, 2021. https://www.yogajournal.com/practice/healing-breath.

"In Vitro Fertilization (IVF)." Mayo Clinic, Mayo Foundation for Medical Education and Research, September 10, 2021. https://www.mayoclinic.org/tests-procedures/in -vitro fertilization/about/pac-20384716.

"The Influence of Direct Mobile Phone Radiation on Sperm Quality." *Central European Journal of Urology* 67, no. 1 (January 15, 2014). https://doi.org/10.5173/ceju.2014.01. art14. "The Role of MTHFR in Infertility and Miscarriages." Naturna, August 15, 2019. https://naturnalife.com/the-role-of-mthfr-in-infertility-and-miscarriages.

"Office of Dietary Supplements: Vitamin E." NIH Office of Dietary Supplements, U.S. Department of Health and Human Services, March 26, 2021. https://ods.od.nih.gov /factsheets/VitaminE-HealthProfessional/#h3.

"Pelvic Inflammatory Disease (PID)." Mayo Clinic, Mayo Foundation for Medical Education and Research, April 23, 2020. https://www.mayoclinic.org/diseases-conditions /pelvic inflammatory-disease/symptoms-causes/syc-20352594.

"Pesticides in Produce Linked with Reduced Fertility in Women." Harvard School of Public Health, June 22, 2018. https://www.hsph.harvard.edu/news/hsph-in-the -news/pesticides produce-fertility-women.

"Pregnenolone: What You Need to Know: USADA." U.S. Anti-Doping Agency, September 2, 2015. https://www.usada.org/spirit-of-sport/education/pregnenolone.

"Press Release: Age Is the Key Factor for Egg Freezing Success Says New HFEA Report, as Overall Treatment Numbers Remain Low." Human Fertilisation and Embryology Authority, December 20, 2018. https://www.hfea.gov.uk/about-us/news-and-press -releases/2018-news-and-press-releases/press-release-age-is-the-key-factor-for-eggfreez ing-success-says-new-hfea-report-as-overall-treatment-numbers-remain-low.

"Reiki: What Is It, and Are There Benefits?" Medical News Today, MediLexicon International. Accessed February 5, 2022. https://www.medicalnewstoday.com/articles /308772#summary.

"Stress: Signs, Symptoms, Management, and Prevention." Cleveland Clinic. Accessed February 7, 2022. https://my.clevelandclinic.org/health/articles/11874-stress.

"Study Reports That High Insulin Levels Are Toxic to Placenta Cells, Potentially Causing Miscarriages." Columbia University Department of Obstetrics and Gynecol-

ogy, April 9, 2019. https://www.columbiaobgyn.org/news/study-reports-high-insulin
-levels-are-toxic placenta-cells-potentially-causing-miscarriages.

"Type 2 Diabetes." Mayo Clinic, Mayo Foundation for Medical Education and Research, January 20, 2021. https://www.mayoclinic.org/diseases-conditions/type-2
-diabetes/symptoms-causes/syc-20351193.

"Vitamin D Levels and IVF Success." Center for Reproductive Medicine. Accessed
February 6, 2022. https://www.ivforlando.com/blog/vitamin-d-levels-and-ivf-success.

Abu-Ouf, Noran M., and Mohammed M. Jan. "The Impact of Maternal Iron Deficiency
and Iron Deficiency Anemia on Child's Health." *Saudi Medical Journal* 36, no. 2
(2015): 146–49. https://doi.org/10.15537/smj.2015.2.10289.

Ağaçayak, Elif, Neval Yaman Görük, Hakan Küsen, Senem Yaman Tunç, Serdar
Başaranoğlu, Mehmet Sait İçen, et al. "Role of Inflammation and Oxidative Stress in
the Etiology of Primary Ovarian Insufficiency." *Journal of Turkish Society of Obstetrics
and Gynecology* 13, no. 3 (September 30, 2016): 109–15. https://doi.org/10.4274
/tjod.00334.

Agarwal, Ashok, Gurpriya Virk, Chloe Ong, and Stefan S. du Plessis. "Effect of Oxidative Stress on Male Reproduction." *World Journal of Men's Health* 32, no. 1 (April 25,
2014): 1. https://doi.org/10.5534/wjmh.2014.32.1.1.

Akmal, Mohammed, J. Q. Qadri, Noori S. Al-Waili, Shahiya Thangal, Afrozul Haq, and
Khelod Y. Saloom. "Improvement in Human Semen Quality after Oral Supplementation of Vitamin C." *Journal of Medicinal Food* 9, no. 3 (September 2006): 440–42.
https://doi.org/10.1089/jmf.2006.9.440.

Aleksic, Ana. "How the Immune System and Digestive System Work Together." Microbiome Plus+. Accessed February 4, 2022. https://microbiomeplus.com/blogs/our-blog
-posts/how-digestive-and-immune-systems-work-together.

Almenning, Ida, Astrid Rieber-Mohn, Kari Margrethe Lundgren, Tone Shetelig Løvvik,
Kirsti Krohn Garnæs, and Trine Moholdt. "Effects of High Intensity Interval Training and Strength Training on Metabolic, Cardiovascular, and Hormonal Outcomes in
Women with Polycystic Ovary Syndrome: A Pilot Study." *PLoS One* 10, no. 9 (2015).
https://doi.org/10.1371/journal.pone.0138793.

Alok, Shashi, Sanjay Kumar Jain, Amita Verma, Mayank Kumar, Alok Mahor, and
Monika Sabharwal. "Plant Profile, Phytochemistry and Pharmacology of Asparagus
Racemosus (Shatavari): A Review." *Asian Pacific Journal of Tropical Disease* 3, no. 3
(April 2013): 242–51. https://doi.org/10.1016/s2222-1808(13)60049-3.

Alukal, Joseph P., and Dolores J. Lamb. "Intracytoplasmic Sperm Injection (ICSI)—
What Are the Risks?" *Urologic Clinics of North America* 35, no. 2 (May 1, 2008):
277–88. https://doi.org/10.1016/j.ucl.2008.01.004.

Ambiye, Vijay R., Deepak Langade, Swati Dongre, Pradnya Aptikar, Madhura Kulkarni,
and Atul Dongre. "Clinical Evaluation of the Spermatogenic Activity of the Root
Extract of Ashwagandha (*Withania somnifera*) in Oligospermic Males: A Pilot Study."
Evidence Based Complementary and Alternative Medicine 2013 (November 28, 2013):
1–6. https://doi.org/10.1155/2013/571420.

Anik Ilhan, G., and B. Yildizhan. "Evaluation of Zonulin, a Marker of Intestinal Permeability as a Novel Biomarker in Polycystic Ovary Syndrome." *Fertility and Sterility* 110, no. 4 (September 1, 2018): E117. https://doi.org/10.1016/j.fertnstert.2018.07.352.

Australian Spinal Research Foundation. "Chronic Stress—The Effects on Your Brain." Australian Spinal Research Foundation, June 30, 2016. https://spinalresearch.com.au /chronic-stress-effects-brain.

Bahadir Koca, Seval, Omer Ongun, Ozlem Ozmen, and Nalan Ozgur Yigit. "Subfertility Effects of Turmeric (*Curcuma longa*) on Reproductive Performance of Pseudotropheus ACEI." *Animal Reproduction Science* 202 (2019): 35–41. https://doi.org/10.1016/j .anireprosci. 2019.01.005.

Balk, Judith, Janet Catov, Brandon Horn, Kimberly Gecsi, and Anthony Wakim. "The Relationship between Perceived Stress, Acupuncture, and Pregnancy Rates among IVF Patients: A Pilot Study." *Complementary Therapies in Clinical Practice* 16, no. 3 (August 2010): 154–57. https://doi.org/10.1016/j.ctcp.2009.11.004.

Balmagambetova, Aru, Gulmira Zhurabekova, Ibrahim A. Abdelazim, and Sapargali Rakhmanov. "Effect of Environmental Factors on Ovarian Reserve of Women Living in Aral Sea Area." *Journal of Infertility and Reproductive Biology* 3, no. 1 (2015):145–49.

Baré, S. N., R. Póka, I. Balogh, and É. Ajzner. "Factor v Leiden as a Risk Factor for Miscarriage and Reduced Fertility." *Australian and New Zealand Journal of Obstetrics and Gynaecology* 40, no. 2 (May 2000): 186–90. https://doi.org/10.1111/j.1479-828x .2000.tb01144.x.

Beck, V., U. Rohr, and A. Jungbauer. "Phytoestrogens Derived from Red Clover: An Alternative to Estrogen Replacement Therapy?" *Journal of Steroid Biochemistry and Molecular Biology* 94, no. 5 (April 2005): 499–518. https://doi.org/10.1016/j .jsbmb.2004.12.038.

Bedaiwy, M. A., A. RezkH. Al Inany, and T. Falcone. "N-Acetyl Cystein Improves Pregnancy Rate in Long Standing Unexplained Infertility: A Novel Mechanism of Ovulation Induction." *Fertility and Sterility* 82, suppl. 2 (September 1, 2004): S228. https://doi.org/10.1016/j.fertnstert.2004.07.604.

Ben-Meir, Assaf, Eliezer Burstein, Aluet Borrego-Alvarez, Jasmine Chong, Ellen Wong, Tetyana Yavorska, et al. "Coenzyme Q10 Restores Oocyte Mitochondrial Function and Fertility during Reproductive Aging." *Aging Cell* 14, no. 5 (June 26, 2015): 887–95. https://doi.org/10.1111/acel.12368.

Bentov, Yaakov, and Robert F. Casper. "The Aging Oocyte—Can Mitochondrial Function Be Improved?" *Fertility and Sterility* 99, no. 1 (January 2013): 18–22. https://doi .org/10.1016/j.fertnstert.2012.11.031.

Bevilacqua, Arturo, and Mariano Bizzarri. "Inositols in Insulin Signaling and Glucose Metabolism." *International Journal of Endocrinology* 2018 (2018): 1–8. https://doi .org/10.1155/2018/1968450.

Bilbao, Aitziber Domingo, Antonio Forgiarini, Emilio Gómez Sánchez, José Luis de Pablo, Maria Arqué, Patricia Recuerda Thomas, et al. "Day 5 vs. Day 3 Embryo Transfer—What Are the Pros & Cons?" inviTRA, August 16, 2021. https://www .invitra.com/en/embryo transfer-on-day-3-or-on-dforday-5.

Block, Gladys, Christopher D. Jensen, Tapashi B. Dalvi, Edward P. Norkus, Mark Hudes, Patricia B. Crawford, et al. "Vitamin C Treatment Reduces Elevated C-

Reactive Protein." *Free Radical Biology and Medicine* 46, no. 1 (January 2009): 70–77. https://doi.org/10.1016/j.freeradbiomed.2008.09.030.

Bold, Justine, and Susan Bedford. *Integrated Approaches to Infertility, IVF, and Recurrent Miscarriage: A Handbook.* London: Singing Dragon, 2016.

Boots, Christina, and Emily Jungheim. "Inflammation and Human Ovarian Follicular Dynamics." *Seminars in Reproductive Medicine* 33, no. 4 (July 1, 2015): 270–75. https://doi.org/10.1055/s-0035-1554928.

Borup, Lissa, Winnie Wurlitzer, Morten Hedegaard, Ulrik S. Kesmodel, and Lone Hvidman. "Acupuncture as Pain Relief during Delivery: A Randomized Controlled Trial." *Birth* 36, no. 1 (March 2009): 5–12. https://doi.org/10.1111/j.1523-536x.2008.00290.x.

Boxmeer, J. C., N. S. Macklon, J. Lindemans, N. G. M. Beckers, M. J. C. Eijkemans, J. S. E. Laven, et al. "IVF Outcomes Are Associated with Biomarkers of the Homocysteine Pathway in Monofollicular Fluid." *Human Reproduction* 24, no. 5 (May 27, 2009): 1059– 66. https://doi.org/10.1093/humrep/dep009.

Brezina, Paul R., Raymond W. Ke, and William H. Kutteh. "Preimplantation Genetic Screening: A Practical Guide." *Clinical Medicine Insights: Reproductive Health* 7 (January 2013): 37–42. https://doi.org/10.4137/cmrh.s10852.

Brocker, Chad, David C. Thompson, and Vasilis Vasiliou. "The Role of Hyperosmotic Stress in Inflammation and Disease." *BioMolecular Concepts* 3, no. 4 (August 1, 2012): 345–64. https://doi.org/10.1515/bmc-2012-0001.

Bukovsky, Antonin, and Michael R. Caudle. "Immunoregulation of Follicular Renewal, Selection, POF, and Menopause in Vivo, vs. Neo-Oogenesis in Vitro, POF and Ovarian Infertility Treatment, and a Clinical Trial." *Reproductive Biology and Endocrinology* 10, no. 1 (November 23, 2012): 97. https://doi.org/10.1186/1477-7827-10-97.

Cabioglu, Mehmet Tugrul. "Role of Acupuncture in Stress Management." *Marmara Pharmaceutical Journal* 2, no. 16 (January 1, 2012): 107–14. https://doi.org/10.12991/201216408.

Cai, X. "Substitution of Acupuncture for HCG in Ovulation Induction." *Journal of Traditional Chinese Medicine* 17, no. 2 (June 1997): 119–21.

Cariati, Federica, Nadja D'Uonno, Francesca Borrillo, Stefania Iervolino, Giacomo Galdiero, and Rossella Tomaiuolo. "Bisphenol a: An Emerging Threat to Male Fertility." *Reproductive Biology and Endocrinology* 17, no. 1 (January 20, 2019). https://doi.org/10.1186/s12958-018-0447-6.

Carp, Howard J. A., Carlo Selmi, and Yehuda Shoenfeld. "The Autoimmune Bases of Infertility and Pregnancy Loss." *Journal of Autoimmunity* 38, no. 2–3 (May 2012): J266–74. https://doi.org/10.1016/j.jaut.2011.11.016.

Center for Food Safety and Applied Nutrition. "Advice about Eating Fish." U.S. Food and Drug Administration. Accessed February 3, 2022. https://www.fda.gov/food/consumers/advice about-eating-fish.

Chang, Eun M., Ji E. Han, Hyun H. Seok, Dong R. Lee, Tae K. Yoon, and Woo S. Lee. "Insulin Resistance Does Not Affect Early Embryo Development but Lowers Implantation Rate in *In Vitro* Maturation–*In Vitro* Fertilization–Embryo Transfer Cycle." *Clinical Endocrinology* 79, no. 1 (April 19, 2013): 93–99. https://doi.org/10.1111/cen.12099.

Chase, Sandra M. "American Institute of Homeopathy." Homeopathy. Accessed February 5, 2022. https://homeopathyusa.org/homeopathic-medicine.html.

Chavarro, J. E., J. W. Rich-Edwards, B. Rosner, and W. C. Willett. "Dietary Fatty Acid Intakes and the Risk of Ovulatory Infertility." *American Journal of Clinical Nutrition* 85, no. 1 (January 1, 2007a): 231–37. https://doi.org/10.1093/ajcn/85.1.231.

———. "A Prospective Study of Dairy Foods Intake and Anovulatory Infertility." *Human Reproduction* 22, no. 5 (February 28, 2007b): 1340–47. https://doi.org/10.1093/humrep/dem019.

———. "A Prospective Study of Dietary Carbohydrate Quantity and Quality in Relation to Risk of Ovulatory Infertility." *European Journal of Clinical Nutrition* 63, no. 1 (September 19, 2007c): 78–86. https://doi.org/10.1038/sj.ejcn.1602904.

———. "Protein Intake and Ovulatory Infertility." *American Journal of Obstetrics and Gynecology* 198, no. 2 (February 2008). https://doi.org/10.1016/j.ajog.2007.06.057.

Chiu, Tony T. Y., Michael S. Rogers, Eric L. K. Law, Christine M. Briton-Jones, L. P. Cheung, and Christopher J. Haines. "Follicular Fluid and Serum Concentrations of Myo-Inositol in Patients Undergoing IVF: Relationship with Oocyte Quality." *Human Reproduction* 17, no. 6 (June 2002): 1591–96. https://doi.org/10.1093/humrep/17.6.1591.

Chiu, Yu-Han, Paige L. Williams, Matthew W. Gillman, Audrey J. Gaskins, Lidia Mínguez-Alarcón, Irene Souter, et al. "Association between Pesticide Residue Intake from Consumption of Fruits and Vegetables and Pregnancy Outcomes among Women Undergoing Infertility Treatment with Assisted Reproductive Technology." *JAMA Internal Medicine* 178, no. 1 (2018):17–26. doi:10.1001/jamainternmed.2017.5038.

Cho, Geum Joon, Sung Won Han, Jung-Ho Shin, and Tak Kim. "Effects of Intensive Training on Menstrual Function and Certain Serum Hormones and Peptides Related to the Female Reproductive System." *Medicine* 96, no. 21 (May 2017): e6876. https://doi.org/10.1097/md.0000000000006876.

Christiane Northrup, M.D. "What Are the Symptoms of Estrogen Dominance?" Christiane Northrup, M.D., March 14, 2017. https://www.drnorthrup.com/estrogen-dominance.

Ciotta, L., M. Stracquadanio, I. Pagano, A. Carbonaro, M. Palumbo, and F. Gulino. "Effects of Myo-Inositol Supplementation on Oocyte's Quality in PCOS Patients: A Double Blind Trial." *European Review for Medical and Pharmacological Sciences* 15, no. 5 (May 2011): 509–14.

Coletta, Jaclyn M., and Stacey J. Bell. "Omega-3 Fatty Acids and Pregnancy." *Reviews in Obstetrics & Gynecology* 3, no. 4 (2010): 163–71.

Crane, Rich. "Enhance Your Sleep Cycles." Alaska Sleep Clinic, September 30, 2016. https://www.alaskasleep.com/blog/enhance-your-sleep-cycles.

Cui, Jia, Shaobai Wang, Jiehui Ren, Jun Zhang, and Jun Jing. "Use of Acupuncture in the USA: Changes over a Decade (2002–2012)." *Acupuncture in Medicine* 35, no. 3 (June 1, 2017): 200–207. https://doi.org/10.1136/acupmed-2016-011106.

da Silva, Fernando Moreira. "Antioxidant Properties of Polyphenols and Their Potential Use in Improvement of Male Fertility: A Review." *Biomedical Journal of Scientific & Technical Research* 1, no. 3 (August 7, 2017). https://doi.org/10.26717/bjstr.2017.01.000259.

Das, Jai K., Rohail Kumar, Rehana A. Salam, and Zulfiqar A. Bhutta. "Systematic Review of Zinc Fortification Trials." *Annals of Nutrition and Metabolism* 62, suppl. 1 (2013): 44– 56. https://doi.org/10.1159/000348262.

Dayani Siriwardene, S. A., L. P. A Karunathilaka, N. D. Kodituwakku, and Y. A. U. D. Karunarathne. "Clinical Efficacy of Ayurveda Treatment Regimen on Subfertility with Poly Cystic Ovarian Syndrome (PCOS)." *AYU (An International Quarterly Journal of Research in Ayurveda)* 31, no. 1 (January 2010): 24–27. https://doi.org/10.4103/0974-8520.68203.

de Lacey, Sheryl, Caroline A. Smith, and Charlotte Paterson. "Building Resilience: A Preliminary Exploration of Women's Perceptions of the Use of Acupuncture as an Adjunct to in Vitro Fertilisation." *BMC Complementary and Alternative Medicine* 9, no. 1 (December 2009). https://doi.org/10.1186/1472-6882-9-50.

de Ziegler, Dominique, Pietro Santulli, Alice Seroka, Christine Decanter, David R. Meldrum, and Charles Chapron. "In Women, the Reproductive Harm of Toxins Such as Tobacco Smoke Is Reversible in 6 Months: Basis for the 'Olive Tree' Hypothesis." *Fertility and Sterility* 100, no. 4 (June 24, 2013): 927–28. https://doi.org/10.1016/j.fertnstert.2013.05.043.

Delli Bovi, Anna Pia, Laura Di Michele, Giuliana Laino, and Pietro Vajro. "Obesity and Obesity Related Diseases, Sugar Consumption and Bad Oral Health: A Fatal Epidemic Mixtures: The Pediatric and Odontologist Point of View." *Translational Medicine @ UniSa* 16 (July 1, 2017): 11–16.

Deville, Lauren. "Vitamin B6 and Your Cycle: Dr. Lauren Deville, Naturopathic Doctor." Dr. Lauren Deville, December 15, 2017. https://www.drlaurendeville.com/articles/vitamin b6-cycle.

Dieterle, Stefan, Gao Ying, Wolfgang Hatzmann, and Andreas Neuer. "Effect of Acupuncture on the Outcome of in Vitro Fertilization and Intracytoplasmic Sperm Injection: A Randomized, Prospective, Controlled Clinical Study." *Fertility and Sterility* 85, no. 5 (May 2006): 1347–51. https://doi.org/10.1016/j.fertnstert.2005.09.062.

Dominguez, Francisco. "Phthalates and Other Endocrine-Disrupting Chemicals: The 21st Century's Plague for Reproductive Health." *Fertility and Sterility* 111, no. 5 (April 8, 2019): 885–86. https://doi.org/10.1016/j.fertnstert.2019.01.029.

Donald, J. M., K. Hooper, and C. Hopenhayn-Rich. "Reproductive and Developmental Toxicity of Toluene: A Review." *Environmental Health Perspectives* 94 (August 1, 1991): 237–44. https://doi.org/10.1289/ehp.94-1567945.

Dongre, Swati, Deepak Langade, and Sauvik Bhattacharyya. "Efficacy and Safety of Ashwagandha (*Withania somnifera*) Root Extract in Improving Sexual Function in Women: A Pilot Study." *BioMed Research International* 2015 (October 4, 2015): 1–9. https://doi.org/10.1155/2015/284154.

Donor Nexus. "Epigenetics Using Donor Eggs or Donor Embryos." Donor Nexus, June 1, 2021. https://donornexus.com/blog/epigenetics-and-donor-eggs.

El-Nemr A., T. Al-Shawaf, L. Sabatini, C. Wilson, A. M. Lower, and J. G. Grudzinskas. "Effect of Smoking on Ovarian Reserve and Ovarian Stimulation in In-Vitro Fertilization and Embryo Transfer." *Human Reproduction* 13, no. 8 (1998): 2192–198. doi:10.1093/humrep/13.8.2192. PMID: 9756295.

Falsig, A.-M. L., C. S. Gleerup, and U. B. Knudsen. "The Influence of Omega-3 Fatty Acids on Semen Quality Markers: A Systematic Prisma Review." *Andrology* 7, no. 6 (May 22, 2019): 794–803. https://doi.org/10.1111/andr.12649.

Fatini, Cinzia, Lucia Conti, Valentina Turillazzi, Elena Sticchi, Ilaria Romagnuolo, Maria Novella Milanini, et al. "Unexplained Infertility: Association with Inherited Thrombophilia." *Thrombosis Research* 129, no. 5 (March 16, 2012): E185–88. https://doi.org/10.1016/j.thromres.2012.02.012.

Favier, Alain Emile. "The Role of Zinc in Reproduction." *Biological Trace Element Research* 32, no. 1–3 (January 1992): 363–82. https://doi.org/10.1007/bf02784623.

Federation of American Societies for Experimental Biology. "Ozone Air Pollution Could Harm Women's Fertility." ScienceDaily, March 29, 2015. http://www.sciencedaily.com/releases/2015/03/150329141015.htm.

Ford, E. S., S. Liu, D. M. Mannino, W. H. Giles, and S. J. Smith. "C-Reactive Protein Concentration and Concentrations of Blood Vitamins, Carotenoids, and Selenium among United States Adults." *European Journal of Clinical Nutrition* 57, no. 9 (2003): 1157–63. https://doi.org/10.1038/sj.ejcn.1601667.

Fouany, Mazen R., and Fady I. Sharara. "Is There a Role for DHEA Supplementation in Women with Diminished Ovarian Reserve?" *Journal of Assisted Reproduction and Genetics* 30, no. 9 (June 5, 2013): 1239–44. https://doi.org/10.1007/s10815-013-0018-x.

Fraga, C. G., P. A. Motchnik, M. K. Shigenaga, H. J. Helbock, R. A. Jacob, and B. N. Ames. "Ascorbic Acid Protects against Endogenous Oxidative DNA Damage in Human Sperm." *Proceedings of the National Academy of Sciences* 88, no. 24 (December 15, 1991): 11003–6. https://doi.org/10.1073/pnas.88.24.11003.

Fulghesu, A. "N-Acetyl-Cysteine Treatment Improves Insulin Sensitivity in Women with Polycystic Ovary Syndrome." *Fertility and Sterility* 77, no. 6 (June 2002): 1128–35. https://doi.org/10.1016/s0015-0282(02)03133-3.

Gameiro, Sofia, Alexandra W. van den Belt-Dusebout, Jesper M. J. Smeenk, Didi D. M. Braat, Flora E. van Leeuwen, and Christianne M. Verhaak. "Women's Adjustment Trajectories during IVF and Impact on Mental Health 11–17 Years Later." *Human Reproduction* 31, no. 8 (2016): 1788–98. https://doi.org/10.1093/humrep/dew131.

Gardella, Jennifer R., and Joseph A. Hill III. "Environmental Toxins Associated with Recurrent Pregnancy Loss." *Seminars in Reproductive Medicine* 18, no. 4 (2000): 407–24. https://doi.org/10.1055/s-2000-13731.

Gil, Y. R. C., R. L. M. Fagundes, E. Santos, M. C. M. Calvo, and J. D. Bernardine. "Relation of Menstrual Cycle and Alimentary Consumption of Women." *e-SPEN, the European e Journal of Clinical Nutrition and Metabolism* 4, no. 5 (October 1, 2009): E257–60. https://doi.org/10.1016/j.eclnm.2009.08.002.

Gleicher, N., V. A. Kushnir, and D. H. Barad. "Worldwide Decline of IVF Birth Rates and Its Probable Causes." *Human Reproduction Open* 2019, no. 3 (August 2019): hoz017. https://doi.org/10.1093/hropen/hoz017.

Goldman, R. H., C. Racowsky, L. V. Farland, S. Munné, L. Ribustello, and J. H. Fox. "Predicting the Likelihood of Live Birth for Elective Oocyte Cryopreservation: A Counseling Tool for Physicians and Patients." *Human Reproduction* 32, no. 4 (February 6, 2017): 853–59. https://doi.org/10.1093/humrep/dex008.

Gonzales, Gustavo F. "Ethnobiology and Ethnopharmacology of *Lepidium meyenii* (Maca), a Plant from the Peruvian Highlands." *Evidence-Based Complementary and Alternative Medicine* 2012 (October 2, 2011): 1–10. https://doi.org/10.1155/2012/193496.

Gorpinchenko, Igor, Oleg Nikitin, Oleg Banyra, and Alexander Shulyak. "The Influence of Direct Mobile Phone Radiation on Sperm Quality." *Central European Journal of Urology* 67, no. 1 (2014): 65–71. doi:10.5173/ceju.2014.01.

Grant, Paul, and Shamin Ramasamy. "An Update on Plant Derived Anti-Androgens." *International Journal of Endocrinology and Metabolism* 10, no. 2 (2012): 497–502. https://doi.org/10.5812/ijem.3644.

Greger, Michael. "How Does Meat Cause Inflammation?" NutritionFacts.org, September 20, 2012. https://nutritionfacts.org/2012/09/20/why-meat-causes-inflammation.

Grindler, Natalia M., Jenifer E. Allsworth, George A. Macones, Kurunthachalam Kannan, Kimberly A. Roehl, and Amber R. Cooper. "Persistent Organic Pollutants and Early Menopause in U.S. Women." *PLoS One* 10, no. 1 (2015). https://doi.org/10.1371/journal.pone.0116057.

Güçel, Funda, Burak Bahar, Canan Demirtas, Setenay Mit, and Cemal Çevik. "Influence of Acupuncture on Leptin, Ghrelin, Insulin and Cholecystokinin in Obese Women: A Randomised, Sham-Controlled Preliminary Trial." *Acupuncture in Medicine* 30, no. 3 (December 2018): 203–7. https://doi.org/10.1136/acupmed-2012-010127.

Gunnars, Kris. "How Blocking Blue Light at Night Helps You Sleep." Healthline Media, May 21, 2020. https://www.healthline.com/nutrition/block-blue-light-to-sleep-better#blue light.

Gupta, Sajal, Jennifer Fedor, Kelly Biedenharn, and Ashok Agarwal. "Lifestyle Factors and Oxidative Stress in Female Infertility: Is There an Evidence Base to Support the Linkage?" *Expert Review of Obstetrics & Gynecology* 8, no. 6 (January 10, 2013): 607–24. https://doi.org/10.1586/17474108.2013.849418.

Gurfinkel, Edson, Agnaldo P. Cedenho, Ysao Yamamura, and Miguel Srougi. "Effects of Acupuncture and Moxa Treatment in Patients with Semen Abnormalities." *Asian Journal of Andrology* 4, no. 5 (2003): 345–48.

Hakansson, Asa, and Goran Molin. "Gut Microbiota and Inflammation." *Nutrients* 3, no. 6 (June 3, 2011): 637–82. https://doi.org/10.3390/nu3060637.

Haller-Kikkatalo, Kadri, Andres Salumets, and Raivo Uibo. "Review on Autoimmune Reactions in Female Infertility: Antibodies to Follicle Stimulating Hormone." *Clinical and Developmental Immunology* 2012 (October 5, 2011): 1–15. https://doi.org/10.1155/2012/762541.

Harakeh, Steve M., Imran Khan, Taha Kumosani, Elie Barbour, Saad B. Almasaudi, Suhad M. Bahijri, et al. "Gut Microbiota: A Contributing Factor to Obesity." *Frontiers in Cellular and Infection Microbiology* 6 (August 30, 2016): 95. https://doi.org/10.3389/fcimb.2016.00095.

Hasan, Mohidul, and Hanhong Bae. "An Overview of Stress-Induced Resveratrol Synthesis in Grapes: Perspectives for Resveratrol-Enriched Grape Products." *Molecules* 22, no. 2 (February 14, 2017): 294. https://doi.org/10.3390/molecules22020294.

Hatırnaz, Şafak, and Mine Kanat Pektaş. "Day 3 Embryo Transfer versus Day 5 Blastocyst Transfers: A Prospective Randomized Controlled Trial." *Journal of Turkish*

Society of Obstetrics and Gynecology 14, no. 2 (June 1, 2017): 82–88. https://doi.org/10.4274/tjod. 99076.

Heese, Inga. "The 'Egg Factor': Using Chinese Herbal Medicine to Improve Fertility in a 45-Year Old Woman." *Journal of Chinese Medicine*, no. 82 (October 2006): 36–41.

Henmi, Hirofumi, Toshiaki Endo, Yoshimitsu Kitajima, Kengo Manase, Hiroshi Hata, and Ryuich Kudo. "Effects of Ascorbic Acid Supplementation on Serum Progesterone Levels in Patients with a Luteal Phase Defect." *Fertility and Sterility* 80, no. 2 (August 1, 2003): 459–61. https://doi.org/10.1016/s0015-0282(03)00657-5.

Heo, Sujeong, Kwan-Il Kim, Junhee Lee, Eunjeong Jeong, and Jaesung Lee. "Effects of Korean Herbal Medicine on Pregnancy Outcomes of Infertile Women Aged over 35: A Retrospective Study." *European Journal of Integrative Medicine* 8, no. 5 (October 2016): 670–75. https://doi.org/10.1016/j.eujim.2016.07.002.

Herbalist, Dalene Barton, Certified. "Is My Adrenal Health Affecting My Fertility?" Natural Fertility Info, July 24, 2021. https://natural-fertility-info.com/is-my-adrenal-health-affecting-my-fertility.html.

Hinks, J., and C. Coulson. "An Assessment of the Demand and Importance of Acupuncture to Patients of a Fertility Clinic during Investigations and Treatment." *Human Fertility* 13, no. 1 (2010): 3–21.

Hirsch, Larissa, ed. "Blood Test: Immunoglobulins (IGA, IGG, IGM) (for Parents)—Nemours Kidshealth." KidsHealth, April 2020. https://kidshealth.org/en/parents/test immunoglobulins.html.

Hollis, NaTasha D., Emily G. Allen, Tiffany Renee Oliver, Stuart W. Tinker, Charlotte Druschel, Charlotte A. Hobbs, et al. "Preconception Folic Acid Supplementation and Risk for Chromosome 21 Nondisjunction: A Report from the National Down Syndrome Project." *American Journal of Medical Genetics—Part A* 161, no. 3 (February 7, 2013): 438–44. https://doi.org/10.1002/ajmg.a.35796.

Hornstein, Mark D. "Lifestyle and IVF Outcomes." *Reproductive Sciences* 23, no. 12 (August 27, 2016): 1626–29. https://doi.org/10.1177/1933719116667226.

Hosseini, Jalil, Azar Mardi Mamaghani, Hani Hosseinifar, Mohammad Ali Sadighi Gilani, Farid Dadkhah, and Mahdi Sepidarkish. "The Influence of Ginger (*Zingiber officinale*) on Human Sperm Quality and DNA Fragmentation: A Double-Blind Randomized Clinical Trial." *International Journal of Reproductive BioMedicine* 14, no. 8 (August 2016): 533–40.

Hotzehealth. "Hypothyroidism: Houston TX." Hotze Health & Wellness Center, November 23, 2021. https://www.hotzehwc.com/hypothyroidism.

Hyman, Mark. *The Blood Sugar Solution 10-Day Detox Diet: Activate Your Body's Natural Ability to Burn Fat and Lose Weight Fast.* London: Yellow Kite Books, 2016.

Inoue, Taketo, Yoshiyuki Ono, Yukiko Yonezawa, Michinobu Oi, Naomi Kobayashi, Junji Kishi, et al. "Oocyte Quality Improvement Using a Herbal Medicine Comprising 7 Crude Drugs." *Open Journal of Obstetrics and Gynecology* 3, no. 1A (February 2013): 195–202. https://doi.org/10.4236/ojog.2013.31a036.

Irandoost, Pardis, Mehrangiz Ebrahimi-Mameghani, and Saeed Pirouzpanah. "Does Grape Seed Oil Improve Inflammation and Insulin Resistance in Overweight or Obese Women?" *International Journal of Food Sciences and Nutrition* 64, no. 6 (2013): 706–10. https://doi.org/10.3109/09637486.2013.775228.

Isoyama, Daniela, Emerson Barchi Cordts, Angela Mara de Souza van Niewegen, Waldemar de Almeida Pereira de Carvalho, Simone Tiemi Matsumura, and Caio Parente Barbosa. "Effect of Acupuncture on Symptoms of Anxiety in Women Undergoing in Vitro Fertilisation: A Prospective Randomised Controlled Study." *Acupuncture in Medicine* 30, no. 2 (June 2012): 85–88. https://doi.org/10.1136/acupmed-2011-010064.

Jain, Seema, Priyamvada Sharma, Shobha Kulshreshtha, Govind Mohan, and Saroj Singh. "The Role of Calcium, Magnesium, and Zinc in Pre-Eclampsia." *Biological Trace Element Research* 133, no. 2 (June 23, 2009): 162–70. https://doi.org/10.1007/s12011-009-8423-9.

Jannatifar, Rahil, Kazem Parivar, Nasim Hayati Roodbari, and Mohammad Hossein Nasr Esfahani. "Effects of N-Acetyl-Cysteine Supplementation on Sperm Quality, Chromatin Integrity and Level of Oxidative Stress in Infertile Men." *Reproductive Biology and Endocrinology* 17, no. 1 (February 16, 2019). https://doi.org/10.1186/s12958-019-0468-9.

Jian-jun, Shi. "A Four Step Protocol for Improving the Effects of Clomiphene in Patients with Ovulatory Dysfunction." *Zhejiang Journal of Chinese Medicine*, no. 7 (2007): 405.

Jinno, Masao, Kenichi Kondou, and Koji Teruya. "Low-Dose Metformin Improves Pregnancy Rate in In Vitro Fertilization Repeaters without Polycystic Ovary Syndrome: Prediction of Effectiveness by Multiple Parameters Related to Insulin Resistance." *Hormones* 9, no. 2 (April 15, 2010): 161–70. https://doi.org/10.14310/horm.2002.1266.

Joseph, Dana, and Shannon Whirledge. "Stress and the HPA Axis: Balancing Homeostasis and Fertility." *International Journal of Molecular Sciences* 18, no. 10 (October 24, 2017): 2224. https://doi.org/10.3390/ijms18102224.

Kachhawa, Garima, Nisha Malik, Alka Kriplani, Nutan Agarwal, Neerja Bhatla, and RajKumar Yadav. "Dehydroepiandrosterone as an Adjunct to Gonadotropins in Infertile Indian Women with Premature Ovarian Aging: A Pilot Study." *Journal of Human Reproductive Sciences* 8, no. 3 (September 11, 2015): 135–41. https://doi.org/10.4103/0974-1208.165142.

Kallen, Caleb B., and Aydin Arici. "Immune Testing in Fertility Practice: Truth or Deception?" *Current Opinion in Obstetrics and Gynecology* 15, no. 3 (June 2003): 225–31. https://doi.org/10.1097/00001703-200306000-00003.

Kaur, Sat Dharam, Mary Danylak-Arhanic, and Carolyn Dean. *The Complete Natural Medicine Guide to Women's Health.* Toronto: Robert Rose, 2005.

Kelly, G. S. "Nutritional and Botanical Interventions to Assist with the Adaptation to Stress." *Alternative Medicine Review* 4, no. 4 (August 1999): 249–65.

Kelly, John R., Paul J. Kennedy, John F. Cryan, Timothy G. Dinan, Gerard Clarke, and Niall P. Hyland. "Breaking Down the Barriers: The Gut Microbiome, Intestinal Permeability and Stress-Related Psychiatric Disorders." *Frontiers in Cellular Neuroscience* 9 (October 14, 2015): 392. https://doi.org/10.3389/fncel.2015.00392.

Keskes-Ammar, L., N. Feki-Chakroun, T. Rebai, Z. Sahnoun, H. Ghozzi, S. Hammami, et al. "Sperm Oxidative Stress and the Effect of an Oral Vitamin E and Selenium Supplement on Semen Quality in Infertile Men." *Archives of Andrology* 49, no. 2 (January 2003): 83–94. https://doi.org/10.1080/01485010390129269.

Kiecolt-Glaser, Janice K., Martha A. Belury, Rebecca Andridge, William B. Malarkey, Beom Seuk Hwang, and Ronald Glaser. "Omega-3 Supplementation Lowers Inflammation in Healthy Middle-Aged and Older Adults: A Randomized Controlled Trial." *Brain, Behavior, and Immunity* 26, no. 6 (August 2012): 988–95. https://doi .org/10.1016/j.bbi. 2012.05.011.

Kim, Gi Young. "What Should Be Done for Men with Sperm DNA Fragmentation?" *Clinical and Experimental Reproductive Medicine* 45, no. 3 (September 30, 2018): 101–9. https://doi.org/10.5653/cerm.2018.45.3.101.

Kim, Keewan, Jean Wactawski-Wende, Kara A. Michels, Karen C. Schliep, Torie C. Plowden, Ellen N. Chaljub, et al. "Dietary Minerals, Reproductive Hormone Levels and Sporadic Anovulation: Associations in Healthy Women with Regular Menstrual Cycles." *British Journal of Nutrition*. U.S. National Library of Medicine, July 2018. https://www.ncbi.nlm.nih.gov/pmc/articles/PMC6019139.

Klonoff-Cohen, Hillary, Phung Lam-Kruglick, and Cristina Gonzalez. "Effects of Maternal and Paternal Alcohol Consumption on the Success Rates of In Vitro Fertilization and Gamete Intrafallopian Transfer." *Fertility and Sterility* 79, no. 2 (February 2003): 330–39. https://doi.org/10.1016/s0015-0282(02)04582-x.

Ko, E. Y., and E. S. Sabanegh. "The Role of Over-the-Counter Supplements for the Treatment of Male Infertility—Fact or Fiction?" *Journal of Andrology* 33, no. 3 (May 19, 2011): 292– 308. https://doi.org/10.2164/jandrol.111.013730.

Krieg, Sacha A., Lora K. Shahine, and Ruth B. Lathi. "Environmental Exposure to Endocrine Disrupting Chemicals and Miscarriage." *Fertility and Sterility* 106, no. 4 (September 15, 2016): 941–47. https://doi.org/10.1016/j.fertnstert.2016.06.043.

Krystal. "Should You Try Seed Cycling to Balance Hormones?" Dishing Up Balance, February 8, 2018. https://dishingupbalance.com/seed-cycling.

Kunc, Michał, Anna Gabrych, and Jacek M Witkowski. "Microbiome Impact on Metabolism and Function of Sex, Thyroid, Growth and Parathyroid Hormones." *Acta Biochimica Polonica* 63, no. 2 (October 26, 2015): 189–201. https://doi.org/10.18388 /abp. 2015_1093.

Kwon, Ohmin, UiMin Jerng, Jun-Young Jo, Seunghoon Lee, and Jin-Moo Lee. "The Effectiveness and Safety of Acupuncture for Poor Semen Quality in Infertile Males: A Systematic Review and Meta-Analysis." *Asian Journal of Andrology* 16, no. 6 (2014): 884–91. https://doi.org/10.4103/1008-682x.129130.

Lafuente, Rafael, Mireia González-Comadrán, Ivan Solà, Gemma López, Mario Brassesco, Ramón Carreras, et al. "Coenzyme Q10 and Male Infertility: A Meta-Analysis." *Journal of Assisted Reproduction and Genetics* 30, no. 9 (August 3, 2013): 1147–56. https://doi.org/10.1007/s10815-013-0047-5.

Laganà, Antonio Simone, Amerigo Vitagliano, Marco Noventa, Guido Ambrosini, and Rosario D'Anna. "Myo-Inositol Supplementation Reduces the Amount of Gonadotropins and Length of Ovarian Stimulation in Women Undergoing IVF: A Systematic Review and Meta-Analysis of Randomized Controlled Trials." *Archives of Gynecology and Obstetrics* 298, no. 4 (August 4, 2018): 675–84. https://doi.org/10.1007 /s00404-018-4861-y.

La Merrill, Michele A., Laura N. Vandenberg, Martyn T. Smith, William Goodson, Patience Browne, Heather B. Patisaul, et al. "Consensus on the Key Characteristics of Endocrine-Disrupting Chemicals as a Basis for Hazard Identification." *Nature Reviews Endocrinology* 16, no. 1 (2020): 45–57.

Lerchbaum, Elisabeth, and Thomas Rabe. "Vitamin D and Female Fertility." *Current Opinion in Obstetrics & Gynecology* 26, no. 3 (June 2014): 145–50. https://doi.org/10.1097/gco. 0000000000000065.

Ley, Sylvia H., Qi Sun, Walter C. Willett, A. Heather Eliassen, Kana Wu, An Pan, et al. "Associations between Red Meat Intake and Biomarkers of Inflammation and Glucose Metabolism in Women." *American Journal of Clinical Nutrition* 99, no. 2 (November 27, 2014): 352–60. https://doi.org/10.3945/ajcn.113.075663.

Li, Hang Wun, Rebecca E. Brereton, Richard A. Anderson, A. Michael Wallace, and Clement K.M. Ho. "Vitamin D Deficiency Is Common and Associated with Metabolic Risk Factors in Patients with Polycystic Ovary Syndrome." *Metabolism* 60, no. 10 (October 2011): 1475–81. https://doi.org/10.1016/j.metabol.2011.03.002.

Li, Lu, Chi Chiu Wang, Lixia Dou, and Ping Chung Leung. "Chinese Herbal Medicines for Threatened Miscarriage." *Cochrane Database of Systematic Reviews*, May 12, 2010. https://doi.org/10.1002/14651858.cd008510.

Liang, F., and D. Koya. "Acupuncture: Is It Effective for Treatment of Insulin Resistance?" *Diabetes, Obesity and Metabolism* 12, no. 7 (May 2010): 555–69. https://doi.org/10.1111/j.1463-1326.2009.01192.x.

Lindtner, Claudia, Thomas Scherer, Elizabeth Zielinski, Nika Filatova, Martin Fasshauer, Nicholas K. Tonks, et al. "Binge Drinking Induces Whole-Body Insulin Resistance by Impairing Hypothalamic Insulin Action." *Science Translational Medicine* 5, no. 170 (January 30, 2013). https://doi.org/10.1126/scitranslmed.3005123.

Liu, Mei-Ju, Ai-Gang Sun, Shi-Gang Zhao, Hui Liu, Shui-Ying Ma, Mei Li, et al. "Resveratrol Improves In Vitro Maturation of Oocytes in Aged Mice and Humans." *Fertility and Sterility* 109, no. 5 (May 2018): 900–907. https://doi.org/10.1016/j.fertnstert. 2018.01.020.

Lynch, C. D., R. Sundaram, J. M. Maisog, A. M. Sweeney, and G. M. Buck Louis. "Preconception Stress Increases the Risk of Infertility: Results from a Couple-Based Prospective Cohort Study—The Life Study." *Human Reproduction* 29, no. 5 (May 2014): 1067–75. https://doi.org/10.1093/humrep/deu032.

MacMillan, Carrie. "Is Egg Freezing Right for You?" Yale Medicine, May 29, 2019. https://www.yalemedicine.org/stories/egg-freezing-fertility.

Maes, Michael, Marta Kubera, and Jean-Claude Leunis. "The Gut-Brain Barrier in Major Depression: Intestinal Mucosal Dysfunction with an Increased Translocation of LPS from Gram Negative Enterobacteria (Leaky Gut) Plays a Role in the Inflammatory Pathophysiology of Depression." *Neuroendocrinology Letters* 29, no. 1 (February 2008): 117–24.

Maher, Brendan. "Lab Disinfectant Harms Mouse Fertility." *Nature* 453, no. 7198 (June 18, 2008): 964. https://doi.org/10.1038/453964a.

Maizes, Victoria, and Andrew Weil. *Be Fruitful: The Essential Guide to Maximizing Fertility and Giving Birth to a Healthy Child.* New York: Scribner, 2013.

Malachi, Rebecca. "16 Fertility Yoga Poses to Boost Your Chances of Conception." MomJunction, February 1, 2022. https://www.momjunction.com/articles/yoga-asanas that-boost-fertility_003039.

Manheimer, Eric, Grant Zhang, Laurence Udoff, Aviad Haramati, Patricia Langenberg, Brian M. Berman, et al. "Effects of Acupuncture on Rates of Pregnancy and Live

Birth among Women Undergoing In Vitro Fertilisation: Systematic Review and Meta-Analysis." *BMJ* 336, no. 7643 (February 7, 2008): 545–49. https://doi.org/10.1136/bmj.39471.430451.be.

Maroon, Joseph Charles, and Jeffrey W. Bost. "Ω-3 Fatty Acids (Fish Oil) as an Anti In-flammatory: An Alternative to Nonsteroidal Anti-Inflammatory Drugs for Discogenic Pain." *Surgical Neurology* 65, no. 4 (April 2006): 326–31. https://doi.org/10.1016/j.surneu.2005.10.023.

Marotta, F., R. Barreto, C. C. Wu, Y. Naito, F. Gelosa, A. Lorenzetti, et al. "Experimental Acute Alcohol Pancreatitis-Related Liver Damage and Endotoxemia: Synbiotics but Not Metronidazole Have a Protective Effect." *Chinese Journal of Digestive Diseases* 6, no. 4 (October 24, 2005): 193–97. https://doi.org/10.1111/j.1443-9573.2005.00230.x.

Masharani, U., C. Gjerde, J. L. Evans, J. F. Youngren, and I. D. Goldfine. "Effects of Controlled Release Alpha Lipoic Acid in Lean, Nondiabetic Patients with Polycystic Ovary Syndrome." *Journal of Diabetes Science and Technology* 4, no. 2 (March 1, 2010): 359–64. https://doi.org/10.1177/193229681000400218.

Maughan, Toni A., and Zhai Xiao-Ping. "The Acupuncture Treatment of Female In-fertility—With Particular Reference to Egg Quality and Endometrial Receptiveness." *Journal of Chinese Medicine* 98, no. 9 (February 2012): 13–21.

Mayo Clinic Staff. "How Much Water Do You Need to Stay Healthy?" Mayo Founda-tion for Medical Education and Research, October 14, 2020. https://www.mayoclinic.org/healthy lifestyle/nutrition-and-healthy-eating/in-depth/water/art-20044256.

Mazidi, M., and H. Vatanparast. "Serum Trans-fatty Acids Level Are Positively As-sociated with Lower Food Security among American Adults." *Nutrition & Diabetes* 8, no. 1 (March 7, 2018): 17. doi:10.1038/s41387-017-0008-7. PMID: 29549245; PMCID: PMC5856754.

McRorie, Johnson W. "Evidence-Based Approach to Fiber Supplements and Clinically Meaningful Health Benefits, Part 1." *Nutrition Today* 50, no. 2 (March 2015): 82–89. https://doi.org/10.1097/nt.0000000000000082.

Messerlian, Carmen, Blair J. Wylie, Lidia Mínguez-Alarcón, Paige L. Williams, Jennifer B. Ford, Irene C. Souter, et al. "Urinary Concentrations of Phthalate Metabolites and Pregnancy Loss among Women Conceiving with Medically Assisted Reproduction." *Epidemiology* 27, no. 6 (2016): 879–88.

Mills, Jesse N., and David F. Yao. "Male Infertility: Lifestyle Factors and Holistic, Com-plementary, and Alternative Therapies." *Asian Journal of Andrology* 18, no. 3 (March 4, 2016): 410–18. https://doi.org/10.4103/1008-682x.175779.

Mingmin, Zhang, Huang Guangying, Lu Fuer, W. E. Paulus, and K. Sterzik. "Influence of Acupuncture on Idiopathic Male Infertility in Assisted Reproductive Technology." *Journal of Huazhong University of Science and Technology [Medical Sciences]* 22, no. 3 (September 2002): 228–30. https://doi.org/10.1007/bf02828187.

Mínguez-Alarcón, Lidia, Russ Hauser, and Audrey J. Gaskins. "Effects of Bisphenol A on Male and Couple Reproductive Health: A Review." *Fertility and Sterility* 106, no. 4 (September 15, 2016): 864–70. https://doi.org/10.1016/j.fertnstert.2016.07.1118.

Mishra, Vikas, Susan L. DiAngelo, and Patricia Silveyra. "Sex-Specific IL-6-Associated Signaling Activation in Ozone-Induced Lung Inflammation." *Biology of Sex Differerences 7 (2016):16. doi:10.1186/s13293-016-0069-7. PMID: 26949510; PMCID: PMC4779258.

Moreno, Inmaculada, Francisco M. Codoñer, Felipe Vilella, Diana Valbuena, Juan F. Martinez-Blanch, Jorge Jimenez-Almazán, et al. "Evidence That the Endometrial Microbiota Has an Effect on Implantation Success or Failure." *American Journal of Obstetrics and Gynecology* 215, no. 6 (2016): 684–703. https://doi.org/10.1016/j.ajog.2016.09.075.

Moslemi, Mohammad Kazem, and Seiied Ali Zargar. "Selenium–Vitamin E Supplementation in Infertile Men: Effects on Semen Parameters and Pregnancy Rate." *International Journal of General Medicine* 4 (January 23, 2011): 99–104. https://doi.org/10.2147/ijgm.s16275.

Mullington, Janet M., Norah S. Simpson, Hans K. Meier-Ewert, and Monika Haack. "Sleep Loss and Inflammation." *Best Practice & Research Clinical Endocrinology & Metabolism* 24, no. 5 (October 2010): 775–84. https://doi.org/10.1016/j.beem.2010.08.014.

Murphy, Carrie. "The Effects of Joy on Your Body." Healthline Media, August 22, 2018. https://www.healthline.com/health/affects-of-joy#6.

Nair, Pradeep. "Naturopathy and Yoga in Ameliorating Multiple Hormonal Imbalance: A Single Case Report." *International Journal of Reproduction, Contraception, Obstetrics and Gynecology* 5, no. 3 (February 2016): 916–18. https://doi.org/10.18203/2320-1770.ijrcog20160612.

National Summary Report. Accessed February 6, 2022. https://www.sartcorsonline.com/rptCSR_PublicMultYear.aspx?reportingYear=2016.

Nehra, Deepika, Hau D. Le, Erica M. Fallon, Sarah J. Carlson, Dori Woods, Yvonne A. White, et al. "Prolonging the Female Reproductive Lifespan and Improving Egg Quality with Dietary Omega-3 Fatty Acids." *Aging Cell* 11, no. 6 (December 19, 2012): 1046–54. https://doi.org/10.1111/acel.12006.

Nimlos, Allison. "How to Measure Insulin Resistance." Type 2 Nation, November 22, 2016. https://www.type2nation.com/treatment/beyond-bmi-and-a1c-measuring-insulin resistance-2.

Noventa, Marco, Michela Quaranta, Amerigo Vitagliano, Vescio Cinthya, Romina Valentini, Tania Campagnaro, et al. "May Underdiagnosed Nutrition Imbalances Be Responsible for a Portion of So-Called Unexplained Infertility? From Diagnosis to Potential Treatment Options." *Reproductive Sciences* 23, no. 6 (December 20, 2015): 812–22. https://doi.org/10.1177/1933719115620496.

Ozkan, Sebiha, Sangita Jindal, Keri Greenseid, Jun Shu, Gohar Zeitlian, Cheryl Hickmon, et al. "Replete Vitamin D Stores Predict Reproductive Success Following in Vitro Fertilization." *Fertility and Sterility*. U.S. National Library of Medicine, September 2010. https://www.ncbi.nlm.nih.gov/pmc/articles/PMC2888852.

Pacchiarotti, Alessandro, Gianfranco Carlomagno, Gabriele Antonini, and Arianna Pacchiarotti. "Effect of Myo-Inositol and Melatonin versus Myo-Inositol, in a Randomized Controlled Trial, for Improving In Vitro Fertilization of Patients with Polycystic Ovarian Syndrome." *Gynecological Endocrinology* 32, no. 1 (October 28, 2015): 69–73. https://doi.org/10.3109/09513590.2015.1101444.

Pahwa, Roma. "Chronic Inflammation." U.S. National Library of Medicine, September 28, 2021. https://www.ncbi.nlm.nih.gov/books/NBK493173/.

Palacios, Cristina, Lia K. Kostiuk, and Juan Pablo Peña-Rosas. "Vitamin D Supplementation for Women during Pregnancy." *Cochrane Database of Systematic Reviews* 7, no. 7 (July 26, 2019): CD008873. https://doi.org/10.1002/14651858.cd008873.pub4.

Palomba, Stefano, Jessica Daolio, Sara Romeo, Francesco Antonino Battaglia, Roberto Marci, and Giovanni Battista La Sala. "Lifestyle and Fertility: The Influence of Stress and Quality of Life on Female Fertility." *Reproductive Biology and Endocrinology* 16, no. 1 (December 2018). https://doi.org/10.1186/s12958-018-0434-y.

Panth, Neelima, Adam Gavarkovs, Martha Tamez, and Josiemer Mattei. "The Influence of Diet on Fertility and the Implications for Public Health Nutrition in the United States." *Frontiers in Public Health* 6 (July 31, 2018): 211. https://doi.org/10.3389/fpubh.2018.00211.

Papaleo, Enrico, Vittorio Unfer, Jean-Patrice Baillargeon, Lucia De Santis, Francesco Fusi, Claudio Brigante, et al. "Myo-Inositol in Patients with Polycystic Ovary Syndrome: A Novel Method for Ovulation Induction." *Gynecological Endocrinology* 23, no. 12 (January 2007): 700–703. https://doi.org/10.1080/09513590701672405.

Papanas, Nikolaos, and Dan Ziegler. "Efficacy of α-Lipoic Acid in Diabetic Neuropathy." *Expert Opinion on Pharmacotherapy* 15, no. 18 (November 10, 2014): 2721–31. https://doi.org/10.1517/14656566.2014.972935.

Paulus, Wolfgang E., Mingmin Zhang, Erwin Strehler, Imam El-Danasouri, and Karl Sterzik. "Influence of Acupuncture on the Pregnancy Rate in Patients Who Undergo Assisted Reproduction Therapy." *Fertility and Sterility* 77, no. 4 (April 2002): 721–24. https://doi.org/10.1016/s0015-0282(01)03273-3.

Pei, Jian, Erwin Strehler, Ulrich Noss, Markus Abt, Paola Piomboni, Baccio Baccetti, et al. "Quantitative Evaluation of Spermatozoa Ultrastructure after Acupuncture Treatment for Idiopathic Male Infertility." *Fertility and Sterility* 84, no. 1 (July 2005): 141–47. https://doi.org/10.1016/j.fertnstert.2004.12.056.

Pelzer, Elise S., John A. Allan, Mary A. Waterhouse, Tara Ross, Kenneth W. Beagley, and Christine L. Knox. "Microorganisms within Human Follicular Fluid: Effects on IVF." *PLoS One* 8, no. 3 (March 12, 2013). https://doi.org/10.1371/journal.pone.0059062.

Peña-Rosas, Juan Pablo, Luz Maria De-Regil, Therese Dowswell, and Fernando E. Viteri. "Daily Oral Iron Supplementation during Pregnancy." *Cochrane Database of Systematic Reviews* 12 (October 12, 2012). https://doi.org/10.1002/14651858.cd004736.pub4.

Peters, E. M., R. Anderson, D. C. Nieman, H. Fickl, and V. Jogessar. "Vitamin C Supplementation Attenuates the Increases in Circulating Cortisol, Adrenaline and Anti-Inflammatory Polypeptides Following Ultramarathon Running." *International Journal of Sports Medicine* 22, no. 7 (October 4, 2001): 537–43. https://doi.org/10.1055/s-2001-17610.

Pizzorno, Joseph. "Toxins from the Gut." *Integrative Medicine* 13, no. 6 (December 2014): 8–11.

Potera, Carol. "Women's Health: Endometriosis and PCB Exposure." *Environmental Health Perspectives* 114, no. 7 (July 2006). https://doi.org/10.1289/ehp.114-a404a.

Pulido, Jesús Miguel, and Melchor Alpizar Salazar. "Changes in Insulin Sensitivity, Secretion and Glucose Effectiveness during Menstrual Cycle." *Archives of Medical Research* 30, no. 1 (1999): 19–22. https://doi.org/10.1016/s0188-0128(98)00008-6.

Qu, Fan, Yan Wu, Yu-Hang Zhu, John Barry, Tao Ding, Gianluca Baio, et al. "The Association between Psychological Stress and Miscarriage: A Systematic Review and Meta Analysis." *Scientific Reports* 7, no. 1 (2017). https://doi.org/10.1038/s41598 -017-01792-3.

Raupp, Aimee E. *Yes, You Can Get Pregnant: Natural Ways to Improve Your Fertility Now and into Your 40s.* New York: Demos Medical Publishing, 2014.

Razavi, M., M. Jamilian, Z. Fakhrieh Kashan, Z. Heidar, M. Mohseni, Y. Ghandi, et al. "Selenium Supplementation and the Effects on Reproductive Outcomes, Biomarkers of Inflammation, and Oxidative Stress in Women with Polycystic Ovary Syndrome." *Hormone and Metabolic Research* 48, no. 3 (August 12, 2015): 185–90. https://doi .org/10.1055/s-0035-1559604.

Redman, Leanne M., Karen Elkind-Hirsch, and Eric Ravussin. "Aerobic Exercise in Women with Polycystic Ovary Syndrome Improves Ovarian Morphology Independent of Changes in Body Composition." *Fertility and Sterility* 95, no. 8 (June 30, 2011): 2696– 99. https://doi.org/10.1016/j.fertnstert.2011.01.137.

Reed, Josh. "You Won't Believe What Turmeric Is Being Used For." Body and Soul, May 24, 2017. https://www.bodyandsoul.com.au/nutrition/you-wont-believe-what -turmeric-is being-used-for/news-story/80d6f9d28dd57246107db9903f4422f0.

Reiki. "What Is Reiki?" Reiki, September 10, 2019. https://www.reiki.org/faqs/what -reiki.

Rhee, Taeho Greg. "Perceived Benefits of Utilising Acupuncture by Reason for Use among US Adults." *Acupuncture in Medicine* 35, no. 6 (December 2017): 460–63. https://doi.org/10.1136/acupmed-2017-011490.

Ried, Karin. "Chinese Herbal Medicine for Female Infertility: An Updated Meta-Analysis." *Complementary Therapies in Medicine* 23, no. 1 (February 2015): 116–28. https:// doi.org/10.1016/j.ctim.2014.12.004.

Rier, Sherry, and Warren G. Foster. "Environmental Dioxins and Endometriosis." *Toxicological Sciences* 70, no. 2 (December 1, 2002): 161–70. https://doi.org/10.1093 /toxsci/70.2.161.

Rizk, Ahmed Y., Mohamed A. Bedaiwy, and Hesham G. Al-Inany. "Clomiphene-Acetyl Cysteine Combination as a New Protocol to a Friendly IVF Cycle." *Middle East Fertility Society Journal* 10, no. 2 (2005): 130–34.

Rodríguez-Morán Martha, and Fernando Guerrero-Romero. "Oral Magnesium Supplementation Improves Insulin Sensitivity and Metabolic Control in Type 2 Diabetic Subjects." *Diabetes Care* 26, no. 4 (2003): 1147–52. https://doi.org/10.2337/dia care.26.4.1147.

Ronnenberg, Alayne G., Scott A. Venners, Xiping Xu, Changzhong Chen, Lihua Wang, Wenwei Guang, et al. "Preconception B-Vitamin and Homocysteine Status, Conception, and Early Pregnancy Loss." *American Journal of Epidemiology* 166, no. 3 (May 2007): 304–12. https://doi.org/10.1093/aje/kwm078.

Rosen, Mitchell P., Shehua Shen, Paolo F. Rinaudo, Heather G. Huddleston, Charles E. McCulloch, and Marcelle I. Cedars. "Fertilization Rate Is an Independent Predictor of Implantation Rate." *Fertility and Sterility* 94, no. 4 (September 2010): 1328–33. https://doi.org/10.1016/j.fertnstert.2009.05.024.

Ruder, Elizabeth H., Terryl J. Hartman, Richard H. Reindollar, and Marlene B. Goldman. "Female Dietary Antioxidant Intake and Time to Pregnancy among Couples Treated for Unexplained Infertility." *Fertility and Sterility* 101, no. 3 (March 2014): 759–66. https://doi.org/10.1016/j.fertnstert.2013.11.008.

Safarinejad, M. R. "Effect of Omega-3 Polyunsaturated Fatty Acid Supplementation on Semen Profile and Enzymatic Anti-Oxidant Capacity of Seminal Plasma in Infertile Men with Idiopathic Oligoasthenoteratospermia: A Double-Blind, Placebo-Controlled, Randomised Study." *Andrologia* 43, no. 1 (December 19, 2010): 38–47. https://doi.org/10.1111/j. 1439-0272.2009.01013.x.

Saldaña, Shaula. "The Importance of the Five Flavors in Ancient Medicine." Birdman Life, June 9, 2020. https://birdmanlife.com/blogs/health-and-nutrition/the-importance-of-the-five flavors-in-ancient-medicine.

Salim, Samina. "Oxidative Stress and Psychological Disorders." *Current Neuropharmacology* 12, no. 2 (March 31, 2014): 140–47. https://doi.org/10.2174/1570159x 11666131120230309.

Schaefer, Ella, and Deborah Nock. "The Impact of Preconceptional Multiple-Micronutrient Supplementation on Female Fertility." *Clinical Medicine Insights: Women's Health* 12 (April 23, 2019). https://doi.org/10.1177/1179562x19843868.

Scher, Jonathan, and Carol Dix. *Preventing Miscarriage: The Good News.* New York: Perennial Currents, 2005.

Schmid, Sebastian M., Manfred Hallschmid, Kamila Jauch-Chara, Jan Born, and Bernd Schultes. "A Single Night of Sleep Deprivation Increases Ghrelin Levels and Feelings of Hunger in Normal-Weight Healthy Men." *Journal of Sleep Research* 17, no. 3 (September 2008): 331–34. https://doi.org/10.1111/j.1365-2869.2008.00662.x.

Schweitzer, Harvey. "Adoption and Foster Care—Resolve: The National Infertility Association." Resolve, August 5, 2020. https://resolve.org/what-are-my-options/adoption/adoption-and-foster-care.

Sears, Margaret E. "Chelation: Harnessing and Enhancing Heavy Metal Detoxification—A Review." *The Scientific World Journal* 2013 (April 18, 2013): 1–13. https://doi.org/10.1155/2013/219840.

Shemek, Lori. "11 Ways You're Inadvertently Causing Inflammation." MindBodyGreen, June 1, 2021. https://www.mindbodygreen.com/0-18643/11-ways-youre-inadvertently -causing inflammation.html.

Singh, N., M. Bhalla, P. De Jager, and M. Gilca. "An Overview on Ashwagandha: A Rasayana (Rejuvenator) of Ayurveda." *African Journal of Traditional, Complementary and Alternative Medicines* 8, no. 5S (May 15, 2011): 208–13. https://doi.org/10.4314 /ajtcam.v8i5s.9.

Singh, Saravjeet. "What Is an Example of Catabolism?" Quora, 2015. https://www .quora.com/What-is-an-example-of-catabolism.

Sirota, Ido, Shvetha Zarek, and James Segars. "Potential Influence of the Microbiome on Infertility and Assisted Reproductive Technology." *Seminars in Reproductive Medicine* 32, no. 1 (January 3, 2014): 35–42. https://doi.org/10.1055/s-0033-1361821.

Siterman, S., F. Eltes, V. Wolfson, H. Lederman, and B. Bartoov. "Does Acupuncture Treatment Affect Sperm Density in Males with Very Low Sperm Count? A Pilot Study." *Andrologia* 32, no. 1 (January 2000): 31–39. https://doi.org/10.1111/j.1439-0272.2000 .tb02862.x.

Smith, Caroline A., Mike Armour, Zewdneh Shewamene, Hsiewe Ying Tan, Robert J. Norman, and Neil P. Johnson. "Acupuncture Performed around the Time of Embryo Transfer: A Systematic Review and Meta-Analysis." *Reproductive BioMedicine Online* 38, no. 3 (March 2019): 364–79. https://doi.org/10.1016/j.rbmo.2018.12.038.

Smith, Kristen W., Irene Souter, Irene Dimitriadis, Shelley Ehrlich, Paige L. Williams, Antonia M. Calafat, et al. "Urinary Paraben Concentrations and Ovarian Aging among Women from a Fertility Center." *Environmental Health Perspectives* 121, no. 11–12 (January 1, 2013): 1299–305. https://doi.org/10.1289/ehp.1205350.

Soares, Fabíola Lacerda Pires, Rafael de Oliveira Matoso, Lílian Gonçalves Teixeira, Zélia Menezes, Solange Silveira Pereira, Andréa Catão Alves, et al. "Gluten-Free Diet Reduces Adiposity, Inflammation and Insulin Resistance Associated with the Induction of PPAR-Alpha and PPAR-Gamma Expression." *Journal of Nutritional Biochemistry*, 2012. http://www.medicinacomplementar.com.br/biblioteca/pdfs /Biomolecular/mb-0416.pdf.

Souter, I., Y.-H. Chiu, M. Batsis, M. C. Afeiche, P. L. Williams, R. Hauser, et al. "The Association of Protein Intake (Amount and Type) with Ovarian Antral Follicle Counts among Infertile Women: Results from the Earth Prospective Study Cohort." *BJOG: An International Journal of Obstetrics & Gynaecology* 124, no. 10 (March 9, 2017): 1547–55. https://doi.org/10.1111/1471-0528.14630.

Souter, Irene, Kristen W. Smith, Irene Dimitriadis, Shelley Ehrlich, Paige L. Williams, Antonia M. Calafat, et al. "The Association of Bisphenol-a Urinary Concentrations with Antral Follicle Counts and Other Measures of Ovarian Reserve in Women Undergoing Infertility Treatments." *Reproductive Toxicology* 42 (December 2013): 224–31. https://doi.org/10.1016/j.reprotox.2013.09.008.

Spann, Marisa N., Jennifer Smerling, Hanna Gustafsson, Sophie Foss, Margaret Altemus, and Catherine Monk. "Deficient Maternal Zinc Intake—but Not Folate—Is Associated with Lower Fetal Heart Rate Variability." *Early Human Development* 91, no. 3 (March 2015): 169–72. https://doi.org/10.1016/j.earlhumdev.2015.01.007.

Spritzler, Franziska. "10 Magnesium-Rich Foods That Are Super Healthy." Healthline Media, August 22, 2018. https://www.healthline.com/nutrition/10-foods-high-in magnesium#section1.

Stener-Victorin, Elisabet, Fariba Baghaei, Göran Holm, Per Olof Janson, Gunilla Olivecrona, Malin Lönn, et al. "Effects of Acupuncture and Exercise on Insulin Sensitivity, Adipose Tissue Characteristics, and Markers of Coagulation and Fibrinolysis in Women with Polycystic Ovary Syndrome: Secondary Analyses of a Randomized Controlled Trial." *Fertility and Sterility* 97, no. 2 (February 2012): 501–8. https://doi .org/10.1016/j.fertnstert.2011.11.010.

Stener-Victorin, E., U. Waldenstrom, S. A. Andersson, and M. Wikland. "Reduction of Blood Flow Impedance in the Uterine Arteries of Infertile Women with Electro-Acupuncture." *Human Reproduction* 11, no. 6 (June 1, 1996): 1314–17. https://doi .org/10.1093/oxfordjournals.humrep.a019378.

Siriwardene S. A., L. P. Karunathilaka, N. D. Kodituwakku, and Y. A. Karunarathne. "Clinical Efficacy of Ayurveda Treatment Regimen on Subfertility with Poly Cystic Ovarian Syndrome (PCOS)." *Ayu* 31, no. 1 (January 2010): 24-27. doi: 10.4103/0974-8520.68203. PMID: 22131680; PMCID: PMC3215317.

Stuefer, Sibilla, Helga Moncayo, and Roy Moncayo. "The Role of Magnesium and Thyroid Function in Early Pregnancy after In-Vitro Fertilization (IVF): New Aspects in Endocrine Physiology." *BBA Clinical* 3 (June 2015): 196–204. https://doi .org/10.1016/j.bbacli. 2015.02.006.

Taguchi, Ayumi, Osamu Wada-Hiraike, Kei Kawana, Kaori Koga, Aki Yamashita, Akira Shirane, et al. "Resveratrol Suppresses Inflammatory Responses in Endometrial Stromal Cells Derived from Endometriosis: A Possible Role of the Sirtuin 1 Pathway." *Journal of Obstetrics and Gynaecology Research* 40, no. 3 (December 10, 2013): 770–78. https://doi.org/10.1111/jog.12252.

Takasaki, Akihisa, Hiroshi Tamura, Ichiro Miwa, Toshiaki Taketani, Katsunori Shimamura, and Norihiro Sugino. "Endometrial Growth and Uterine Blood Flow: A Pilot Study for Improving Endometrial Thickness in the Patients with a Thin Endometrium." *Fertility and Sterility* 93, no. 6 (April 2010): 1851–58. https://doi .org/10.1016/j.fertnstert. 2008.12.062.

Tamura, Hiroshi, Akihisa Takasaki, Toshiaki Taketani, Manabu Tanabe, Lifa Lee, Isao Tamura, et al. "Melatonin and Female Reproduction." *Journal of Obstetrics and Gynaecology Research* 40, no. 1 (October 7, 2013): 1–11. https://doi.org/10.1111/jog.12177.

Tan, Li, Yao Tong, Stephen Cho Sze, Mei Xu, Yang Shi, Xin-yang Song, et al. "Chinese Herbal Medicine for Infertility with Anovulation: A Systematic Review." *Journal of Alternative and Complementary Medicine* 18, no. 12 (December 2012): 1087–100. https://doi.org/10.1089/acm.2011.0371.

Tangvoranuntakul, P., P. Gagneux, S. Diaz, M. Bardor, N. Varki, A. Varki, and E. Muchmore. "Human Uptake and Incorporation of an Immunogenic Nonhuman Dietary Sialic Acid." *PNAS* 100, no. 21 (October 1, 2003): 12045–50. https://doi .org/10.1073/pnas.2131556100. PMID: 14523234; PMCID: PMC218710.

Tersigni, C., S. D'Ippolito, F. Di Nicuolo, R. Marana, V. Valenza, V. Masciullo, et al. "Recurrent Pregnancy Loss Is Associated to Leaky Gut: A Novel Pathogenic Model of Endometrium Inflammation?" *Journal of Translational Medicine* 16, no. 1 (April 17, 2018): 102. https://doi.org/10.1186/s12967-018-1482-y.

Trister, Renata. "Nutritional Influences on Estrogen Metabolism." Vernon Integrative Medical Group, October 19, 2013. http://jontristermd.com/for-patients/nutritional -influences-on-estrogen metabolism.

Trout, Kimberly K., Michael R. Rickels, Mark H. Schutta, Maja Petrova, Ellen W. Freeman, Nancy C. Tkacs, et al. "Menstrual Cycle Effects on Insulin Sensitivity in Women with Type 1 Diabetes: A Pilot Study." *Diabetes Technology & Therapeutics* 9, no. 2 (2007): 176–82. https://doi.org/10.1089/dia.2006.0004.

Turi, Angelo, Stefano Raffaele Giannubilo, Francesca Brugè, Federica Principi, Silvia Battistoni, Fabrizia Santoni, et al. "Coenzyme Q10 Content in Follicular Fluid and Its Relationship with Oocyte Fertilization and Embryo Grading." *Archives of Gynecology and Obstetrics* 285, no. 4 (December 3, 2011): 1173–76. https://doi.org/10.1007 /s00404-011-2169-2.

Unterreiner, Alison. "The Gut-Brain Connection." Alison Unterreiner Acupuncture, May 11, 2020. https://alisonunterreiner.com/blog-alisonunterreinerlac/2020/5/9/the -gut-brain connection.

Ushiroyama, Takahisa, Noriko Yokoyama, Midori Hakukawa, Kou Sakuma, Fumio Ichikawa, and Satoshi Yoshida. "Clinical Efficacy of Macrophage-Activating Chinese Mixed Herbs (Mach) in Improvement of Embryo Qualities in Women with Long-Term Infertility of Unknown Etiology." *American Journal of Chinese Medicine* 40, no. 1 (January 2012): 1–10. https://doi.org/10.1142/s0192415x12500012.

Uusitalo, Ulla, Xiang Liu, Jimin Yang, Carin Andrén Aronsson, Sandra Hummel, Martha Butterworth, et al. "Association of Early Exposure of Probiotics and Islet Autoimmunity in the Teddy Study." *JAMA Pediatrics* 170, no. 1 (January 1, 2016): 20. https://doi.org/10.1001/jamapediatrics.2015.2757.

Vabre, Pauline, Nicolas Gatimel, Jessika Moreau, Véronique Gayrard, Nicole Picard-Hagen, Jean Parinaud, et al. "Environmental Pollutants, a Possible Etiology for Premature Ovarian Insufficiency: A Narrative Review of Animal and Human Data." *Environmental Health* 16, no. 1 (April 7, 2017). https://doi.org/10.1186/s12940-017-0242-4.

Vega, Mario, Maurizio Mauro, and Zev Williams. "Direct Toxicity of Insulin on the Human Placenta and Protection by Metformin." *Fertility and Sterility* 111, no. 3 (2019):489–496.

Veleva, Z., A. Tiitinen, S. Vilska, C. Hyden-Granskog, C. Tomas, H. Martikainen, et al. "High and Low BMI Increase the Risk of Miscarriage after IVF/ICSI and FET." *Human Reproduction* 23, no. 4 (January 31, 2008): 878–84. https://doi.org/10.1093 /humrep/den017.

Vitale, Salvatore Giovanni, Paola Rossetti, Francesco Corrado, Agnese Maria Rapisarda, Sandro La Vignera, Rosita Angela Condorelli, et al. "How to Achieve High-Quality Oocytes? The Key Role of Myo-Inositol and Melatonin." *International Journal of Endocrinology* 2016 (August 29, 2016): 1–9. https://doi.org/10.1155/2016/4987436.

Vujkovic, Marijana, Jeanne H. de Vries, Jan Lindemans, Nick S. Macklon, Peter J. van der Spek, Eric A. P. Steegers, et al. "The Preconception Mediterranean Dietary Pattern in Couples Undergoing in Vitro Fertilization/Intracytoplasmic Sperm Injection Treatment Increases the Chance of Pregnancy." *Fertility and Sterility* 94, no. 6 (November 2010): 2096–101. https://doi.org/10.1016/j.fertnstert.2009.12.079.

Wald, N., and J. Sneddon. "Prevention of Neural Tube Defects: Results of the Medical Research Council Vitamin Study." *Lancet* 338, no. 8760 (July 1991): 131. https:// www.sjsu.edu/faculty/gerstman/hs261/Lancet1991-338-8760-131-137.htm.

Wallace, Ian R., Michelle C. McKinley, Patrick M. Bell, and Steven J. Hunter. "Sex Hormone Binding Globulin and Insulin Resistance." *Clinical Endocrinology* 78, no. 3 (2013): 321–29. https://doi.org/10.1111/cen.12086.

Wang, H. Joe. "Alcohol, Inflammation, and Gut-Liver-Brain Interactions in Tissue Damage and Disease Development." *World Journal of Gastroenterology* 16, no. 11 (March 21, 2010): 1304. https://doi.org/10.3748/wjg.v16.i11.1304.

Warren, M. P., and N. E. Perlroth. "The Effects of Intense Exercise on the Female Reproductive System." *Journal of Endocrinology* 170, no. 1 (2001): 3–11. https://doi .org/10.1677/joe. 0.1700003.

Weiss, Gerson, Laura T. Goldsmith, Robert N. Taylor, Dominique Bellet, and Hugh S. Taylor. "Inflammation in Reproductive Disorders." *Reproductive Sciences* 16, no. 2 (February 2009): 216–29. https://doi.org/10.1177/1933719108330087.

Wennborg, H. "Solvent Use and Time to Pregnancy among Female Personnel in Biomedical Laboratories in Sweden." *Occupational and Environmental Medicine* 58, no. 4 (April 1, 2001): 225–31. https://doi.org/10.1136/oem.58.4.225.

West, Helen. "What Are Essential Oils, and Do They Work?" Healthline Media, September 30, 2019. https://www.healthline.com/nutrition/what-are-essential-oils#what-they-are.

West, Zita. *Zita West's Guide to Fertility and Assisted Conception: Essential Advice on Preparing Your Body for IVF and Other Fertility Treatments.* London: Vermilion, 2010.

Westphal, L. M., M. L. Polan, and A. Sontag Trent. "Double-Blind, Placebo-Controlled Study of Fertilityblend: A Nutritional Supplement for Improving Fertility in Women." *Clinical and Experimental Obstetrics & Gynecology* 33, no. 4 (2006): 205–8.

Westphal, Lynn M., Mary Lake Polan, Aileen Sontag Trant, and Stephen B. Mooney. "A Nutritional Supplement for Improving Fertility in Women: a Pilot Study." *Journal of Reproductive Medicine* 49, no. 4 (April 2004): 289–93.

Whitaker, B. D., S. J. Casey, and R. Taupier. "The Effects of N-Acetyl-L-Cysteine Supplementation on in Vitro Porcine Oocyte Maturation and Subsequent Fertilisation and Embryonic Development." *Reproduction, Fertility and Development* 24, no. 8 (April 10, 2012): 1048. https://doi.org/10.1071/rd12002.

Whitaker, B. D., and J. W. Knight. "Effects of N-Acetyl-Cysteine and N-Acetyl-Cysteine-Amide Supplementation on In Vitro Matured Porcine Oocytes." *Reproduction in Domestic Animals* 45, no. 5 (October 2010): 755–59. https://doi.org/10.1111/j.1439-0531.2009.01344.x.

Whitbread, Daisy. "Top 10 Foods Highest in Zinc." My Food Data, January 14, 2022. https://www.myfooddata.com/articles/high-zinc-foods.php.

Wright, C., S. Milne, and H. Leeson. "Sperm DNA Damage Caused by Oxidative Stress: Modifiable Clinical, Lifestyle and Nutritional Factors in Male Infertility." *Reproductive Biomedicine Online* 28, no. 6 (2014): 684–703. doi:10.1016/j.rbmo.2014.02.004. PMID: 24745838.

Yang, Bao-Zhi, Wei Cui, and Jing Li. "Effects of Electroacupuncture Intervention on Changes of Quality of Ovum and Pregnancy Outcome in Patients with Polycystic Ovarian Syndrome." *Acupuncture Research* 40, no. 2 (April 2015): 151–56.

Yang, Qing. "Gain Weight by 'Going Diet?' Artificial Sweeteners and the Neurobiology of Sugar Cravings." *Yale Journal of Biology and Medicine* 82, no. 2 (June 2010): 101–8.

Young, Alison, and Mark Nichols. "Beyond Flint: Excessive Lead Levels Found in Almost 2,000 Water Systems across All 50 States." Gannett Satellite Information Network, March 27, 2017. https://www.usatoday.com/story/news/2016/03/11/nearly-2000-water-systems-fail lead-tests/81220466.

Yu, W., B. Horn, B. Acacio, D. Ni, R. Quintero, and M. Nouriani. "A Pilot Study Evaluating the Combination of Acupuncture with Sildenafil on Endometrial Thickness." *Fertility and Sterility* 87, no. 4, suppl. 2 (April 1, 2007): S23. https://doi.org/10.1016/j.fertnstert.2007.01.203.

Zadek, Sarah. "Fertility Nutrition & Protein | Blog | Conceive Health." Conceive Health, November 25, 2019. https://conceivehealth.com/blog/how-protein-affects-fertility/#:~:text=That's%20why%20a%20woman's%20protein,and%20other%20cell%2Dsignalli ng%20molecules.

Zangeneh, Farideh Zafari, Mina Jafarabadi, Mohammad Mehdi Naghzadeh, Nasrine Abedinia, and Fedyeh Haghollahi. "Psychological Distress in Women with Polycystic Ovary Syndrome from Imam Khomeini Hospital, Tehran." *Journal of Reproduction & Infertility* 13, no. 2 (April 2012): 111–15.

Zhang, Weidong, Yong Zhao, Pengfei Zhang, Yanan Hao, Shuai Yu, Lingjiang Min, et al. "Decrease in Male Mouse Fertility by Hydrogen Sulfide and/or Ammonia Can Be Inheritable." *Chemosphere* 194 (March 2018): 147–57. https://doi.org/10.1016/j.chemosphere.2017.11.164.

Zhao, Jiamin, Beibei Fu, Wei Peng, Tingchao Mao, Haibo Wu, and Yong Zhang. "Melatonin Protect the Development of Preimplantation Mouse Embryos from Sodium Fluoride Induced Oxidative Injury." *Environmental Toxicology and Pharmacology* 54 (September 2017): 133–41. https://doi.org/10.1016/j.etap.2017.06.014.

Zheng, Cui Hong, Ming Min Zhang, Guang Ying Huang, and Wei Wang. "The Role of Acupuncture in Assisted Reproductive Technology." *Evidence-Based Complementary and Alternative Medicine* 2012 (July 2, 2012): 1–15. https://doi.org/10.1155/2012/543924.

Zhong, Li-Xia, Mo-Li Wu, Hong Li, Jia Liu, and Li-Zhu Lin. "Efficacy and Safety of Intraperitoneally Administered Resveratrol against Rat Orthotopic Ovarian Cancers." *Cancer Management and Research* 11 (July 2019): 6113–24. https://doi.org/10.2147/cmar.s206301.

Zhou, Zejun, Chuanxiu Bian, Zhenwu Luo, Constance Guille, Elizabeth Ogunrinde, Jiapeng Wu, et al. "Progesterone Decreases Gut Permeability through Upregulating Occludin Expression in Primary Human Gut Tissues and Caco-2 Cells." *Scientific Reports* 9, no. 1 (June 10, 2019). https://doi.org/10.1038/s41598-019-44448-0.

Zhu, Guanghui, Chunhua Jiang, Xin Yan, Shu Zhao, Dingjie Xu, and Ying Cao. "Shaofu Zhuyu Decoction Regresses Endometriotic Lesions in a Rat Model." *Evidence-Based Complementary and Alternative Medicine* 2018 (2018): 1–7. https://doi.org/10.1155/2018/3927096.

Zijlstra, Freek J., Ineke van den Berg-de Lange, Frank J. Huygen, and Jan Klein. "Anti Inflammatory Actions of Acupuncture." *Mediators of Inflammation* 12, no. 2 (April 2003): 59–69. https://doi.org/10.1080/0962935031000114943.

Index

Note: Page numbers in *italics* refer to tables and figures.

216; vitamin D, 65, 80, 86, 157, 213, 232; vitamin E, 150, 164, 165–66, *166*, 216, 232. *See also* vitamin B

walking as exercise, 174, 176, 181
warm foods, 109, 124–25, 153, 158, 164, 242
Warm the Valley Decoction (Wen Jing Tang), 86, 227, 252–53
Washington State University studies, 114
water filters, 110
water intake, 68, 84, 124, 126
water sautéing, 66
weight issues: fertility and, 175–76; gaining weight, 61; insatiable hunger, 64; losing weight, 140; PCOS and, 30
weight training, 174

Wen Jing Tang (Warm the Valley Decoction), 86, 227, 252–53
Western botanical boosters, 208–9
Williams, Zev, 75, 77–78
workforce statistics, xi
workplace exposures, 279
World Naturopathic Federation, 225, 244

xenoestrogens, 6, 35, 47, 108, 113

yeast, 16, 167
yin and yang, 93, 155, 169–71, 176–77
yoga, 128, 138, 177–78, 188, 190. *See also* meditation; mindfulness
You Gui Wan, 18

zinc, 65, 160–61, *161*, 213

Praise for *The Ultimate Fertility Guidebook*

"The infertility journey is a scary, emotionally challenging process for women and couples. Amid a process with variables beyond anyone's control, *The Ultimate Fertility Guidebook* is an invaluable resource that provides guidance on the things one can control to optimize health." —**Eric J. Forman**, MD, HCLD, medical and laboratory director for Columbia University Fertility Center

"Christina Burns demystifies, distills, and delivers the practical advice every woman looking to get pregnant needs. She lays out a step-by-step process for understanding, evaluating, and improving the internal and external factors that lead to successful baby-making. And best of all, she wraps it up in a book that's easy to follow and a delightfully fun read." —**Carey Davidson**, author of *The Five Archetypes: Discover Your True Nature and Transform Your Life and Relationships*